T0263222

Top Topics in Child and Adolescent Psychiatry

Editor

HARSH K. TRIVEDI

CHILD AND ADOLESCENT PSYCHIATRIC CLINICS OF NORTH AMERICA

www.childpsych.theclinics.com

Consulting Editor
HARSH K. TRIVEDI

January 2015 • Volume 24 • Number 1

ELSEVIER

1600 John F. Kennedy Boulevard • Suite 1800 • Philadelphia, Pennsylvania, 19103-2899

http://www.theclinics.com

**CHILD AND ADOLESCENT PSYCHIATRIC CLINICS OF NORTH AMERICA Volume 24, Number 1
January 2015 ISSN 1056–4993, ISBN-13: 978-0-323-35816-3**

Editor: Joanne Husovski
Developmental Editor: Stephanie Carter

© 2015 Elsevier Inc. All rights reserved.

This periodical and the individual contributions contained in it are protected under copyright by Elsevier, and the following terms and conditions apply to their use:

Photocopying
Single photocopies of single articles may be made for personal use as allowed by national copyright laws. Permission of the Publisher and payment of a fee is required for all other photocopying, including multiple or systematic copying, copying for advertising or promotional purposes, resale, and all forms of document delivery. Special rates are available for educational institutions that wish to make photocopies for non-profit educational classroom use. For information on how to seek permission visit www.elsevier.com/permissions or call: (+44) 1865 843830 (UK)/(+1) 215 239 3804 (USA).

Derivative Works
Subscribers may reproduce tables of contents or prepare lists of articles including abstracts for internal circulation within their institutions. Permission of the Publisher is required for resale or distribution outside the institution. Permission of the Publisher is required for all other derivative works, including compilations and translations (please consult www.elsevier.com/permissions).

Electronic Storage or Usage
Permission of the Publisher is required to store or use electronically any material contained in this periodical, including any article or part of an article (please consult www.elsevier.com/permissions). Except as outlined above, no part of this publication may be reproduced, stored in a retrieval system or transmitted in any form or by any means, electronic, mechanical, photocopying, recording or otherwise, without prior written permission of the Publisher.

Notice
No responsibility is assumed by the Publisher for any injury and/or damage to persons or property as a matter of products liability, negligence or otherwise, or from any use or operation of any methods, products, instructions or ideas contained in the material herein. Because of rapid advances in the medical sciences, in particular, independent verification of diagnoses and drug dosages should be made.

Although all advertising material is expected to conform to ethical (medical) standards, inclusion in this publication does not constitute a guarantee or endorsement of the quality or value of such product or of the claims made of it by its manufacturer.

Child and Adolescent Psychiatric Clinics of North America (ISSN 1056-4993) is published quarterly by Elsevier Inc., 360 Park Avenue South, New York, NY 10010-1710. Months of issue are January, April, July, and October. Business and Editorial Offices: 1600 John F. Kennedy Boulevard, Suite 1800, Philadelphia, PA 19103-2899. Periodicals postage paid at New York, NY and additional mailing offices. Subscription prices are $310.00 per year (US individuals), $491.00 per year (US institutions), $155.00 per year (US students), $360.00 per year (Canadian individuals), $598.00 per year (Canadian institutions), $200.00 per year (Canadian students), $430.00 per year (international individuals), $598.00 per year (international institutions), and $200.00 per year (international students). International air speed delivery is included in all *Clinics* subscription prices. All prices are subject to change without notice. **POSTMASTER:** Send address changes to *Child and Adolescent Psychiatric Clinics of North America*, Elsevier Health Sciences Division, Subscription Customer Service, 3251 Riverport Lane, Maryland Heights, MO 63043. **Customer Service: 1-800-654-2452 (U.S. and Canada); 314-447-8871 (outside U.S. and Canada). Fax: 314-447-8029. E-mail: JournalsCustomer Service-usa@elsevier.com (for print support) or journalsonlinesupport-usa@elsevier.com (for online support).**

Reprints. For copies of 100 or more of articles in this publication, please contact the Commercial Reprints Department, Elsevier Inc., 360 Park Avenue South, New York, New York 10010-1710 Tel.: 212-633-3874; Fax: 212-633-3820, E-mail: reprints@elsevier.com.

Child and Adolescent Psychiatric Clinics of North America is covered in *MEDLINE/PubMed (Index Medicus), ISI, SSCI, Research Alert, Social Search, Current Contents,* and *EMBASE/Excerpta Medica.*

Contributors

CONSULTING EDITOR

HARSH K. TRIVEDI, MD, MBA
Executive Director and Chief Medical Officer; Behavioral Health Vice Chair for Clinical Affairs; Associate Professor of Psychiatry, Vanderbilt University School of Medicine, Nashville, Tennessee

CONSULTING EDITOR EMERITUS

ANDRÉS MARTIN, MD, MPH

FOUNDING CONSULTING EDITOR

MELVIN LEWIS, MBBS, FRCPSYCH, DCH

EDITOR

HARSH K. TRIVEDI, MD, MBA
Executive Director and Chief Medical Officer; Behavioral Health Vice Chair for Clinical Affairs; Associate Professor of Psychiatry, Vanderbilt University School of Medicine, Nashville, Tennessee

AUTHORS

KEVIN M. ANTSHEL, PhD
Director of Clinical Psychology Program; Associate Professor, Department of Psychology, Syracuse University, Syracuse, New York

TERESA BAKER, MD
Associate Professor of Obstetrics and Gynecology, Texas Tech University School of Medicine, Amarillo, Texas

SCOTT BELLINI, PhD
Director, Social Skills Research Clinic; Associate Professor of School Psychology, Indiana University, Bloomington, Indiana

JEANNE FUNK BROCKMYER, PhD
Distinguished University Professor-Emeritus, Department of Psychology, University of Toledo, Toledo, Ohio

THOMAS H. CHUN, MD, MPH
Associate Professor, Department of Emergency Medicine; Department of Pediatrics, Alpert Medical School of Brown University, Providence, Rhode Island

SUSAN J. DUFFY, MD, MPH
Associate Professor, Department of Emergency Medicine; Department of Pediatrics, Alpert Medical School of Brown University, Providence, Rhode Island

NANCY FOLDVARY-SCHAEFER, DO
Head, Section of Sleep Medicine, Department of Neurology, Cleveland Clinic, Cleveland, Ohio

RUTH S. GERSON, MD
Director, Bellevue Hospital Children's Comprehensive Psychiatric Emergency Program; Clinical Assistant Professor, Department of Child and Adolescent Psychiatry, NYU School of Medicine, New York, New York

MADELEINE M. GRIGG-DAMBERGER, MD
Professor, Department of Neurology, University of New Mexico School of Medicine, Albuquerque, New Mexico

THOMAS W. HALE, PhD
Professor, Department of Pediatrics, Texas Tech University School of Medicine, Amarillo, Texas

BEATE HERPERTZ-DAHLMANN, MD
Professor, Department of Child and Adolescent Psychiatry, Psychosomatics, and Psychotherapy, RWTH Aachen University, Aachen, Germany

SUSAN L. HYMAN, MD
Professor of Pediatrics, Neurodevelopmental and Behavioral Pediatrics, Golisano Children's Hospital, School of Medicine and Dentistry, University of Rochester Medical Center, Rochester, New York

EMILY R. KATZ, MD
Clinical Assistant Professor, Department of Psychiatry and Human Behavior, Alpert Medical School of Brown University, Providence, Rhode Island

AARON N. LEETCH, MD
Assistant Professor of Emergency Medicine/Pediatrics, University of Arizona, Tucson, Arizona

JOHN LEIPSIC, MD
Assistant Professor of Psychiatry and Child and Adolescent Psychiatry, Tucson, Arizona

SUSAN E. LEVY, MD, MPH
Associate Professor of Pediatrics, Division of Developmental & Behavioral Pediatrics, The Children's Hospital of Philadelphia, Perelman School of Medicine, University of Pennsylvania, Philadelphia, Pennsylvania

ANNA C. MERRILL, BA
Department of Counseling and Educational Psychology, School Psychology Doctoral Program, Indiana University, Bloomington, Indiana

TIFFANY L. OTERO, MSEd
Department of Counseling and Educational Psychology, School Psychology Doctoral Program, Indiana University, Bloomington, Indiana

HILARY ROWE, BSc(Pharm), PharmD, ACPR
Clinical Pharmacy Specialist, Department of Pharmacy, Fraser Health Authority, Surrey, British Columbia, Canada

ROCHELLE B. SCHATZ, MSEd
Department of Counseling and Educational Psychology, School Psychology Doctoral Program, Indiana University, Bloomington, Indiana

DALE P. WOOLRIDGE, MD, PhD
Professor of Emergency Medicine/Pediatrics, University of Arizona, Tucson, Arizona

Contents

Attention-deficit/hyperactivity disorder (ADHD) is the most common reason for referral to child and adolescent psychiatry clinics. Although stimulant medications represent an evidence-based approach to managing ADHD, psychosocial interventions for child/adolescent ADHD target functional impairments as the intervention goal, and rely heavily on behavioral therapy techniques and operant conditioning principles. Evidence-based psychosocial interventions for managing pediatric ADHD include behavioral parent training, school-based interventions relying on behavioral modification, teaching skills, and operant conditioning principles, and intensive summer treatment programs. The use of conjoint psychosocial treatments with ADHD medications may enable lower doses of each form of treatment.

In 2008, Bellini and Peters conducted a review of empirically based social skills training procedures for youth with autism spectrum disorders. The results of this review suggested that targeted intervention using social skills training programs that were intensive and implemented in a child's natural setting were best suited to meet the needs of children with autism spectrum disorders. In the current article, a review of the most recent meta-analyses is included. Detailed investigation regarding the effectiveness of 8 social skills training procedures is updated and reviewed. Finally, a discussion of assessment strategies is included.

There are many treatments in current use for core and associated symptoms of autism spectrum disorders (ASD). This review discusses the complementary and alternative medical (CAM) treatments commonly added to conventional interventions for children with ASD, including natural products, mind and body practices, and other biomedical treatments. The article focuses on factors associated with use of CAM, the empirical evidence for the most frequently used treatments, and how clinicians work with families who choose CAM treatments. Some treatments have been ineffective, some have unacceptable potential side effects, and others require more study in depth.

The questions facing clinicians with patients with sleep disorder and epilepsy are addressed in this article. Both adult and child epilepsy are discussed in the context of the most typical questions a clinician would have, such as "Are parasomnias more common in people with epilepsy?", "Is sleep architecture abnormal in children with epilepsy", along with outcomes of numerous questionnaire-based, case-based, and double-blind placebo studies on such aspects as sleep duration, daytime sleepiness, anxiety and fears, limb movement, nocturnal seizures, agitation, behavioral disorders, and learning disorders.

Beate Herpertz-Dahlmann

The prevalence of eating disorders among adolescents continues to increase. The starvation process itself is often associated with severe alterations of central and peripheral metabolism, affecting overall health during this vulnerable period. This article aims to convey basic knowledge on these frequent and disabling disorders, and to review new developments in classification issues resulting from the transition to DSM-5. A detailed description is given of the symptomatology of each eating disorder that typically manifests during adolescence. New data on epidemiology, and expanding knowledge on associated medical and psychiatric comorbidities and their often long-lasting sequelae in later life, are provided.

CHILD AND ADOLESCENT PSYCHIATRIC CLINICS

RELATED INTEREST
Pediatric Obesity
Holterman MJ, Holterman A-XL, and Browne AF, *Authors*
in
Pediatric Surgery, June 2012 (Vol. 92, No. 3, Pages 559–582)
Surgical Clinics
Azarow KS and Cusick RA, *Editors*

AACAP Members: Please go to www.jaacap.org for information on access to the Child and Adolescent Psychiatric Clinics. *Resident* Members of AACAP: Special access information is available at www.childpsych.theclinics.com.

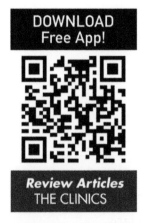

DOWNLOAD Free App!

Review Articles
THE CLINICS

NOW AVAILABLE FOR YOUR iPhone and iPad

Preface

Top Topics in Child and Adolescent Psychiatry

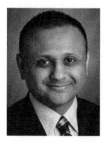

Harsh K. Trivedi, MD, MBA
Editor

The field of medicine is changing. The sheer volume of newly published research is growing. There seem to be new open source journals flooding our e-mail account on a daily basis. Even the methods by which we access information have changed. Long gone are the days of pulling out thick volumes of the *Index Medicus.*

As we look at our own publication, we have noticed both the on-going appeal of topically based issues and the appeal of certain articles electronically. While reading a collection of articles may be helpful to gain a broader and deeper understanding of a topic, the ease of accessing data electronically wherever you may be is undeniable.

An analysis of our data showed that there were distinct articles that stood out as those that were accessed time and again. The concerning part of our analysis was that some of those articles were starting to get dated. While the entire issue was not up for publication, we wanted to find a way to get the most accurate and useful information to you, our readers. With that, I also want to reassure you that we are not moving away from the topical nature of this series.

Welcome to the "Top Topics" issue of the *Child and Adolescent Psychiatric Clinics of North America*. This is a first for this publication and hopefully you will agree that this is something that should be done from time to time. The issue presents a set of articles delving into the interface between psychiatry and medicine; from breastfeeding to sleep disorders in epilepsy, to issues in the emergency assessment of youth. Readers will find a timely article regarding video games and desensitization to violence. We then shift our focus to specific clinical issues that readers always seem to ask more information about: eating disorders, attention deficit hyperactivity disorder, and autism.

I want to thank our wonderful publisher at Elsevier who has had the flexibility and foresight to support this issue, Joanne Husovski. We ask for your feedback on this presentation of select topics that have engendered much interest. Let us know whether you find this useful in advancing your knowledge. We welcome your feedback and

Child Adolesc Psychiatric Clin N Am 24 (2015) ix–x
http://dx.doi.org/10.1016/j.chc.2014.10.001
1056-4993/15/$ – see front matter © 2015 Elsevier Inc. All rights reserved.

hope to use your ideas as we keep *Child and Adolescent Psychiatric Clinics of North America* timely, clinically meaningful, and relevant to you.

Harsh K. Trivedi, MD, MBA
Vanderbilt University School of Medicine
Nashville, TN 37212, USA

E-mail address:
harsh.k.trivedi@vanderbilt.edu

Maternal Medication, Drug Use, and Breastfeeding

Hilary Rowe, BSc(Pharm), PharmD, ACPR[a], Teresa Baker, MD[b], Thomas W. Hale, PhD[b,*]

KEYWORDS

- Breastfeeding • Medications • Infant exposure • Antidepressants • Antipsychotics

KEY POINTS

- Drugs transfer into milk as a function of molecular weight. The higher the molecular weight, the less the drug transfers into human milk.
- Drugs transfer into human milk as a function of the maternal plasma level. The higher the plasma level, the higher the transfer into human milk.
- Drugs with poor oral bioavailability seldom produce significant clinical levels in human milk, and are generally poorly absorbed by the infant as well.
- Drugs that transfer into the brain compartment also likely transfer into human milk, although this does not mean that levels in milk are clinically high or even clinically relevant.
- The transfer of drugs into human milk is one of the purest forms of compartment pharmacokinetics. A good knowledge of the kinetics and chemistry of a medication aids in predicting levels in human milk. However, nothing betters a well-conducted clinical trial in a human model.

INTRODUCTION

The rates of breastfeeding have continued to increase in the United States; according to the Centers for Disease Control and Prevention, approximately 76.5% of infants born in 2013 were breastfed and about 49% were continuing to breastfeed by 6 months of age, with approximately 16.4% of these infants still exclusively receiving breast milk at 6 months.[1] Although there are many social factors that lead to this high rate of discontinuation, the use of medications must be considered. The average number of different medications (excluding iron, minerals, folic acid, and vitamins) taken per mother in a small American study was 4 throughout lactation (0.9 medications per month).[2]

This article is reproduced for psychiatric professionals; it originally appeared in *Pediatric Clinics of North America*, volume 60, issue 1.

[a] Department of Pharmacy, Fraser Health Authority, Surrey, British Columbia, Canada; [b] Texas Tech University School of Medicine, 1400 Coulter Street, Amarillo, Texas 79106, USA
* Corresponding author. Department of Pediatrics, Texas Tech University School of Medicine, 1400 Coulter Street, Amarillo, Texas 79106.
E-mail address: Thomas.Hale@ttuhsc.edu

Child Adolesc Psychiatric Clin N Am 24 (2015) 1–20
http://dx.doi.org/10.1016/j.chc.2014.09.005
1056-4993/15/$ – see front matter © 2015 Elsevier Inc. All rights reserved.

With so many women using drug therapy during lactation, pediatricians and obstetricians are faced with the challenge of determining which medications are suitable for breastfeeding mothers. Although there is more literature available about the transfer of medications into breast milk, this is often not communicated to students and clinicians; therefore, many women are advised to stop breast-feeding or avoid drug therapy based on information obtained from product monographs.

Even without specific medication data from human studies, a good understanding of kinetic principles and mechanisms of medication entry into breast milk can help a clinician make an informed decision that often allows the mother to continue breast-feeding while treating her medical condition. This article discusses the most impor-tant concepts in understanding how medications enter breast milk so as to aid in clinical decision making, and highlights suitable medications for breastfeeding mothers.

KEY CONCEPTS OF MEDICATION ENTRY INTO BREAST MILK

Although all medications enter milk to some degree, clinically relevant levels are seldom attained. Most drugs simply transfer in and out of the milk compartment by passive diffusion from a region of high concentration to a region of low con-centration. While some active transport systems exist for immunoglobulins, elec-trolytes, and particularly iodine, facilitated transport systems are rather limited. The authors know of fewer than 10 drugs that are selectively transported into hu-man milk.

Medications that enter breast milk will often share certain physicochemical charac-teristics.[3] These agents are generally low in molecular weight (<500 Da), often attain higher maternal plasma levels, are generally poorly bound to plasma proteins, and have a higher pK_a (pH at which drug is equally ionic and nonionic; polar or ionic med-ications are less likely to leave the breast milk compartment). Human milk has a lower pH (7–7.2), which causes some medications with a higher pK_a (>7.2) to become ionized and trapped in milk.

In addition, clinicians also need to consider the oral bioavailability of the drug in the infant's gastrointestinal tract. Many drugs simply are not absorbed in the gastrointes-tinal tract of infants. The stage of lactation is important. Although more medication can enter breast milk in the colostral phase, only minimal doses are transferred to the infant during this phase, owing to the limited volume of colostrum. With mature milk there is a larger volume, but less medication enters breast milk because of tight cell-to-cell junctions.

CALCULATING INFANT EXPOSURE

Perhaps the most useful tool in clinical practice is to calculate the actual dose received by the infant. To do so, one must know the actual concentration of medication in the milk and the volume of milk transferred. Though not always available, data on milk levels for many drugs do exist.

More recent studies now calculate the average area under the curve (AUC) value for the medication (C_{ave}).[4] This methodology accurately estimates the average daily level of the drug in milk, and hence the average intake by the infant.

The volume of milk ingested is highly variable, and depends on the age of the in-fant and the extent to which the infant is exclusively breastfed. Many clinicians use the 150 mL/kg/d value to estimate the amount of milk ingested by the infant. The most useful and accurate measure of exposure is to calculate the relative infant dose (RID):

$$\text{Relative Infant Dose (RID)} = \frac{\text{Dose.infant}\left(\frac{mg/kg}{day}\right)}{\text{Dose.mother}\left(\frac{mg/kg}{day}\right)}$$

where Dose.infant is dose in infant per day and Dose.mother is dose in mother per day.

The RID is generally expressed as a percentage of the mother's dose, and provides a standardized method of relating the infant's dose in milk to the maternal dose. Bennett[5] was the first to recommend that a RID of greater than 10% should be the theoretic "level of concern" for most medications. Regardless, the 10% level of concern is relative, and each situation should be individually evaluated according to the overall toxicity of the medication.

UNIQUE INFANT FACTORS

To evaluate the risk of the medication, infants should be categorized as at low, moderate, or high risk. Infants at low risk are generally older (6–18 months) and receive lower volumes of breast milk, but in addition are able to metabolize and handle drugs more efficiently. Mothers in the terminal stage of lactation (>1 year) often produce relatively lower quantities of milk. Thus, the absolute clinical dose transferred is often very low.

Infants at moderate risk are term infants who are 2 weeks to less than 6 months old. Those at higher risk are premature, newborns, or infants with acute or chronic medical conditions that may be affected by the medication or may impair the clearance of medications in the infant (eg, renal dysfunction).

PSYCHIATRIC CONDITIONS

Recent data from 17 American states indicate that postpartum depression affects 12% to 20% of women.[6] Fortunately for practitioners, there is increasing information available about the use of antidepressants during lactation that support the treatment of the condition while breastfeeding (**Table 1**). The selective serotonin reuptake inhibitors (SSRIs) are presently the mainstay of antidepressant therapy in breastfeeding women. **Table 1** provides the RID of common SSRIs. Clinical studies in breastfeeding patients consuming sertraline, fluvoxamine, and paroxetine clearly suggest that the transfer of these medications into human milk is low and uptake by the infant is even lower.[7–9] Thus far, no or minimal untoward effects have been reported following the use of these 3 agents in breastfeeding mothers. Sertraline is overwhelmingly favored, as more than 50 mother-infant pairs have been evaluated in numerous studies, and milk and infant plasma levels are low to undetectable.

Fluoxetine also has been studied in more than 50 mother-infant pairs, and transfers into human milk in relatively higher concentrations, ranging to as high as 9% of the maternal dose.[10] Because of its long half-life and active metabolite, clinically relevant plasma levels in infants have been reported, but without major

Table 1
Antidepressants and reported levels in breast milk

Antidepressant	Relative Infant Dose (RID) %	Comments
Selective Serotonin Reuptake Inhibitors (SSRIs)		
Citalopram	3.6[90]	Compatible: SSRIs are recommended first-line agents
Escitalopram	5.3[95]	for depression and anxiety, and are suitable when
Fluvoxamine	1.6[8]	breastfeeding. There have been 2 cases of excessive
Fluoxetine	5–9[93,94]	somnolence, decreased feeding, and weight loss with
Sertraline	0.54[7]	citalopram; however, most new data suggest these
Paroxetine	1.4[9]	side effects are rare.[91,92] Fluoxetine has been
		reported to cause colic, fussiness, and crying[93,94]
Serotonin Norepinephrine Reuptake Inhibitors		
Venlafaxine	8.1[96]	Compatible: No adverse events reported in breastfed
Desvenlafaxine	6.8[97]	infants with these 3 medications
Duloxetine	0.1[98]	

complications. Long-term studies, however, are not yet available. Owing to a higher RID, fluoxetine is perhaps less preferred unless lower doses are used during pregnancy and early postpartum. However, in reality the incidences of untoward effects are probably remote, and mothers who cannot tolerate other SSRIs should be maintained on the product that works best for them. In essence, if a product works, it is not advisable to change breastfeeding mothers to another product. Although almost all tricyclic antidepressants produce low RIDs and are well tolerated by the infant, they are seldom used because of intolerable anticholinergic side effects in the mother.

Benzodiazepines are often used with antidepressants to help with anxiety, or can be used as sleep aids for short periods of time (when nondrug measures have failed). Kelly and colleagues[11] conducted a prospective study to determine rates of adverse events in infants exposed to benzodiazepines via breast milk. The 3 most commonly used benzodiazepines in this study were lorazepam (52%), clonazepam (18%), and midazolam (15%).[11] Of 124 women taking benzodiazepines, only 1.6% (2 of 124) of their infants (2–24 months old) were found to have central nervous system (CNS) depression.[11] There was no correlation between sedation and the benzodiazepine dose or the duration of breastfeeding.[11] Of the two mothers who reported sedation, one was taking alprazolam occasionally while the other was taking 2 benzodiazepines (clonazepam and flurazepam) chronically.[11] If these agents are used, choose a product with a short half-life and use the lowest effective dose for the shortest duration to minimize exposure.[12]

Other medications used for sedation include the first-generation antihistamines, the most commonly used medications being diphenhydramine, dimenhydrinate, and doxylamine. Dimenhydrinate's active ingredient is diphenhydramine, and doxylamine has a structure similar to that of diphenhydramine; therefore, the RID for diphenhydramine (RID 0.7%–1.5%) is often extrapolated to all 3 of these drugs, and it is thought that none of them readily enter breast milk.[13]

There are 2 medications that are not part of the benzodiazepine family but are indicated for insomnia, namely zopiclone and zolpidem. A study of 12 mothers who took zopiclone 7.5 mg orally, 2 to 6 days postpartum for sleep, found that the RID was approximately 1.4% of the maternal dose, and no adverse effects were reported in the infants.[14] Monitoring the infant for sedation and the ability to breastfeed is recommended with all sedating medications.

Atypical antipsychotics are another class of medications that are being used more commonly for many disorders such as psychosis, bipolar disorder, and depression. Three of the most commonly used atypical antipsychotics are risperidone (RID 4.3%), quetiapine (RID 0.09%), and olanzapine (1.6%), these medications have low RIDs and are thought to be more suitable in breastfeeding than the older antipsychotics (phenothiazines), which have been associated with drowsiness and lethargy.[15–18]

Methylphenidate (RID 0.2%) and dextroamphetamine (RID 5.7%) have relatively low penetration into breast milk and have no history of causing adverse effects in breastfed infants. Regardless, all breastfeeding mothers on stimulants require monitoring of their infant for irritability, weight loss, or poor weight gain.[19,20]

Clinicians are often faced with the decision of whether antiepileptic or mood stabilizer medications are suitable while breastfeeding. If a mother is stable on a drug, vigilant monitoring of the infant can be carried out to evaluate safety, such as drug levels or monitoring signs of sedation. **Table 2** provides the RID of most antiepileptic and mood-stabilizing drugs.

Valproic acid levels in milk are fairly low, with a RID of approximately 1.4% to 1.7%.[21] In a study of 16 patients receiving 300 to 2400 mg/d, valproic acid concentrations in milk ranged from 0.4 to 3.9 mg/L (mean 1.9 mg/L).[21] Although it is generally agreed that the amount of valproic acid transferring to the infant via milk is low, the somewhat high risk of pregnancy in women early postpartum and the high risk of teratology of valproic acid suggest that this drug should probably be avoided in women early postpartum, and certainly in women at high risk of pregnancy.

Lamotrigine has been studied in at least 26 individual breastfeeding mothers. Levels in milk appear quite significant, with RIDs ranging from 9.2% to 18.3%.[22,23] The use of lamotrigine in breastfeeding mothers produces significant plasma levels in some breastfed infants, although they are apparently not high enough to produce side effects. Some investigators suggest it is advisable to monitor the infant's plasma levels if the infant is symptomatic to ensure safety.[22] Premature infants should be closely monitored for apnea, sedation, and weakness. The maternal use of lamotrigine is probably compatible with breastfeeding of premature and full-term breastfeeding infants as long as the infant is closely observed for untoward symptoms.

The transfer of topiramate into human milk is significant. In a study of 3 women who received topiramate (150–200 mg/d) at 3 weeks postpartum, the RID ranged from 3% to 23% of the maternal daily dose.[24] Plasma levels were detectable in 2 of the 3 infants and were low, 10% to 20% of the maternal plasma level. At 4 weeks, the milk/plasma ratio dropped to 0.69 and infant plasma levels were less than 0.9 μM and 2.1 μM, respectively. It should be noted that the breast milk and plasma levels were drawn 10 to 15 hours after the last topiramate dose, which would underestimate the amount found in breast milk. Because the plasma levels found in breastfeeding infants were significantly less than in maternal plasma, the risk of topiramate in breastfeeding mothers is probably acceptable. Close observation, including plasma levels in symptomatic infants, is advised.

RECREATIONAL DRUGS

Alcohol readily transfers into human milk, with an average milk/plasma ratio of approximately 1.0; however, the clinical dose of alcohol in human milk is not necessarily high. In a well-controlled study of 12 women who ingested 0.3 g/kg of ethanol, the mean

Table 2
Seizure and mood stabilizer medications and reported levels in breast milk

Drug	Relative Infant Dose (RID) %	Comments
Valproic acid	1.4–1.7[21]	Probably compatible: In a study of 16 patients receiving 300–2400 mg/d of valproic acid, breast milk concentrations ranged from 0.4 to 3.9 mg/L (mean = 1.9 mg/L)[21]
		One case report of a 3-mo-old breastfed infant who developed thrombocytopenia, petechiae, a minor hematoma, and anemia 6 wk after his mother's valproic acid dose was doubled. The investigators report the onset of symptoms occurred near a minor cold but believe the adverse events were not related to a viral illness[99]
		NEAD study demonstrated adverse cognitive effects from valproic acid exposure in utero. In a 3-year follow up study, 42% of children were breastfed; IQs for breastfed children did not differ from non-breastfed children. Although this study did not show adverse effects, there are many confounding variables; until further trials are published the long-term effects on cognitive development are unknown[100]
Carbamazepine	5.9[101]	Compatible: Levels in milk are reported to be low (2.8–4.5 mg/L), the estimated infant dose is <0.68 mg/kg/d. One report of elevated liver function tests occurred in a 9-d-old infant[101]
Lithium	30.1[102]	Compatible with close observation: Because the RID for lithium is variable, this medication should only be used if found to be the most suitable mood stabilizer for the mother and the infant is full term and healthy. Studies suggest monitoring serum creatinine, BUN, and thyroid function in the infant[102,103]
Lamotrigine	9.2[23]	Compatible: Reports of significant plasma levels have occurred in some breastfed infants, although none have been high enough to produce side effects. It may be helpful to monitor the infant's plasma levels[23,104]
Topiramate	24.5[24]	Compatible: Levels in infants are 10%–20% of mothers; no adverse effects have been reported in breastfed infants[24]
Phenytoin	7.7[105]	Compatible: Low amounts enter breast milk; monitoring for sedation and infant levels can be done if symptoms occur

Abbreviations: BUN, blood urea nitrogen; NEAD, Neurodevelopmental Effects of Antiepileptic Drugs.

maximum concentration of ethanol in milk was only 320 mg/L.[25] In an interesting study of the effect of alcohol on milk ingestion by infants, the rate of milk consumption by infants during the 4 hours immediately after exposure to alcohol (0.3 g/kg) in 12 mothers was significantly less.[26] Reduction of letdown is apparently dose-dependent and requires alcohol consumption of 1.5 to 1.9 g/kg.[27] Other studies have suggested psychomotor delay in infants of moderate drinkers (>2 drinks daily). These reports also suggest that alcohol suppresses milk production significantly, which is secondary to alcohol suppression of oxytocin release. Adult metabolism of alcohol is approximately 30 mL in 3 hours, so mothers who ingest alcohol in moderate amounts may return to breastfeeding after waiting for approximately 2 hours for each drink consumed.[28] Thus, mothers should avoid consuming alcohol or avoid breast-feeding during and for at least 2 hours per drink after consuming alcohol. Chronic or heavy consumers of alcohol should not breastfeed.

Studies concerning the use of cannabis in pregnant women appear to be somewhat inconsistent. Commonly called marijuana, the active component Δ-9-tetrahydrocan-nabinol (THC) is rapidly distributed to the brain and adipose tissue. It is stored in fat tissues for long periods (weeks to months). Small to moderate secretion into breast milk has been documented.[29] These investigators reported that in one mother who consumed marijuana 7 to 8 times daily, milk levels of THC were 340 µg/L.[29]

In one mother who consumed marijuana once daily, milk levels were reportedly 105 µg/L.[29] Analysis of breast milk in a chronic heavy user revealed an 8-fold accumu-lation in breast milk compared with plasma, although the dose received is apparently insufficient to produce significant side effects in the infant. Studies have shown signif-icant absorption and metabolism in infants, although long-term sequelae are conflict-ing. In one study of 27 women who smoked marijuana routinely during breastfeeding, no differences were noted in outcomes on growth, mental, and motor development.[30] In another study, maternal use of marijuana was shown to be associated with a slight decrease in infant motor development at 1 year of age, especially when used during the first month of lactation.[31] This study's data were confounded by the use of mari-juana during the first trimester of pregnancy. Interestingly in this study, maternal use of marijuana during pregnancy and lactation had no detectable effect on infant mental development at 1 year of age.

There are few documented hazards reported following the limited use of marijuana in breastfeeding. Recent data suggest significant changes in the endocannabinoid sys-tem after fetal exposure to marijuana.[32] This system has a major role in the develop-ment of the CNS and is involved in mood, cognition, reward, and goal-directed behavior. Both animal and human data strongly suggest that marijuana exposure in pregnancy, and potentially lactation, may lead to neurobehavioral complications. Until further data can confirm these studies, use of this drug should be strongly discouraged.

Cigarette smoking not only exposes breastfed infants to nicotine and its metabolite cotinine, but also exposes the infant to toxic xenobiotics in the cigarette and environ-mental cigarette smoke. A study by Ilett and colleagues[33] assessed the difference in nicotine and cotinine exposure from smoking cigarettes or using nicotine patches in breastfeeding mothers. This study enrolled 15 women, who smoked an average of 17 cigarettes a day, into an 11-week smoking cessation program using nicotine patches (21 mg/d weeks 1–6, 14 mg/d in weeks 7–8, 7 mg/d patch in weeks 9–10, weaning around week 11). The results showed that the absolute infant dose (in nico-tine equivalents) decreased by approximately 70% by the time the mother was using the 7-mg patch compared with the dose generated by smoking. In addition, the breast milk concentrations of nicotine and cotinine also decreased by 50% and 66%. The average nicotine equivalents in µg/kg/d for infants exposed via breast milk were 25.2, 23, 15.8, and 7.5 for smoking, 21-mg patch, 14-mg patch, and 7-mg patch, respectively. Therefore, as the mother progresses through the patch strengths, the transfer of nicotine equivalents to the infant via breast milk is significantly decreased and the exposure to other toxins from cigarettes is eliminated.

It is not recommended that women smoke near their infants, in the home or before breastfeeding; therefore, should a mother who smokes wish to breastfeed, it would be suitable to recommend nicotine replacement therapy to help her quit while also continuing to breastfeed.

Caffeine is a naturally occurring CNS stimulant in many foods and drinks. Whereas the half-life in adults is 4.9 hours, the half-life in neonates is as high as 97.5 hours. The half-life decreases with age to 14 hours at 3 to 5 months and 2.6 hours at 6 months and older. The average cup of coffee contains 100 to 150 mg of caffeine depending on preparation and country of origin.

Peak levels of caffeine are found in breast milk 60 to 120 minutes after ingestion. In a study of 5 patients following an ingestion of 150 mg caffeine, peak concentrations of caffeine in serum ranged from 2.39 to 4.05 μg/mL and peak concentrations in milk ranged from 1.4 to 2.41 mg/L, with a milk/serum ratio of 0.52.[34] The average milk concentration at 30, 60, and 120 minutes after ingestion was 1.58, 1.49, and 0.926 mg/L, respectively. Another study was conducted in 7 breastfeeding mothers who consumed 750 mg caffeine daily for 5 days, and were 11 to 22 days postpartum. The average milk concentration was 4.3 mg/L,[35] and the mean concentration of caffeine in serum of the infants on day 5 was 1.4 μg/mL.

The occasional use of coffee or tea is not contraindicated, but persistent, chronic use may lead to high plasma levels in the infant, particularly during the neonatal period.

PAIN/ANALGESIA

Analgesics are one of the most commonly used medications in breastfeeding. Options for pain control include acetaminophen, nonsteroidal anti-inflammatory drugs (NSAIDs), and opioids. Most NSAIDs are used to reduce pain and inflammation, and are generally a suitable choice in breastfeeding women. Ibuprofen, acetaminophen, and naproxen are probably the most commonly used analgesics in North America. Their RID in milk ranges from 0.65% for ibuprofen,[36] to 8.81% for acetaminophen,[37] to 3.3% for naproxen.[38]

Opioids are often used for acute pain after cesarean section or for other procedures in breastfeeding mothers. Hydromorphone is a suitable opioid used in breastfeeding mothers because of its low RID of less than 1%.[39] Hydrocodone is another suitable alternative; its active metabolite is hydromorphone, and its RID ranges from 0.2% to 9% (average 2.4%).[40] It should be noted that there have been 2 reports of adverse events with infants exposed to hydrocodone via breast milk.[41,42] In the first case, both mother and infant were sedated after the mother took 2 hydrocodone 10 mg/ acetaminophen 650 mg tablets every 4 hours for mastitis. Once the dose was reduced to 1 tablet every 3 hours, the sedation resolved.[41] The second infant required intubation after exposure to a combination of opioids his mother had taken for a migraine (hydrocodone and methadone).[42] Morphine is also a suitable alternative for short-term treatment of acute pain; however, its large RID of 9% to 35% makes it a less desirable agent.[43]

The use of codeine has started to decline since the death of an infant whose mother was taking codeine while breastfeeding in 2005.[44] Both codeine and oxycodone are less favorable opioids because they have unpredictable metabolism (CYP 2D6 enzyme) that produces active metabolites and data showing CNS depression in infants.[45] In a cohort of mothers using oxycodone, codeine, and acetaminophen for pain during lactation, the reports of infant sedation were 20.1%, 16.7%, and 0.5%, respectively.[45]

All opioids should be used with caution in breastfeeding mothers, using low doses and short courses, avoiding combinations with other opioids, continuous monitoring of the mother and child for sedation/side effects, and constant reevaluation of the need for the opioid. When possible, treating the cause of the underlying pain and using acetaminophen/NSAIDs is recommended.

HYPERTENSION

There are a variety of medications used to treat hypertension, including diuretics, β-adrenergic blockers, calcium-channel blockers (CCBs), angiotensin-converting enzyme inhibitors (ACEIs), and angiotensin receptor blockers (ARBs). Fortunately, many of these medications are suitable in breastfeeding; however, some in the β-blocker family are known to cause problems for breastfed infants. The β-blockers of choice are metoprolol (RID 1.4%) and propranolol (RID 0.3%), neither of which has been associated with any infant adverse events.[46,47] In addition, labetalol has not been associated with any adverse effects in infants and has a low RID of 0.6%.[48] Although rarely, atenolol and acebutolol have both been associated with infant adverse effects such as cyanosis, tachypnea, bradycardia, hypotension, and low body temperature, and are not preferred agents.[49,50] At present there is no information about the transfer of carvedilol or bisoprolol into breast milk. In summary, monitoring the infant for hypotension, bradycardia, and lethargy is suggested when using β-blockers in lactation.

The most common CCBs are amlodipine, felodipine, nifedipine, verapamil, and diltiazem. Studies on nifedipine suggest a low RID of 2.3%, 1 hour after a 30-mg dose.[51] In a patient who took verapamil 80 mg 3 times per day, the average steady-state milk concentration of verapamil was 25.8 µg/L, no drug was found in the infant's plasma, and the RID was estimated to be 0.15%.[52] There is one report of a patient who received diltiazem 60 mg 4 times per day; in this case the RID was low (RID 0.9%).[53] There have been no reports of adverse events in breastfed infants exposed to nifedipine, verapamil, or diltiazem.[51-53]

ACEIs are not only used for hypertension, having numerous other indications such as heart failure, myocardial infarction, diabetes, and kidney disease. The 2 ACEIs with the most breastfeeding data are captopril and enalapril. In a study of 12 women who took captopril 100 mg 3 times daily, breast milk levels were approximately 4.7 µg/L 4 hours after the dose, the estimated RID was 0.002%, and no adverse effects were found.[54] In a study where 5 mothers were given a single 20-mg dose of enalapril, the average maximum milk concentrations of enalapril and its active metabolite enalaprilat were 1.74 and 1.72 µg/L, respectively; the RID was estimated to be approximately 0.175%.[55] Although there are many ACEIs on the market, captopril and enalapril are preferred until there are data to confirm the safety of others in breastfed infants.

At present there are no data available concerning the use of the ARBs in breastfeeding mothers. Until this information becomes available, ACEIs should be used instead of ARBs (candesartan, irbesartan, losartan, and so forth).

Diuretics are often used to help lower blood pressure and decrease edema. There are no published data on the amount of furosemide that enters breast milk. There is one case report of a woman who received hydrochlorothiazide 50 mg daily.[56] On day 28 the mean milk concentration of hydrochlorothiazide was 80 ng/mL, resulting in a total infant daily dose of 0.05 mg hydrochlorothiazide.[56] Plasma levels of hydrochlorothiazide in this infant were undetectable, and no adverse events were reported.[56]

Despite suggestions in the past that diuretics may suppress milk production,[57] no further details of this study or other studies have been published that confirm this controversy; at this time there is no substantial evidence to suggest that diuretics reduce milk volume or that diuretics are contraindicated in breastfeeding.

LIVER/GASTROINTESTINAL

The use of histamine-2 (H2) antagonists and proton-pump inhibitors (PPIs) for gastroesophageal reflux disease (GERD) and nausea/vomiting in pregnancy is increasing.

Famotidine is a preferred H2 antagonist. In a study of 8 women who were given 40 mg famotidine daily, the RID was estimated to be the lowest of the H2 antagonists, at 1.9%.[58] Although ranitidine has a high milk to plasma ratio, it is also a preferred agent, the amount of ranitidine that enters breast milk is still low, the RID ranges between 1.3% and 4.6%, and the total daily infant dose is approximately 0.4 mg/kg/d.[59] Cimetidine has a high milk to plasma ratio and RID between 9.8% and 32.6%, with a total daily infant dose of approximately 5.58 mg/kg/d. Although this dose is lower than the pediatric therapeutic dose, the other 2 drugs are more suitable than cimetidine for breastfeeding.[58] The use of PPIs poses little risk to the infant because all of the current PPIs are unstable at low pH and, thus, little is absorbed by the infant orally. In addition, the RIDs of these medications are very low, demonstrating minimal drug transfer into breast milk (omeprazole RID 1.1%, pantoprazole RID 0.95%).[60,61]

NAUSEA

The 3 medications that are considered most suitable for short-term treatment of nausea and vomiting during lactation are dimenhydrinate (see the section on sleep aid for more information), ondansetron, and metoclopramide. Although the milk levels of ondansetron are unknown, it is a preferred agent because it is commonly used during pregnancy and in young infants without any major reports of safety concerns.[62,63] Metoclopramide is an alternative for short-term use (owing to maternal side effects), with a low RID of 4.7%.

INFECTIOUS DISEASE

Most of the antibiotics such as the penicillins and cephalosporins have been well studied and are compatible with breastfeeding because of their poor entry into breast milk (**Table 3**).[64] Although side effects are uncommon, those reported in infants exposed to antibiotics in breast milk are usually self-limiting, such as diarrhea and rash.[65] Two classes of antibiotics that have known complications in children, and are generally perceived by clinicians and patients as contraindicated in breastfeeding mothers, are the tetracyclines and the fluoroquinolones.[66–68] The tetracyclines are known to cause permanent dental staining that is dose and time dependent, and reduced bone growth in children following deposition of the drug in the epiphyseal plate.[69] Short-term use (<3 weeks) of doxycycline and tetracycline are considered suitable in breastfeeding mothers, as the transfer of these medications into milk is low.[66,70] Tetracycline enters milk poorly because it binds with calcium in breast milk and cannot be absorbed (absolute infant dose 0.17 mg/kg/d, RID 0.6%).[70] Doxycycline absorption is delayed but more complete, and it too has a low RID of 4.2% (absolute infant dose 0.12 mg/kg/d).[66]

Although the fluoroquinolones have caused arthrotoxicity (blisters, fissures, and erosions in cartilage) in animal studies using beagle dogs aged 13 to 16 weeks and have been associated with reversible musculoskeletal adverse effects in children and adults, there have been few reports of arthropathy in human infants and children; therefore, these medications are generally not contraindicated in breastfeeding mothers.[67,71] Although metronidazole has been associated with mutagenicity and carcinogenicity in rodents, this risk has remained theoretic and has not been reported in humans.[72] Topical and vaginal forms are suitable in breastfeeding mothers because they have little systemic absorption.[72] The use of oral metronidazole produces a relatively high RID of 9% to 13% when 1200 mg/d is taken by the mother. No adverse effects have been reported other than a metallic taste of the milk, which may not be palatable to some infants.[73] If larger single doses of metronidazole are used (2 g),

Table 3
Antibiotics and reported levels in breast milk

Antibiotics	Relative Infant Dose (RID) %	Comments
Penicillins		
Amoxicillin	1[64]	Compatible: The penicillins are a class of medication that
Ampicillin	0.3[106]	minimally transfer into human milk; they have been
Ampicillin + sulbactam	0.5[107]	used for years in lactating mothers and have not had any serious adverse events reported in infants. There is no specific information about the quantity of clavulanate that enters breast milk[65]
Aminoglycosides		
Gentamicin	2.1[108]	Compatible: Gentamicin produced measurable blood
Tobramycin	0–2.6[109,110]	levels (0.41 µg/mL) in 5 of 10 infants in a study where women were given gentamicin 80 mg intramuscularly every 8 h.[108] The expected intake for an infant was negligible, at 307 µg/d.[108] Of note, oral absorption is thought to be low (<1%) except in premature neonates; however, this study showed oral absorption did occur in half of their population of full-term infants[108]
Cephalosporins		
Cefazolin	0.8[111]	Compatible: The cephalosporins are also suitable in
Cephalexin	0.5[112]	lactation, as they have low RIDs, and no major adverse
Cefuroxime	0.6[113]	effects in infants have been reported after many years
Ceftriaxone	4.1[114]	of use. In a case report when cephalothin and then
Cefotaxime	0.3[115]	cephalexin+probenecid was administered to the
Ceftazidime	0.9[116]	mother, the infant had green liquid stools, which resolved without dehydration when the infant was supplemented (15% of intake) with goat's milk[112]
Carbapenems		
Meropenem	0.18[117]	Compatible: Currently there is little information about the use of carbapenems in breastfeeding mothers. One published case report found the average and maximum meropenem concentrations in milk to be 0.48 µg/mL and 0.64 µg/mL; this estimated the infant daily dose to be 97 µg/kg/d[117]

breastfeeding should be delayed for 12 to 24 hours to reduce the infant's exposure to this medication.[74]

HEMATOLOGY

The use of antiplatelet and anticoagulant medications is increasing in women for prevention of cardiovascular disease, treatment of venous thrombosis during pregnancy, prevention of procedural-related thrombosis, and numerous other indications (**Table 4**). Older studies of aspirin are somewhat poor and were done using relatively high doses, as opposed to the doses of 81 to 325 mg used today. In the older studies and using a 1-g oral dose the RID was reported as 9.4%.[75] Thus, the risk in using 81-mg or even 325-mg daily doses is probably relatively low. At present there are no data available on the use of clopidogrel, one of the most commonly used drugs in this field.

Table 4
Hematologic medications and reported levels in breast milk

Coagulation Medications	Relative Infant Dose (RID) %	Comments
Aspirin	10.8[118]	Compatible: Use of low-dose aspirin (81 mg) is probably safe; however, little information is known about the relationship between the dose and risk of Reye syndrome in infants. Watch for thrombocytopenia and petechiae in infants[118]
Warfarin		Compatible: In a study of 13 mothers, none of them had detectable levels in breast milk and no adverse events were reported in breastfed infants[119]
Heparin		Compatible: Large molecular weight 12,000–15,000 Da, unlikely to enter breast milk, and most likely destroyed by infant's gastrointestinal tract[120]
Dalteparin sodium (LMWH)		Compatible: In a study of 15 patients at a mean of 5.7 d post cesarean, dalteparin levels in breast milk were <0.005–0.037 IU/mL. Oral absorption is unlikely, and its possible levels in "mature" milk could be lower[121]
Clopidogrel		Probably compatible: To date there are no data on human breast milk. The plasma half-life is 6–8 h, and its metabolite (thiol derivative) covalently bonds to platelet receptors with a half-life of 11 d. Because it produces an irreversible inhibition of platelet aggregation, any drug in milk could inhibit an infant's platelet function for a prolonged period. Given the moderate molecular weight of 420 Da, low protein binding, and 50% oral bioavailability, this drug would not be the drug of choice in breastfeeding, but if required should not be a contraindication[122]

Abbreviation: LMWH, low molecular weight heparin.

ENDOCRINE

The rate of diabetes is increasing, and more mothers are requiring insulin and oral hypoglycemics in pregnancy and throughout lactation. One of the first-line medications used for type 2 diabetes mellitus is metformin. This medication is part of the biguanide class of antidiabetic medications, and has been studied in 5 lactating women and 3 infants.[76] The average peak and trough concentrations in breast milk for metformin were 0.42 μg/mL and 0.39 μg/mL, resulting in an RID of 0.65%.[76] In this study, 3 infants had their blood glucose monitored and no hypoglycemia occurred; therefore, metformin should be compatible with breastfeeding.[76]

Glyburide is a second-generation sulfonylurea that is also one of the first-line therapies used for type 2 diabetes. In a study of 6 mothers given a single dose of glyburide 5 mg, and 2 mothers given a single dose of 10 mg, the drug was undetectable in breast milk at both doses (limit of detection 0.005 μg/mL).[77] In a group of 5 mothers who received daily doses of glyburide 5 mg or glipizide 5 mg, the same results were found, and both medications were undetectable in breast milk.[77] In this study the infant plasma glucose levels were normal, which would be expected if no medication had been consumed by the infant.

Insulin is used in the management of multiple endocrine diseases such as diabetes mellitus types 1 and 2, gestational diabetes, and diabetic ketoacidosis. Insulin is a large peptide molecule that is not secreted into human milk; however, if it were to enter breast milk it would have no or very little absorption, because the infant's gastrointestinal tract would destroy it.[78] Therefore, there is no contraindication to using insulin while breastfeeding.

CONTRACEPTIVES

It is hypothesized that the withdrawal of progesterone in the early postpartum period initiates lactogenesis.[79] Consequently, it has been suggested that if a mother begins progesterone or combined oral contraceptives (COCs) early postpartum (the first few days), it may interrupt the establishment of breastfeeding.[79]

A recently published double-blind randomized trial compared the effect of initiating progesterone-only contraceptives (0.35 mg norethindrone) with COCs (0.035 mg ethinyl estradiol + 1 mg norethindrone) at 2 weeks postpartum.[80] This study found that there was no difference in continuation of breastfeeding between the 2 groups at 8 weeks (64.1% combined pills vs 63.5% progestin only) or 6 months.[80] In both groups, women who supplemented their infants with formula or had concerns of inadequate milk supply were more likely to stop breastfeeding.[80] It should be noted that there was no comparison of discontinuation rates of breastfeeding with a placebo group, so it is unknown whether progesterone itself increased the rates of discontinuation, and only the mother's perception of changes in milk volume, not actual volume measurements, were analyzed.[80]

Although this new study is interesting, an older study with 330 women who used nonhormonal contraceptives (NHC), COCs, and copper intrauterine devices (Cu IUDs) found more infants were weaned at 6 and 8 months in the oral contraceptive group (16.3% COC, 9% NHC, 4.7% Cu IUD at 6 months).[81] However, by the end of 1 year an equivalent number of women (~40%) in each of the 3 groups were no longer breastfeeding.[81]

Therefore, any hormonal product, estrogen or progestin, may suppress lactation at any time (early postpartum or after establishment). NHCs should always be an alternative discussed with breastfeeding mothers, and the potential risk of a hormonal contraceptive should be understood before choosing such a product. Finally, if mothers prefer to use hormonal contraception, they should be advised to avoid contraceptive products for at least the first 4 weeks postpartum to allow the establishment of breastfeeding and to avoid increasing their risk of thrombosis in the postpartum period.[79,80,82]

DRUGS THAT STIMULATE MILK PRODUCTION

During gestation, prolactin levels reach as high as 400 ng/mL. After delivery and over the first 6 months postpartum, maternal prolactin levels steadily drop to approximately 75 ng/mL at 6 months, even though milk production is unchanged.[83] In many mothers who are unable to produce adequate breast milk, prolactin levels are thought to have fallen below adequate levels (less than 75 ng/mL). Therefore, milk production may in some cases be recovered with the use of dopamine antagonists (galactagogues), which stimulate the release of prolactin.

The 2 most common dopamine antagonists used for this purpose are metoclopramide (Reglan) and domperidone (Motilium). Metoclopramide is prescribed most frequently in the United States because domperidone is not approved by the Food and Drug Administration (FDA). Prolactin release as stimulated by metoclopramide is clearly dose related. Ten to 15 mg administered 3 times daily has been demonstrated to be most beneficial.[84] The dose of metoclopramide present in human milk is small, 6 to 24 µg/kg/d for children studied in early postpartum and 1 to 13 µg/kg/d for those studied after 8 to 12 weeks postpartum.[85] Side effects of this medication are severe, and include depression, extrapyramidal symptoms, gastric cramping, and tardive dyskinesia. However, none were reported in this study when mothers were given meto-clopramide 10 mg 3 times daily for a limited duration.[85]

Domperidone is another dopamine antagonist used to stimulate prolactin levels. It is only available in the United States from compounding pharmacies, as it has never been approved for use in the United States. Even though the FDA has issued a black-box warning regarding the risk of QTc prolongation, cardiac arrest, and sudden death, domperidone remains the primary galactagogue used worldwide.[86] Prescribers should be aware that many other medications, especially those used for psychiatric conditions, can also prolong the QTc interval; therefore this medication should not be prescribed to those taking other medications that also prolong this interval (eg, quetiapine, citalopram).[87]

A study of domperidone used a dose of 10 mg 3 times daily for 7 days in mothers of premature infants, and found a mean milk volume increase of 44.5%. Milk levels of domperidone were low in this study at 1.2 ng/mL; consequently the infant dose was also low, less than 0.2 μg/kg/d, and no adverse effects were reported in the infant.[88]

Because breast milk production depends on persistent and elevated prolactin levels produced by the dopamine antagonist, a slow withdrawal of either domperidone or metoclopramide over several weeks to a month is suggested to prevent loss of milk supply.

Fenugreek is the most commonly used herbal for increasing the production of breast milk. There are numerous studies with conflicting data. The most recent placebo-controlled study published as an abstract in 2011 suggested that fenugreek had no effect on either prolactin levels or volume of breast milk.[89] This study included 26 mothers of premature infants who took fenugreek 1725 mg 3 times daily for 3 weeks. Although no adverse effects were noted in the study, herbal products are not controlled by the FDA, so the quality and consistency of the product chosen would be unknown and may put the mother and/or infant at risk of unknown adverse effects. Fenugreek is not recommended to improve the production of breast milk.

SUMMARY

The number of new medications available to breastfeeding mothers requiring drug therapy is expanding on a daily basis, which makes it difficult for clinicians to assess the safety of medications in breast milk. However, knowing how to assess key factors that influence a medication's suitability in breastfeeding allows clinicians to make collaborative clinical decisions with their patients to encourage breastfeeding. In reality, women can breastfeed safely while ingesting most, but not all, medications. Clinicians should become more aware of this area of research to help them better care for breastfeeding mothers and support breastfeeding.

REFERENCES

1. Division of Nutrition, Physical Activity, and Obesity, National Center for Chronic Disease Prevention and Health Promotion. Breastfeeding report card, United States 2013. Centers for Disease Control Report Card [Internet]. 2013. p. 1–8. Available at: http://www.cdc.gov/breastfeeding/pdf/2013 breastfeedingreportcard.pdf. Accessed July 26, 2014.
2. Stultz EE, Stokes JL, Shaffer ML, et al. Extent of medication use in breastfeeding women. Breastfeed Med 2007;2(3):145–51.

3. Hale TW. Medication and mothers' milk. 14th edition. Amarillo (TX): Hale Publishing; 2010.
4. Hale TW, Hartmann PE. Textbook of human lactation. Amarillo (TX): Hale Publishing LPL; 2007.
5. Bennett PN. Drugs and human lactation. Amsterdam: Elsevier; 1996.
6. Centers for Disease Control and Prevention (CDC). Prevalence of self-reported postpartum depressive symptoms—17 states, 2004-2005. MMWR Morb Mortal Wkly Rep 2008;57(14):361–6.
7. Stowe ZN, Hostetter AL, Owens MJ, et al. The pharmacokinetics of sertraline excretion into human breast milk: determinants of infant serum concentrations. J Clin Psychiatry 2003;64(1):73–80.
8. Hagg S, Granberg K, Carleborg L. Excretion of fluvoxamine into breast milk. Br J Clin Pharmacol 2000;49(3):286–8.
9. Ohman R, Hagg S, Carleborg L, et al. Excretion of paroxetine into breast milk. J Clin Psychiatry 1999;60(8):519–23.
10. Kristensen JH, Ilett KF, Hackett LP, et al. Distribution and excretion of fluoxetine and norfluoxetine in human milk. Br J Clin Pharmacol 1999;48(4):521–7.
11. Kelly LE, Poon S, Madadi P, et al. Neonatal benzodiazepines exposure during breastfeeding. J Pediatr 2012;161:448–51.
12. Kanto JH. Use of benzodiazepines during pregnancy, labour and lactation, with particular reference to pharmacokinetic considerations. Drugs 1982;23(5): 354–80.
13. Rindi V. La eliminazione degli antistaminici di sintesi con il latte e l'azione latto-goga de questi. Riv Ital Ginecol 1951;34:147–57.
14. Matheson I, Sande HA, Gaillot J. The excretion of zopiclone into breast milk. Br J Clin Pharmacol 1990;30(2):267–71.
15. Hill RC, McIvor RJ, Wojnar-Horton RE, et al. Risperidone distribution and excretion into human milk: case report and estimated infant exposure during breast-feeding. J Clin Psychopharmacol 2000;20(2):285–6.
16. Croke S, Buist A, Hackett LP, et al. Olanzapine excretion in human breast milk: estimation of infant exposure. Int J Neuropsychopharmacol 2002;5(3):243–7.
17. Rampono J, Kristensen JH, Ilett KF, et al. Quetiapine and breast feeding. Ann Pharmacother 2007;41:711–4.
18. Wiles DH, Orr MW, Kolakowska T. Chlorpromazine levels in plasma and milk of nursing mothers. Br J Clin Pharmacol 1978;5(3):272–3.
19. Hackett LP, Kristensen JH, Hale TW, et al. Methylphenidate and breast-feeding. Ann Pharmacother 2006;40(10):1890–1.
20. Ilett KF, Hackett LP, Kristensen JH, et al. Transfer of dexamphetamine into breast milk during treatment for attention deficit hyperactivity disorder. Br J Clin Pharmacol 2006. http://dx.doi.org/10.1111/j.1365-2125.2006.02767.x.
21. von Unruh GE, Froescher W, Hoffmann F, et al. Valproic acid in breast milk: how much is really there? Ther Drug Monit 1984;6(3):272–6.
22. Tomson T, Ohman I, Vitols S. Lamotrigine in pregnancy and lactation: a case report. Epilepsia 1997;38(9):1039–41.
23. Newport DJ, Pennell PB, Calamaras MR, et al. Lamotrigine in breast milk and nursing infants: determination of exposure. Pediatrics 2008;122(1):e223–31.
24. Ohman I, Vitols S, Luef G, et al. Topiramate kinetics during delivery, lactation, and in the neonate: preliminary observations. Epilepsia 2002;43(10):1157–60.
25. Mennella JA, Beauchamp GK. The transfer of alcohol to human milk. Effects on flavor and the infant's behavior [see comments]. N Engl J Med 1991;325(14): 981–5.

26. Mennella JA. Regulation of milk intake after exposure to alcohol in mothers' milk. Alcohol Clin Exp Res 2001;25(4):590–3.
27. Cobo E. Effect of different doses of ethanol on the milk-ejecting reflex in lactating women. Am J Obstet Gynecol 1973;115(6):817–21.
28. Ho E, Collantes A, Kapur BM, et al. Alcohol and breast feeding: calculation of time to zero level in milk. Biol Neonate 2001;80(3):219–22.
29. Perez-Reyes M, Wall ME. Presence of delta9-tetrahydrocannabinol in human milk [letter]. N Engl J Med 1982;307(13):819–20.
30. Tennes K, Avitable N, Blackard C, et al. Marijuana: prenatal and postnatal exposure in the human. NIDA Res Monogr 1985;59:48–60.
31. Astley SJ, Little RE. Maternal marijuana use during lactation and infant development at one year. Neurotoxicol Teratol 1990;12(2):161–8.
32. Jutras-Aswad D, DiNieri J, Harkany T, et al. Neurobiological consequences of maternal cannabis on human fetal development and its neuropsychiatric outcome. Eur Arch Psychiatry Clin Neurosci 2009;259:395–412.
33. Ilett KF, Hale TW, Page-Sharp M, et al. Use of nicotine patches in breast-feeding mothers: transfer of nicotine and cotinine into human milk. Clin Pharmacol Ther 2003;74(6):516–24.
34. Tyrala EE, Dodson WE. Caffeine secretion into breast milk. Arch Dis Child 1979; 54(10):787–800.
35. Ryu JE. Caffeine in human milk and in serum of breast-fed infants. Dev Pharmacol Ther 1985;8(6):329–37.
36. Weibert RT, Townsend RJ, Kaiser DG, et al. Lack of ibuprofen secretion into human milk. Clin Pharm 1982;1(5):457–8.
37. Bitzen PO, Gustafsson B, Jostell KG, et al. Excretion of paracetamol in human breast milk. Eur J Clin Pharmacol 1981;20(2):123–5.
38. Jamali F, Stevens DR. Naproxen excretion in milk and its uptake by the infant. Drug Intell Clin Pharm 1983;17(12):910–1.
39. Edwards JE, Rudy AC, Wermeling DP, et al. Hydromorphone transfer into breast milk after intranasal administration. Pharmacotherapy 2003;23(2):153–8.
40. Sauberan JB, Anderson PO, Lane JR, et al. Breast milk hydrocodone and hydromorphone levels in mothers using hydrocodone for postpartum pain. Obstet Gynecol 2011;117(3):611–7.
41. Bodley V, Powers D. Long-term treatment of a breastfeeding mother with fluconazole-resolved nipple pain caused by yeast: a case study. J Hum Lact 1997;13(4):307–11.
42. Meyer D, Tobias JD. Adverse effects following the inadvertent administration of opioids to infants and children. Clin Pediatr 2005;44:499–503.
43. Feilberg VL, Rosenborg D, Broen CC, et al. Excretion of morphine in human breast milk. Acta Anaesthesiol Scand 1989;33(5):426–8.
44. Koren G, Cairns J, Chitayat D, et al. Pharmacogenetics of morphine poisoning in a breastfed neonate of a codeine-prescribed mother. Lancet 2006;368(9536):704.
45. Lam J, Kelly L, Ciszkowski C, et al. Central nervous system depression of neonates breastfed by mothers receiving oxycodone for postpartum analgesia. J Pediatr 2012;160:33–7.
46. Sandstrom B, Regardh CG. Metoprolol excretion into breast milk. Br J Clin Pharmacol 1980;9(5):518–9.
47. Taylor EA, Turner P. Anti-hypertensive therapy with propranolol during pregnancy and lactation. Postgrad Med J 1981;57:427–30.

48. Lunell NO, Kulas J, Rane A. Transfer of labetalol into amniotic fluid and breast milk in lactating women. Eur J Clin Pharmacol 1985;28(5):597–9.
49. Schimmel MS, Eidelman AI, Wilschanski MA, et al. Toxic effects of atenolol consumed during breast feeding. J Pediatr 1989;114:476–8.
50. Boutroy MJ, Bianchetti G, Dubruc C, et al. To nurse when receiving acebutolol: is it dangerous for the neonate? Eur J Clin Pharmacol 1986;30(6):737–9.
51. Ehrenkranz RA, Ackerman BA, Hulse JD. Nifedipine transfer into human milk. J Pediatr 1989;114(3):478–80.
52. Anderson P, Bondesson U, Mattiasson I, et al. Verapamil and norverapamil in plasma and breast milk during breast feeding. Eur J Clin Pharmacol 1987;31: 625–7.
53. Okada M, Inoue H, Nakamura Y, et al. Excretion of diltiazem in human milk. N Engl J Med 1985;312(15):992–3.
54. Devlin RG. Selective resistance to the passage of captopril into human milk. Clin Pharmacol Ther 1980;27:250.
55. Redman CW, Kelly JG, Cooper WD. The excretion of enalapril and enalaprilat in human breast milk. Eur J Clin Pharmacol 1990;38(1):99.
56. Miller ME, Cohn RD, Burghart PH. Hydrochlorothiazide disposition in a mother and her breast-fed infant. J Pediatr 1982;101(5):789–91.
57. Healy M. Suppressing lactation with oral diuretics. Lancet 1961;277(1790): 1353–4.
58. Courtney TP, Shaw RW. Excretion of famotidine in breast milk. Br J Clin Pharmacol 1988;26:639.
59. Kearns GL, McConnell RF Jr, Trang JM, et al. Appearance of ranitidine in breast milk following multiple dosing. Clin Pharm 1985;4(3):322–4.
60. Marshall JK, Thompson AB, Armstrong D. Omeprazole for refractory gastro-esophageal reflux disease during pregnancy and lactation. Can J Gastroenterol 1998;12(3):225–7.
61. Plante L, Ferron GM, Unruh M, et al. Excretion of pantoprazole in human breast. J Reprod Med 2004;49(10):825–7.
62. Guikontes E, Spantideas A, Diakakis J. Ondansetron and hyperemesis gravida-rum. Lancet 1992;340:1223.
63. Khalil SN, Roth AG, Cohen IT, et al. A double-blind comparison of intravenous ondansetron and placebo for preventing postoperative emesis in 1 to 24 month old pediatric patients after surgery under general anesthesia. Anesth Analg 2005;101:356–61.
64. Kafetzis DA, Siafas CA, Georgakopoulos PA, et al. Passage of cephalosporins and amoxicillin into the breast milk. Acta Paediatr Scand 1981;70(3):285–8.
65. Benyamini L, Merlob P, Stahl B, et al. The safety of amoxicillin/clavulanic acid and cefuroxime during lactation. Ther Drug Monit 2005;27:499–502.
66. Morganti G, Ceccarelli G, Ciaffi G. Comparative concentrations of a tetracycline antibiotic in serum and maternal milk. Antibiotica 1968;6(3):216–23 [in Multiple languages].
67. Ghaffar F, McCracken GH. Quinolones in pediatrics. In: Hooper DC, Rubinstein E, editors. Quinolone antimicrobial agents. 3rd edition. Washington, DC: ASM Press; 2003. p. 343–54.
68. Giamarellou H, Kolokythas E, Petrikkos G, et al. Pharmacokinetics of three newer quinolones in pregnant and lactating women. Am J Med 1989;87(5A): 49S–51S.
69. Shetty AK. Tetracyclines in pediatrics revisited. Clin Pediatr 2002;41:203–9.

70. Posner AC, Prigot A, Konicoff NG. Further observations on the use of tetracycline hydrochloride in prophylaxis and treatment of obstetric infections. In: Antibiotics annual 1954-1955. New York: Medical Encyclopedia; 1955.

71. von Keutz E, Ruhl-Fehlert C, Drommer W, et al. Effects of ciprofloxacin on joint cartilage in immature dogs immediately after dosing and after a 5-month treatment-free period. Arch Toxicol 2004;78:418–24.

72. Schwebke JR. Metronidazole: utilization in the obstetric and gynecologic patient. Sex Transm Dis 1995;22(6):370–6.

73. Passmore CM, McElnay JC, Rainey EA, et al. Metronidazole excretion in human milk and its effect on the suckling neonate. Br J Clin Pharmacol 1988;26(1):45–51.

74. Erickson SH, Oppenheim GL, Smith GH. Metronidazole in breast milk. Obstet Gynecol 1981;57(1):48–50.

75. Putter J, Satravaha P, Stockhausen H. Quantitative analysis of the main metabolites of acetylsalicylic acid. Comparative analysis in the blood and milk of lactating women (author's transl). Z Geburtshilfe Perinatol 1974;178(2):135–8 [in German].

76. Briggs GG, Ambrose PJ, Nageotte MP, et al. Excretion of metformin into breast milk and the effect on nursing infants. Obstet Gynecol 2005;105(6):1437–41.

77. Feig DS, Briggs GG, Kraemer JM, et al. Transfer of glyburide and glipizide into breast milk. Diabetes Care 2005;28(8):1851–5.

78. Novo Nordisk Canada Inc. Pharmaceutical manufacturer product monograph: human insulin Novolin ge. 2011.

79. Kennedy KI, Short RV, Tully MR. Premature introduction of progestin-only contraceptive methods during lactation. Contraception 1997;55(6):347–50.

80. Espey E, Ogburn T, Leeman L, et al. Effect of progestin compared with combined oral contraceptive pills on lactation. Obstet Gynecol 2012;119(1):5–13.

81. Croxatto HB, Diaz S, Peralta O, et al. Fertility regulation in nursing women: IV. Long-term influence of a low-dose combined oral contraceptive initiated at day 30 postpartum upon lactation and infant growth. Contraception 1983;27(1):13–25.

82. Queenan J. Exploring contraceptive options for breastfeeding mothers. Obstet Gynecol 2012;119(1):1–2.

83. Cox DB, Owens RA, Hartmann PE. Blood and milk prolactin and the rate of milk synthesis in women. Exp Physiol 1996;81(6):1007–20.

84. Kauppila A, Kivinen S, Ylikorkala O. A dose response relation between improved lactation and metoclopramide. Lancet 1981;1(8231):1175–7.

85. Kauppila A, Arvela P, Koivisto M, et al. Metoclopramide and breast feeding: transfer into milk and the newborn. Eur J Clin Pharmacol 1983;25:819–23.

86. US Food and Drug Administration. FDA talk paper: FDA warns against women using unapproved drug, domperidone, to increase milk production 2004. Available at: http://www.fda.gov/drugs/drugsafety/informationbydrugclass/ucm173886.htm. Accessed July 25, 2014.

87. Lexi-Interact [Internet]. Lexi-Comp, Inc. Accessed July 25, 2014.

88. da Silva OP, Knoppert DC, Angelini MM, et al. Effect of domperidone on milk production in mothers of premature newborns: a randomized, double-blind, placebo-controlled trial. CMAJ 2001;164(1):17–21.

89. Reeder C, Legrand A, O'Conner-Von S. The effect of fenugreek on milk production and prolactin levels in mothers of premature infants [abstract]. J Hum Lact 2011;27:74.

90. Rampono J, Kristensen JH, Hackett LP, et al. Citalopram and demethylcitalopram in human milk; distribution, excretion and effects in breast fed infants. Br J Clin Pharmacol 2000;50(10):263–8.
91. Schmidt K, Olesen OV, Jensen PN. Citalopram and breast-feeding: serum concentration and side effects in the infant. Biol Psychiatry 2000;47(2):164–5.
92. Frannsen EJ. Citalopram serum and milk levels in mother and infant during lactation. Ther Drug Monit 2006;28(1):2–4.
93. Taddio A, Ito S, Koren G. Excretion of fluoxetine and its metabolite, norfluoxetine, in human breast milk. J Clin Pharmacol 1996;36(1):42–7.
94. Lester BM, Cucca J, Andreozzi L, et al. Possible association between fluoxetine hydrochloride and colic in an infant. J Am Acad Child Adolesc Psychiatry 1993; 32(6):1253–5.
95. Rampono J, Hackett LP, Kristensen JH, et al. Transfer of escitalopram and its metabolite demethylescitalopram into breast milk. Br J Clin Pharmacol 2006; 62(3):316–22.
96. Newport DJ, Ritchie JC, Knight BT, et al. Venlafaxine in human breast milk and nursing infant plasma: determination of exposure. J Clin Psychiatry 2009;70(9): 1304–10.
97. Rampono J, Teoh S, Hackett LP, et al. Estimation of desvenlafaxine transfer into milk and infant exposure during its use in lactating women with postnatal depression. Arch Womens Ment Health 2011;14(1):49–53.
98. Lobo ED, Loghin C, Knadler MP, et al. Pharmacokinetics of duloxetine in breast milk and plasma of healthy postpartum women. Clin Pharmacokinet 2008;47(2): 103–9.
99. Stahl MM, Neiderud J, Vinge E. Thrombocytopenic purpura and anemia in a breast-fed infant whose mother was treated with valproic acid. J Pediatr 1997; 130:1001–3.
100. Meador KJ, Baker GA, Browning N, et al. Effects of breastfeeding in children of women taking antiepileptic drugs. Neurology 2010;75(22):1954–60.
101. Shimoyama R, Ohkubo T, Sugawara K. Monitoring of carbamazepine and carbamazepine 10,11-epoxide in breast milk and plasma by high-performance liquid chromatography. Ann Clin Biochem 2000;37(Pt 2):210–5.
102. Moretti ME, Koren G, Verjee Z, et al. Monitoring lithium in breast milk: an individualized approach for breast-feeding mothers. Ther Drug Monit 2003;25(3): 364–6.
103. Viguera AC, Newport DJ, Ritchie J, et al. Lithium in breast milk and nursing infants: clinical implications. Am J Psychiatry 2007;164(2):342–5.
104. Ohman I, Vitols S, Tomson T. Lamotrigine in pregnancy: pharmacokinetics during delivery, in the neonate, and during lactation. Epilepsia 2000;41(6): 709–13.
105. Steen B, Rane A, Lonnerholm G, et al. Phenytoin excretion in human breast milk and plasma levels in nursed infants. Ther Drug Monit 1982;4(4):331–4.
106. Matsuda S. Transfer of antibiotics into maternal milk. Biol Res Pregnancy Perinatol 1984;5(2):57–60.
107. Foulds G, Miller RD, Knirsch AK, et al. Sulbactam kinetics and excretion into breast milk in postpartum women. Clin Pharmacol Ther 1985;38(6):692–6.
108. Celiloglu M, Celiker S, Guven H, et al. Gentamicin excretion and uptake from breast milk by nursing infants. Obstet Gynecol 1994;84(2):263–5.
109. Festini F, Ciuti R, Taccetti G, et al. Breast-feeding in a woman with cystic fibrosis undergoing antibiotic intravenous treatment. J Matern Fetal Neonatal Med 2006; 19(6):375–6.

110. Uwaydah M, Bibi S, Salman S. Therapeutic efficacy of tobramycin–a clinical and laboratory evaluation. J Antimicrob Chemother 1975;1(4):429–37.

111. Yoshioka H, Cho K, Takimoto M, et al. Transfer of cefazolin into human milk. J Pediatr 1979;94(1):151–2.

112. Ilett KF, Hackett LP, Ingle B, et al. Transfer of probenecid and cephalexin into breast milk. Ann Pharmacother 2006;40(5):986–9.

113. Takase Z, Shirofuji H, Uchida M. Fundamental and clinical studies of cefuroxime in the field of obstetrics and gynecology. Chemotherapy (Tokyo) 1979;27(Suppl 6): 600–2.

114. Bourget P, Quinquis-Desmaris V, Fernandez H. Ceftriaxone distribution and protein binding between maternal blood and milk postpartum. Ann Pharmacother 1993;27(3):294–7.

115. Kafetzis DA, Lazarides CV, Siafas CA, et al. Transfer of cefotaxime in human milk and from mother to foetus. J Antimicrob Chemother 1980;6(Suppl A):135–41.

116. Blanco JD, Jorgensen JH, Castaneda YS, et al. Ceftazidime levels in human breast milk. Antimicrob Agents Chemother 1983;23(3):479–80.

117. Sauberan J, Bradley J, Blumer J, et al. Transmission of meropenem in breast milk. Pediatr Infect Dis J 2012;31:832–4.

118. Bailey DN, Weibert RT, Naylor AJ, et al. A study of salicylate and caffeine excretion in the breast milk of two nursing mothers. J Anal Toxicol 1982;6:64–8.

119. Orme ML, Lewis PJ, De Swiet M, et al. May mothers given warfarin breast-feed their infants? Br Med J 1977;1(6076):1564–5.

120. McEvoy GE, editor. AFHS drug information. 1992. p. 417–26.

121. Richter C, Sitzmann J, Lang P, et al. Excretion of low molecular weight heparin in human milk. Br J Clin Pharmacol 2001;52(6):708–10.

122. Sanofi-Aventis Canada Inc. Pharmaceutical manufacturer prescribing information: clopidogrel. 2012.

Challenges of Managing Pediatric Mental Health Crises in the Emergency Department

Thomas H. Chun, MD, MPH[a,b],*, Emily R. Katz, MD[c],
Susan J. Duffy, MD, MPH[a,b], Ruth S. Gerson, MD[d]

KEYWORDS

- Psychiatric emergency • Pediatric • Autism • Developmental disorders

KEY POINTS

- Children and adolescents presenting to emergency departments with psychiatric crises are burgeoning; optimal care of these patients includes close collaboration between emergency medicine and psychiatry physicians.
- The evaluation and management of aggressive and/or violent patients, requires a range of skills and knowledge, including verbal de-escalation as well as knowledge of safe chemical and physical restraint practices.
- Children with autism spectrum or other developmental disorders in the emergency department also require specialized skills for communication, transition planning, and calming and soothing the patient.

Conflict of Interest: The authors have no conflicts of interest to disclose.

Grant Support: Supported in part by "Teen Alcohol Screening in the Pediatric Emergency Care Applied Research Network", U03 MC22685, National Institute for Alcohol Abuse and Alcoholism, R01 AA021900 (T.H. Chun).

This article has been revised and updated from an article originally published in *Pediatric Clinics of North America* by Chun, Katz, and Duffy in 2013, entitled "Pediatric Mental Health Emergencies and Special Health Care Needs."

[a] Department of Emergency Medicine, Alpert Medical School of Brown University, 222 Richmond Street, Providence, RI 02903, USA; [b] Department of Pediatrics, Alpert Medical School of Brown University, 222 Richmond Street, Providence, RI 02903, USA; [c] Department of Psychiatry and Human Behavior, Alpert Medical School of Brown University, 222 Richmond Street, Providence, RI 02903, USA; [d] Bellevue Hospital Children's Comprehensive Psychiatric Emergency Program, Department of Child and Adolescent Psychiatry, NYU School of Medicine, 462 1st Avenue, New York, NY 10016, USA

* Corresponding author. Department of Emergency Medicine, Rhode Island Hospital, Claverick 243, 593 Eddy Street, Providence, RI 02903.

E-mail address: Thomas_Chun@brown.edu

http://dx.doi.org/10.1016/j.chc.2014.09.003
childpsych.theclinics.com
1056-4993/15/$ – see front matter © 2015 Elsevier Inc. All rights reserved.

COMMENTARY: CRISIS IN THE EMERGENCY ROOM: MANAGING PEDIATRIC MENTAL HEALTH CRISES IN THE EMERGENCY DEPARTMENT

The constriction of inpatient and outpatient services for children's mental health treatment, coupled with an increased awareness of the potentially disastrous consequences of untreated suicidality and aggression in children and adolescents, has led to a dramatic increase in youth presenting to the Emergency Room (ER) for psychiatric care. This article, updated from an article published in the *Pediatrics Clinics of North America* in 2013, highlights the key features of appropriate emergency evaluation and treatment of youth in psychiatric crisis. The article's description of detailed and structured risk assessment, involvement of family and other key caregivers, careful use of de-escalation strategies to ensure safety in the ER, and connection to appropriate inpatient or outpatient services provides a much-needed standard for high-quality emergency psychiatric care for children.

Unfortunately, too many children and adolescents in psychiatric crisis do not receive such care. Emergency programs, due to lack of funding, support, and training, have not kept pace with the escalating demand for emergency psychiatric care. Most children and adolescents in psychiatric crisis are seen in general pediatric or medical ERs, which are crowded, noisy, high-stimulation environments, often with long wait times and little available private or quiet space.[1,2] For agitated, paranoid, traumatized, or autistic youth, this can be disastrous, often ending in restraints or seclusions that might have been avoided in a quieter, calmer setting. Adding to the difficulty of managing these patients in ERs, most young people presenting with a psychiatric crisis are treated by pediatric emergency clinicians and staff who lack psychiatric training, or by adult psychiatric clinicians who lack training in the diagnosis and treatment of children and adolescents. In a statewide survey in California, only 10% of emergency programs had child psychiatrists available for consultation (and most who did were academic centers, not community hospitals); less than 35% had general psychiatrists available, only 15% had a psychiatric nurse present, and less than 50% programs had a social worker (and not necessarily a psychiatric social worker) to assist in evaluation or disposition.[3] Medical providers see most young people presenting to ERs in psychiatric crisis, but only a third of these providers have ever had any training in treating psychiatric patients.[4] More than half of the youth presenting to the ER after a suicide attempt or other episode of deliberate self-harm never receive any mental health evaluation.[5] Of youth presenting with mental health complaints (including self-harm and suicide attempts) to the ER, two-thirds are discharged, but only about a third of patients are given a referral for any psychiatric follow-up care.[1,5] Clinicians may lack sufficient training to recognize the need for a hospitalization or outpatient referral; there may not be inpatient beds or outpatient services available; or insurance may balk at paying for psychiatric treatment (particularly inpatient or intensive treatment). When an outpatient referral is made, there are often long wait lists to be seen in community clinics, and in most communities, acute care outpatient services such intensive outpatient programs, partial hospitalization programs, and home-based crisis services are either unavailable or prohibitively expensive.

To ensure that every child and adolescent presenting to an ER in psychiatric crisis receives the standard of care described below would require a broad investment and collaboration between child and adolescent psychiatrists and pediatricians. Together, the following must be advocated for:

1. Development of clear standards of care for emergency evaluation and treatment
2. Increased training for emergency medical providers and pediatricians in identification and treatment of child mental illness, as well as in de-escalation and crisis management

3. Greater collaboration between emergency providers and child psychiatrists for consultation around high-risk cases
4. Greater availability and accessibility of high-quality inpatient and acute care outpatient services for youth in crisis
5. Coordination of research and program-development efforts to identify and disseminate efficacious and cost-effective models of crisis care, both ER-based and community-based, for children and adolescents.

Development of clear standards of care for emergency evaluation and treatment. The lack of consensus guidelines or standards of care for management of pediatric psychiatric emergencies means there is no metric by which hospitals can measure their performance. Child psychiatrists and pediatricians should collaborate to develop standards for evaluation, risk assessment, and management of agitation (including both nonpharmacologic and pharmacologic interventions), as well as for the staffing and physical space requirements for appropriate management of children in psychiatric crisis.

Increased training for emergency medical providers and pediatricians in identification and treatment of child mental illness as well as in de-escalation and crisis management. A few training programs for pediatricians, nurse practitioners, emergency medicine physicians, and other disciplines now offer opportunities for exposure to acute-care child psychiatry; these should be standardized and expanded. ER staff should undergo in-service training on identification and management of suicidality, perhaps including the use of suicide screening tools (either interview-based or computer-based) that have been shown to be effective in ER settings.[2] Staff training in verbal de-escalation and crisis management techniques will also help avoid unnecessary restraints of child psychiatric patients in the ER.

Greater collaboration between emergency providers and child psychiatrists for consultation around high-risk cases. With the national workforce shortage of child psychiatrists, it is crucial to find ways to extend the reach of child psychiatry through consultation. Telepsychiatry programs and phone consultation programs similar to the Child and Adolescent Psychiatry for Primary Care (CAP-PC) program for pediatricians and primary care physicians should be developed for ERs, to allow pediatricians greater access to child psychiatry consultation. Another innovation, used in Massachusetts and some other states, is the use of mobile psychiatric evaluation teams that can move from one hospital ER to another to provide expert evaluation and treatment of kids when a child psychiatrist or other specialized provider is not available.

Greater availability and accessibility of high-quality inpatient and acute care outpatient services for youth in crisis. Several innovative programs have been developed across the country to enhance quick access to crisis services. These programs include enhanced emergency programs such as the Comprehensive Psychiatric Emergency Program model developed in New York State, in which an inpatient crisis stabilization unit and crisis outpatient services are embedded within the ER; crisis clinics within outpatient clinics or attached to psychiatric ERs; and mobile crisis programs and emergency screening units that allow youth to receive emergency evaluations in the community rather than in a medical ER.

Coordination of research and program-development efforts to identify and disseminate efficacious and cost-effective models of crisis care, both ER-based and community-based, for children and adolescents. The innovations described demonstrate potential solutions to the challenges of managing child psychiatric patients in the ER, but they must be rigorously studied (both regarding efficacy and cost-effectiveness), standardized, and disseminated. The Pediatric Emergency Care

Applied Research Network's mental health interest group has led several large-scale research studies to identify best practices for mental health treatment in pediatric ERs, but a broader research effort is needed to evaluate consultation and telepsychiatry programs as well as the care of children in psychiatric ERs and community-based crisis services.

The emergency department has become the de facto safety net for children in psychiatric crisis, but ERs must be equipped to catch them. With collaboration and advocacy, it can be ensured that all children in crisis receive the kind of excellent care described later, and that they leave the ER with the clinical and social supports and services that will put them on the path to recovery.

INTRODUCTION

Visits for mental health problems to both pediatric primary care settings and pediatric emergency departments have skyrocketed in recent decades and now account for up to 25% to 50% of primary care and 5% of pediatric emergency department visits.[6-11] Both pediatricians[12] and pediatric emergency physicians[13-15] identify lack of training in and lack of confidence in their ability to care for mental health problems as barriers to caring for these patients. Child and adolescent psychiatrists can play a significant role and be an important resource for pediatric clinicians who care for these patients. This article includes the 2 most common pediatric mental health emergencies, both of which involve threats to safety:

1. Suicide, where there is risk of harm to the patient, and
2. Homicide or aggression, where there is risk of harm to others.

In addition, the challenges of caring for children with autism or other developmental disabilities in medical settings are also discussed. The foci of this article are the key elements and practical suggestions for pediatric providers, when caring for these populations.

SUICIDAL IDEATION AND SUICIDE ATTEMPTS
Key Points

- Suicide is one of the leading causes of death in pediatric patients.
- Constant observation is necessary to ensure patient safety during suicide evaluation and crisis stabilization.
- Evaluation includes assessment for potential underlying or associated medical conditions.
- Laboratory and/or imaging should be obtained on an as-needed basis.
- High-risk patients should be referred directly for inpatient psychiatric admission.
- Less-intensive treatment options may be considered for patients who are able to maintain their safety in outpatient settings.
- Although no medications directly treat suicidality, there are safe and effective treatments for most of the associated psychiatric conditions.
- All evaluations of patients in the setting of suicidal ideation or suicide attempts should include a thorough discussion of safety planning, including means restriction and indications for seeking emergency care.

Introduction

Suicide is the third leading cause of death among persons aged 10 to 24, accounting for more than 4000 deaths per year.[16] Approximately 16% of teenagers report having seriously considered suicide in the past year; 12.8% report having planned a suicide attempt, and 7.8% report having attempted suicide in the past year. Although only a small percentage of suicide attempts lead to medical attention,[17] suicide attempts still account for a significant number of emergency visits.[18]

Risk factors

Female teenagers are more likely to consider and attempt suicide, but male teenagers are more than 5 times more likely to complete suicide. This difference is primarily accounted for their use of more lethal means: male teenagers are more likely to attempt via firearms and hanging, whereas female teenagers are more likely to attempt via overdose.[17] Other risk factors for attempting and/or completing suicide include the following[19-27]:

- History of previous suicide attempts
- Impulsivity, mood, or behavior disorders
- Recent psychiatric hospitalizations
- Substance abuse
- Family history of suicide
- History of physical or sexual abuse
- Homelessness/runaways
- Identification as lesbian, gay, bisexual, or transsexual.

Evaluation

Identifying at-risk patients

Some patients will identify themselves as being suicidal with suicidal ideation or suicide attempt as their chief complaint. However, many may not proactively report their suicidality to providers.[28] Given the prevalence of suicidal ideation and attempts as well as the morbidity and mortality associated with attempts, pediatric providers are encouraged to screen all of their teen patients for suicidality.[29-31] Screens may be brief and focused directly on suicide risk[32] or more extensive/part of a broader mental health screening tool, such as the Pediatric Symptom Checklist. All patients presenting with mood symptoms, substance abuse, ingestions, acute intoxication, single-car motor vehicle crashes, self-inflicted or accidental gunshot wounds, and falls from significant heights should be screened for the presence of suicidal ideation.

Ensuring safety

First and foremost, providers must ensure the safety of the patient, their family, and health care staff during the course of the evaluation. Whenever concern for suicidal ideation or attempt is present, patients should be constantly monitored. They should not be left unobserved, as they are at risk for further injuring themselves or eloping. Patients should undergo a persons-and-belongings search. In some cases, it may be desirable to ask them to change into an examination gown, to decrease risk of harm and elopement. Patients should be placed in as safe a setting as possible, ideally one without access to medical equipment, which could be used for self-harm.

Confidentiality

When a physician is concerned that the patient may be at imminent risk for harm to self or others, confidentiality requirements no longer apply. Physicians may disclose information gathered by patients to caregivers and they may obtain information from others (including friends, family members, school personnel, and other caregivers) without obtaining consent from the patient or guardians.

Interview

Patients and caregivers should be interviewed both together and alone. It is essential that providers obtain collateral information from caregivers, because patients frequently minimize the severity of their symptoms or the intention behind their acts. It is paramount to ask patients directly about suicidality. Asking patients about suicidal ideation and attempts does not increase suicidal behaviors. In fact, it may have the opposite effect, as having an open, honest conversation about their suicidal thoughts may provide patients with a sense of safety and relief. This conversation may in turn enable them to fully disclose their suicidality and engage in treatment.

In addition to obtaining routine historical data, both medical and mental health histories, clinicians should obtain thorough details of the events and symptoms leading up to patient's presentation. Specific attention should be paid to the following:

- Recent psychosocial stressors, for example
  - Family conflict
  - Break-up of a romantic relationship
  - Bullying
  - Academic difficulties
  - Disciplinary actions/legal troubles
- Depression
- Mania
- Anxiety
- Psychosis
- Impulsivity
- Aggression
- Substance abuse
- Access to lethal means
  - Firearms
  - Knives
  - Medications
- Access to a responsible, supportive adult to whom they could turn if they had suicidal thoughts.

Younger patients tend to be triggered more often by family conflict, whereas older adolescents are more likely to cite peer or romantic conflicts.[33]

When discussing suicidal ideation, clinicians should inquire about a patient's reasons for considering/attempting suicide, and what—if any—their reasons are for living. Where were they, and what was happening immediately before the attempt? Was the attempt planned or impulsive? Did they do anything to avoid discovery? What was their expectation of the outcome? It should be noted that adolescents are typically poor judges of the dangerousness of their acts.[34,35] Although patients with low-lethality attempts may not be at significant medical risk, the *patient's* understanding of the potential lethality of their actions should be the basis of the suicide risk assessment.

Patients may deny that their behaviors constituted a suicide attempt and instead report that they "did it without thinking," or that they were just trying to go to sleep or get high or get a break from their feelings. Clinicians should be wary of accepting these explanations at face value and should probe for any signs of ambiguity or ambivalence. For example, in the setting of an overdose, it may be useful to ask if the patient questioned the safety of their ingestion beforehand. Was there any part of them that thought it might endanger their life? If so, it may be helpful to wonder out loud whether there was a part of them that would not have cared if they did not wake up from the ingestion. If the patient acknowledges any ambivalence, the clinician should follow up by exploring what parts of them would not have cared, and how, in the face of awareness of the potential lethality of their planned ingestion, they arrived at the decision to carry it out.

If the patient responds by steadfastly denying any suicidal thoughts and/or maintaining that they did not consider the consequences of their actions, it may be that there truly was not intent for self-harm. However, there are some circumstances in which there is enough evidence supporting suicidal intent (such as statements to family and friends or postings on social media) that is concerning enough to overcome any potential reassurance from a patient's denial of intent for self-harm. There may also be circumstances in which a patient may not have had any intent to harm themselves, but their lack of judgment about the dangerousness of their actions could be considered life-threatening and still necessitate intensive psychiatric treatment.

Family interview

Parents should be questioned about recent signs, symptoms, and stressors as well as the details of the any events that may have led to the patient's presentation. In addition, pediatricians should inquire about the patient's access to lethal means, the level of the caregiver's knowledge of/concern for the patient's safety and well-being, their willingness/ability to monitor the patient, their level of openness to psychiatric treatment, and any barriers that might impede engagement in care. Clinicians should also work to identify areas of competence in both the patient and the family. These areas of strength form the basis for a successful treatment plan that enables the family to respond effectively to the crisis at hand.

Physical Examination

There are several purposes to the medical examination in suicidal patients. Clinicians should evaluate the patient for any evidence of injury or ingestion. Specific attention should be paid to the skin examination to look for evidence of cutting and also for signs suggestive of a toxidrome. Clinicians should examine the patient for any signs suggestive of an underlying medical cause for the patient's psychiatric symptoms or for any medical conditions that would require treatment beyond the initial medical evaluation.

Laboratory Testing

Many patients, particularly those with pre-existing psychiatric diagnoses and who have normal vital signs, a normal physical examination, and no "red flags" for medical illness on history and review of systems, do not require routine laboratory or radiologic testing.[36–38] Decisions to obtain laboratory testing should be based on the patient's presenting medical and mental health condition. Clinicians should have a low threshold, however, for obtaining toxicology screens and pregnancy screening. In addition, patients with an acute change in psychiatric symptoms, especially if psychosis or alterations in mental health status, typically require at least some laboratory evaluation.

Pharmacologic Considerations

There are no medications whose primary indication is the prevention or treatment of suicide. Pediatricians may consider starting a selective serotonin reuptake inhibitor (SSRI) for patients with a significant depressive episode or an anxiety disorder. If SSRIs are initiated, these patients and their caregivers should receive extensive education about and be closely monitored for worsening suicidal ideation.[39]

Pediatricians should be wary of prescribing disinhibiting medications such as benzo-diazepines to suicidal patients and use extreme caution in prescribing medications that could be lethal in overdose (eg, tricyclic antidepressants or narcotics). If such medications are necessary, special care should be taken to ensure the safety of their administration, such as dispensing a week's worth of medicine at a time and/or having a responsible caregiver lock up and directly administer the medication.

Nonpharmacologic Strategies

One of the primary roles of a pediatrician managing a suicidal patient and their family is to provide psychoeduation about the need and support for engaging in adequate treatment. Caregivers may need help in recognizing the seriousness of the child's symptoms. They may also harbor negative feelings and/or misunderstandings about mental health diagnoses and their management options. Pediatricians should try to impress on patients and families the many dangers of untreated mental illness and/or unaddressed psychological stressors (including family discord) and that there are safe, confidential, and effective treatments available. It may be useful to inform care-givers that patients are at the highest risk of reattempting suicide in the months following the initial attempt[40–42] and that, while treatment may take time to help, they should do everything they can to help support the patient in adhering to recom-mended care.

Determining Level of Care

There are no validated criteria available to guide a pediatrician in assessing level of risk for subsequent suicide and determining level of care needs. However, it is generally agreed that criteria for immediate referral for an inpatient psychiatric admission include any the following:

- Continued desire to die
- Severe hopelessness
- Ongoing agitation
- Inability to engage in a discussion around safety planning
- Inadequate support system/ability to adequate monitoring and follow-up
- High lethality attempt or an attempt with clear expectation of death.

Under certain circumstances, pediatricians must insist on admission to a psychiatric inpatient unit over the objections of patients and/or their guardians. Every state in the United States has laws governing involuntary admission (ie, a "psychiatric hold") for inpatient psychiatric hospitalization. Laws vary from state to state; however, in most cases, physicians are able to admit a patient against his or her will for a brief period of time. Pediatricians should familiarize themselves with the relevant statutes and involuntary commitment procedures in the states where they practice.

Patients who do not meet criteria for inpatient psychiatric hospitalization should be referred for subsequent mental health intervention. Partial hospital programs, inten-sive outpatient services, or in-home treatment/crisis stabilization interventions should be considered when a patient needs more intensive or urgent treatment than weekly counseling. It should be noted that even patients who are deemed to be at relatively low risk of future suicidal or self-injurious acts still warrant at least some outpatient follow-up. Unfortunately, outpatient mental health providers are not always readily accessible. In those circumstances, primary care providers may need to play an ongoing treatment role, by providing frequent follow-up, bridging care, and/or in-office counseling.[43]

Safety Planning

Although having a patient sign a no-suicide contract has not been shown to prevent subsequent suicides,[44] pediatricians should still engage in a safety-planning discussion. Safety plans typically include elements such as identification of[45]

1. Warning signs and potential triggers for recurrence of suicidal ideation
2. Coping strategies the patient could use
3. Healthy activities that could provide distraction or suppression of suicidal thoughts
4. Responsible social supports to which the patient could turn should suicidal urges return
5. Contact information for professional supports, including instructions on how and when to reaccess emergency services
6. Means restriction.

"Means restriction" refers to counseling families about restricting access to potentially lethal methods. Because a large percentage of suicide attempts are impulsive in nature, educating caregivers about "suicide-proofing" their home is critical. One study of patients aged 13 to 34 who had near-lethal attempts found that 24% of patients went from deciding to attempt suicide to implementing their plan within 0 to 5 minutes, and another 47% took between 6 minutes and 1 hour.[46] Several studies have demonstrated that patients usually misjudge the lethality of their attempts.[34,35,47] There is also a wide variation in the case-fatality rates of common methods of suicide attempt, ranging from 85% for gunshot wounds to 2% for ingestions and 1% for cutting.[48] It thus follows that interventions that decrease access to more lethal means and/or increase the amount of time and effort it would take for someone to carry out their suicidal plan are likely to have a positive effect.

Means restriction education should include recommendations for securing knives, locking up medicines, and removing firearms. It is important to note that parents often underestimate their children's abilities to locate and access firearms[49] and that a gun in the home has been shown to double the risk of youth suicide.[50] Families who are reluctant to permanently remove firearms from the home may be open to temporarily relocating them until the child is in a better emotional state. If families insist on keeping firearms in the home, they should be counseled to secure them with trigger locks, to store them unloaded in a specialized or tamper-proof safe, to separately lock or temporarily remove ammunition, and ensure that minors do not have access to keys or lock combinations. Given the rates of drug and alcohol intoxication among attempts and completers, physicians may also want to recommend restricting access to alcohol and drugs, as well as referral for substance abuse treatment.

Instill Hope

At the conclusion of the visit, the pediatrician should review with the patient their reasons for living. Many patients may need help in generating this list. Pediatricians should highlight any of the patient's stated goals for the future and the ways in which the recommended treatment plan is designed to help the patient not only to survive but also to thrive.

HOMICIDAL IDEATION, AGGRESSION, AND RESTRAINT
Key Points

- Aggression is the final common pathway for a variety of medical and mental health conditions.

- Similar to the approach to the suicidal patient, careful evaluation for potential medical causes that may be the underlying cause and/or may complicate treatment of the aggression is vital.
- Mandatory federal and regulatory standards should guide the use of restraints with children and adolescents, including using the least restrictive methods as possible, frequent reassessment of the need for continued versus discontinuing restraint, and offering of food, drink, and bathroom facilities.
- Physical and chemical restraint may have significant adverse effects and require careful planning, administration, and monitoring.

Introduction

Aggressive, violent behavior is not a diagnosis unto itself but is the result of an underlying medical, toxicologic, or mental problem, or a combination of these conditions. Symptoms vary widely, depending on the patient's age, developmental level, and physical condition, and may include restlessness, hyperactivity, confusion, disorientation, verbal threats, and frank violence toward property, others, or oneself. It is a frequent cause of injury to both patients and medical staff.[51,52] As the evaluation of homicidal ideation and aggression shares many of the priorities and strategies of the evaluation of the suicidal patient, this section focuses primarily on the management of aggressive patients.

Risk factors

Risk factors for aggressive, violent behavior are presented in **Box 1**.

Evaluation

Strategies and priorities for evaluating the aggressive patient are the same as those detailed in the evaluation of the suicidal patient. The first priority is ensuring the safety of the patient and the medical staff. One critical difference with these patients regards the potential victim or victims of future violence. If a potential victim or victims of an aggressive patient are identified, there is an established legal precedent and duty to

---

Box 1
Aggression/violence risk factors

History of violence (especially recent)

Possession of weapons

Intoxication

Command hallucinations

Impulse control disorders

Concurrent psychosocial stressors

Verbal/physical threats

Psychomotor agitation

Paranoia

Impaired executive functioning

History of antisocial behavior

Concrete plans to harm others

warn the victims of the possibility of future violence.[53] Similar to the situation with the suicidal patient, this duty supersedes patient confidentiality.

When interviewing an aggressive patient, one should use the same techniques as discussed with the suicidal patient. Asking directly about homicidal ideation, thoughts or plans of violence, probing ambiguous or ambivalent statements, obtaining a comprehensive medical, mental health, substance abuse, legal/law enforcement history, inquiring about past and current psychosocial stressors, and access to weapons, from both the patient and the caregivers, should be used. The goal of the physical examination and any laboratory workup is to evaluate for potential medical causes of the patient's aggression as well as to detect any potential injuries or illnesses.

Management Goals

In 1998, the *Hartford Courant* published a series of articles detailing deaths of psychiatric patients, which, it was thought, were attributed to the use of physical restraint.[54] In response to these articles, the Centers for Medicare and Medicaid Services (CMS), and subsequently the Joint Commission for the Accreditation of Hospital Organizations, adopted regulations governing the use of and monitoring requirements for restraint (CMS-3018-F [42 CFR Part 482, RIN 0938-AN30]).[55] Key features of these regulations can be found in **Table 1**.

Nonpharmacologic Strategies

Verbal restraint and staff training in restraint reduction and de-escalation strategies have been shown to be effective at reducing the need for chemical and physical restraint.[56] Common verbal restraint strategies can be found in **Box 2**.[57] The presence of family members, caregivers, and friends is usually calming to a patient, although in some situations they may escalate a patient's agitation. In these situations, asking that person to temporarily leave the room is advisable.

Physical restraint has been associated with adverse outcomes including death. Recommended physical restraint approaches are listed in **Box 3**. Physical restraint should be applied with a minimum of 5 staff, 1 to control each limb and 1 for the patient's head. Restraints made of sturdy (eg, leather) materials should be used, whereas those of less durable construction (eg, "soft restraints") should be avoided. Once a patient has calmed, removal of restraints should be considered. Restraint removal will be dictated by the severity of the patient's condition. In some cases, they may be removed all at

Table 1	
Centers for Medicare and Medicaid Services restraint regulations	
Regulations apply to both physical and chemical restraint	
Must document need for and monitoring of restraint on 100% of patients	
Restraint Order Time Limit (Time to Renew)	**Monitoring/Basic Care Requirements**
Under 9 y: every 1 h	Visual check: every 15 min or constant observation
9–17 y: every 2 h	Release a restraint: every 2 h (may reapply if needed)
Above 18 y: every 4 h	Neurovascular check: every 2 h
	Offer food/water/bathroom: every 2 h
	Behavior check: every 2 h
	Respiratory status check: every 2 h
	Change physical position: every 2 h

Box 2
Verbal restraint strategies

Introduce oneself, staff

Prepare patient for what will happen

Respect patient autonomy

Offer food and liquids

Empathetic listening

Ask about patient requests/preferences

Honor reasonable requests

Nonpunitive limit setting

Simple direct language, soft voice

Decrease environmental stimulation

Allow patient to walk/move in room

Reassure patient that they will be safe

Offer distraction (eg, toy/books/movie)

Nonthreatening movement/posture

Remove breakable objects, equipment

---

once; in others, they may need to be removed one at a time with reassessment of the patient's agitation after the removal of each restraint. In every case, the same number of personnel that were present during the placement of the restraints should be available during removal of restraints, in case the restraints need to be reapplied.

Pharmacologic Strategies

Although many first-generation and second-generation antipsychotics have been approved by the Food and Drug Administration for use in children with autistic, mood, psychotic and tic disorders, none have been approved for use in agitation or aggression.[58] There is a growing body of literature on the use of benzodiazepines and antipsychotics for agitated adults in emergency department and psychiatric settings.[59–62] However, very few children were included in these studies and there are no high-quality pediatric trials. In addition, most pediatric agitation studies are from inpatient psychiatric settings, which may not be generalizable to the ED. For both adults and children, agitation in the ED is more likely to be undifferentiated or due to intoxication. These limitations aside, most psychiatric and emergency medicine experts

---

Box 3
Physical restraint recommendations

Supine position preferred

Avoid pressure on neck/back/chest

Mandatory staff training on restraint

Avoid covering patient's face/mouth/nose

Elevate head of bed, if possible

think that these medications are both efficacious and safe, with rare but easily treated adverse reactions.

Table 2 lists commonly used medications and starting doses for pediatric chemical restraint. If a patient is already on one of these medications, administering their usual or an increased dose of that medication is acceptable. Regarding which medication should be used as the first-line agent, most experts recommend tailoring the choice of medication to the severity and underlying cause of the agitation (**Table 3**). An important caveat is that younger patients and children with autism and other developmental disabilities may have an atypical, idiosyncratic response to benzodiazepines. These patients may become disinhibited and/or their agitation may worsen when given a benzodiazepine.

The most common adverse effects of chemical restraint medications are cardiorespiratory and central nervous system depression, and extrapyramidal reactions. The former are usually easily treated with simple supportive measures, and the latter are usually easily treated with anticholinergics (eg, diphenhydramine, benztropine, or trihexyphenidyl). Rarely are invasive or aggressive treatment measures needed. The most serious acute, adverse effects of antipsychotics are arrhythmias due to QT_c prolongation. These events are rare and are most likely to occur in patients receiving other QT_c prolonging medications and/or with underlying cardiac conditions. Continuous cardiorespiratory monitoring is thus recommended for patients receiving chemical restraint.

CARE OF CHILDREN WITH AUTISM AND DEVELOPMENTAL DISORDERS
Key Points

- Children with autism and other developmental disorders span a wide range of symptoms of severities, ranging from very high functioning with minimal disabilities to profoundly impaired.
- Accordingly, such children may have unique and idiosyncratic communication methods, interaction styles, and responses to sensory stimuli.
- Parents and caregivers are the pediatricians' greatest allies in planning and delivering optimal treatment for their children.

Table 2
Medications for pediatric chemical restraint

Medication	Initial Dose	Onset (min)	Half-life (h)
Diphenhydramine	1.25 mg/kg Teen: 50 mg	20–30 (PO) 5–15 (IM)	2–8
Lorazepam	0.05–0.1 mg/kg Teen: 2–4 mg	20–30 (PO) 5–15 (IM)	12
Midazolam	0.05–0.15 mg/kg Teen: 2–4 mg	20–30 (PO) 5–15 (IM)	3–4
Haloperidol	0.1 mg/kg Teen: 2–4 mg	30–60 (PO) 15–30 (IM)	21
Risperidone	<12 y: 0.5 mg Teen: 1 mg	45–60 (PO)	20
Olanzapine	<12 y: 2.5 mg Teen: 5–10 mg	45–60 (PO) 30–60 (IM)	30
Ziprasidone	<12 y: 5 mg Teen: 10–20 mg	60 (PO) 30–60 (IM)	2–7
Aripiprazole	<12 y: 1–2 mg Teen: 2–5 mg	60–180 (PO) 30–120 (IM)	75

Table 3
Choice of initial chemical restraint agent

Etiology of Agitation	Symptom Severity	
	Mild/Moderate	Severe
Medical	Benzodiazepine	Benzodiazepine or antipsychotic
Psychiatric	Benzodiazepine or antipsychotic	Antipsychotic

Note. Benzodiazepines may disinhibit and/or worsen agitation in young children and patients with autism or other developmental disabilities.

- Several simple strategies, such as communication adjuncts, transition planning, sensory and environmental modification, and distraction techniques, may be useful in caring for these patients.

Introduction

The incidence of autism spectrum disorders (ASD) is increasing, for a multitude of reasons, many of which are still unclear.[63] The 3 cardinal features of ASD are impaired communication, impaired social interaction, and repetitive/restrictive areas of interest. The severity of these symptoms and the degree of impairment vary greatly and include people who have obtained PhDs (eg, Temple Grandin) to people who are nonverbal and cannot communicate nor care for themselves. In addition, each person may have specific and distinctive interaction patterns and response to stimuli. For all these reasons, caring for these children can be extremely challenging.

Regarding effective treatment strategies for children with ASD, many previous studies suffer from methodologic limitations, such as small sample size, generalizability, lack of blinding or control groups, and so on.[64] Most treatment recommendations, including those in this article, have been based on expert consensus opinion. Fortunately, in recent years, there has been a growth in more rigorously designed studies, including randomized control trials.[65–68]

Children with other developmental disorders (DD) similarly span a wide range of symptoms, severity, and disabilities, too numerous to list and beyond the scope of this article. As the strategies for caring for these children are similar to those used in caring for children with ASD, for the purposes of this article, the term ASD/DD will be used to collectively refer to all these children.

Evaluation

One of the most challenging aspects of caring for children with ASD/DD is interpreting the unique meaning of their behaviors, as well as discovering the optimal methods for interacting with and caring for the child. Fortunately, most of these children are accompanied by an expert in these areas, namely their parent(s) and/or caregiver(s). Time spent asking them about the child is likely to be time well spent, increasing the efficiency with which care is delivered and the patient's, family's, and clinician's satisfaction with the encounter. Suggested topics to discuss with the parent/caregiver are listed as follows:

- What is your child's level of communication, cognitive, and psychosocial functioning?
- How does your child communicate?
- When your child does (behavior), what does it mean?
- What upsets or scares your child? What calms/soothes them?
- Is your child sensitive to light, sound, or other stimuli?

- What's the best way to prepare your child for something new?
- Does your child like to be touched? If so, what types of tactile sensations do they like?
- Are there things (eg, toys, a favorite object, electronic devices) that are good distractions for your child?

Transition Planning

Preparing a child with ASD for what is about to happen is one of the most common strategies used by their caregivers. In ideal cases, the parent/caregiver begins talking to the child about what to expect while en route to the medical setting. Once there, it is worthwhile discussing what will occur during the visit and determining a plan for how to prepare the child for the visit.

Transition planning may also include planned breaks for the child. Some children with ASD/DD are able to stay on task or remain in one location for only brief periods of time. Building rest periods, distractions, bathroom breaks, and so forth into the visit may be an important component to a successful visit. Finally, a method for signaling transitions and/or new activities may also be helpful. A transition cue may be auditory (eg, certain words or phrases, ringing a bell), visual (eg, pointing to a picture, turning on a light, showing the child a certain object), or tactile (eg, a touch with a specific object).

Sensory/Environmental Modification and Distraction

Some patients may be very sensitive to environmental stimuli, such as light, noise, crowds of people, complex/cluttered environments. If a child has such sensitivities, altering their environment and visit may be helpful. For example, instead of sitting in a busy, noisy waiting room, have the child wait in a quiet office or counseling area. Turning the lights in a room off or down, or lighting a room with a single lamp, may help a child who is sensitive to light. A rocking chair or rocking toy (with supervision) may soothe a child who prefers motion. For children who respond to tactile stimulation, a weighted blanket (available through occupational therapy vendors), a radiology leaded vest, or a "bean-bag" chair can all serve to provide the sensation of a heavy touch. Those who prefer the sensation of a light touch may respond to gentle massage (manual or mechanical devices) or stroking the skin with a soft object (eg, a cotton ball, gauze pad, soft blanket). Any toy or electronic device that holds the child's attention and distracts them may assist in caring for the child.

Communication Adjuncts

Visual communication systems, both print and electronic versions, have demonstrated efficacy in improving communication with children with ASD/DD.[68–71] Not only may such a system improve communication with the child, more importantly, it may be the only way the child can communicate with the clinicians. There are a large number of both free and commercial products that are readily available. Alternatively, a system customized to a particular setting can easily be made with digital photographs and/or computerized clip art. A custom visual communication tool has the advantage of containing pictures specific to the site. The disadvantage of such a system, however, is that the patient may not be familiar with it.

REFERENCES

1. Case SD, Case BG, Olfson M, et al. Length of stay of pediatric mental health emergency department visits in the United States. J Am Acad Child Adolesc Psychiatry 2011;50(11):1110–9.

2. Dolan MA, Fein JA, Committee on Pediatric Emergency Medicine. Pediatric and adolescent mental health emergencies in the emergency medical service system. Pediatrics 2011;127(5):e1356–66.

3. Baraff LJ, Janowicz N, Asarnow JR. Survey of California emergency departments about practices for management of suicidal patients and resources available for their care. Ann Emerg Med 2006;48(4):452–8.

4. Santucci KA, Sather J, Baker MD. Emergency medicine training programs' educational requirements in the management of psychiatric emergencies: current perspective. Pediatr Emerg Care 2003;19(3):154–6.

5. Bridge JA, Marcus SC, Olfson M. Outpatient care of young people after emergency treatment of deliberate self-harm. J Am Acad Child Adolesc Psychiatry 2012;51(2):213–22.

6. Grupp-Phelan J, Harman JS, Kelleher KJ. Trends in mental health and chronic condition visits by children presenting for care at U.S. emergency departments. Public Health Rep 2007;122(1):55–61.

7. Kessler RC, Demler O, Frank RG, et al. Prevalence and treatment of mental disorders, 1990 to 2003. N Engl J Med 2005;352(24):2515–23. http://dx.doi.org/10.1056/NEJMsa043266.

8. Lewis M. Child psychiatric consultation in pediatrics. Pediatrics 1978;62(3):359–64.

9. Sills MR, Bland SD. Summary statistics for pediatric psychiatric visits to US emergency departments, 1993-1999. Pediatrics 2002;110(4):e40.

10. Wang PS, Demler O, Olfson M, et al. Changing profiles of service sectors used for mental health care in the United States. Am J Psychiatry 2006;163(7):1187–98. http://dx.doi.org/10.1176/appi.ajp.163.7.1187.

11. Cooper S, Valleley RJ, Polaha J, et al. Running out of time: physician management of behavioral health concerns in rural pediatric primary care. Pediatrics 2006;118(1):e132–8. http://dx.doi.org/10.1542/peds.2005-2612.

12. Heneghan A, Garner AS, Storfer-Isser A, et al. Pediatricians' role in providing mental health care for children and adolescents: do pediatricians and child and adolescent psychiatrists agree? J Dev Behav Pediatr 2008;29(4):262–9. http://dx.doi.org/10.1097/DBP.0b013e31817dbd97.

13. Hoyle JD Jr, White LJ. Treatment of pediatric and adolescent mental health emergencies in the United States: current practices, models, barriers, and potential solutions. Prehosp Emerg Care 2003;7(1):66–73.

14. Hoyle JD Jr, White LJ. Pediatric mental health emergencies: summary of a multidisciplinary panel. Prehosp Emerg Care 2003;7(1):60–5.

15. Sivakumar S, Weiland TJ, Gerdtz MF, et al. Mental health-related learning needs of clinicians working in Australian emergency departments: a national survey of self-reported confidence and knowledge. Emerg Med Australas 2011;23(6): 697–711. http://dx.doi.org/10.1111/j.1742-6723.2011.01472.x.

16. Centers for Disease Control and Prevention. Leading causes of death 1999-2010. Atlanta (GA): Centers for Disese Control and Prevention; 2012.

17. Eaton DK, Kann L, Kinchen S, et al. Youth risk behavior surveillance - United States, 2011. MMWR Surveill Summ 2012;61(4):1–162.

18. Ting SA, Sullivan AF, Boudreaux ED, et al. Trends in US emergency department visits for attempted suicide and self-inflicted injury, 1993-2008. Gen Hosp Psychiatry 2012;34(5):557–65. http://dx.doi.org/10.1016/j.genhosppsych.2012.03.020.

19. Brown J, Cohen P, Johnson JG, et al. Childhood abuse and neglect: specificity of effects on adolescent and young adult depression and suicidality. J Am Acad Child Adolesc Psychiatry 1999;38(12):1490–6. http://dx.doi.org/10.1097/00004583-199912000-00009.

20. Esposito-Smythers C, Spirito A. Adolescent substance use and suicidal behavior: a review with implications for treatment research. Alcohol Clin Exp Res 2004;28(Suppl 5):77S–88S.
21. Foley DL, Goldston DB, Costello EJ, et al. Proximal psychiatric risk factors for suicidality in youth: the Great Smoky Mountains study. Arch Gen Psychiatry 2006;63(9):1017–24. http://dx.doi.org/10.1001/archpsyc.63.9.1017.
22. Lewinsohn PM, Rohde P, Seeley JR. Psychosocial risk factors for future adolescent suicide attempts. J Consult Clin Psychol 1994;62(2):297–305.
23. McDaniel JS, Purcell D, D'Augelli AR. The relationship between sexual orientation and risk for suicide: research findings and future directions for research and prevention. Suicide Life Threat Behav 2001;31(Suppl):84–105.
24. McKeown RE, Garrison CZ, Cuffe SP, et al. Incidence and predictors of suicidal behaviors in a longitudinal sample of young adolescents. J Am Acad Child Adolesc Psychiatry 1998;37(6):612–9. http://dx.doi.org/10.1097/00004583-199806000-00011.
25. Shaffer D, Craft L. Methods of adolescent suicide prevention. J Clin Psychiatry 1999;60(Suppl 2):70–4 [discussion 75-6], 113–6.
26. Shaffer D, Gould MS, Fisher P, et al. Psychiatric diagnosis in child and adolescent suicide. Arch Gen Psychiatry 1996;53(4):339–48.
27. Smart RG, Walsh GW. Predictors of depression in street youth. Adolescence 1993;28(109):41–53.
28. Brent DA, Emslie GJ, Clarke GN, et al. Predictors of spontaneous and systematically assessed suicidal adverse events in the treatment of SSRI-resistant depression in adolescents (TORDIA) study. Am J Psychiatry 2009;166(4):418–26. http://dx.doi.org/10.1176/appi.ajp.2008.08070976.
29. Committee on Pathophysiology and Prevention of Adolescent and Adult Suicide, Board on Neuroscience and Behavioral Health, Institute of Medicine. Reducing suicide: a national imperative. Washington, DC: The National Academies Press; 2002.
30. Williams SB, O'Connor EA, Eder M, et al. Screening for child and adolescent depression in primary care settings: a systematic evidence review for the US Preventive Services Task Force. Pediatrics 2009;123(4):e716–35. http://dx.doi.org/10.1542/peds.2008-2415.
31. Foy JM, Kelleher KJ, Laraque D. Enhancing pediatric mental health care: strategies for preparing a primary care practice. Pediatrics 2010;125(Suppl 3):S87–108. http://dx.doi.org/10.1542/peds.2010-0788E.
32. Wintersteen MB. Standardized screening for suicidal adolescents in primary care. Pediatrics 2010;125(5):938–44. http://dx.doi.org/10.1542/peds.2009-2458.
33. Overholser JC. Predisposing factors in suicide attempts: life stressors. In: Spirito A, Overholser JC, editors. Evaluating and treating adolescent suicide attempters: from research to practice. New York: Academic Press; 2002. p. 42–54.
34. Swahn MH, Potter LB. Factors associated with the medical severity of suicide attempts in youths and young adults. Suicide Life Threat Behav 2001;32(Suppl 1):21–9.
35. Brown GK, Henriques GR, Sosdjan D, et al. Suicide intent and accurate expectations of lethality: predictors of medical lethality of suicide attempts. J Consult Clin Psychol 2004;72(6):1170–4. http://dx.doi.org/10.1037/0022-006X.72.6.1170.
36. Santillanes G, Donofrio JJ, Lam CN, et al. Is medical clearance necessary for pediatric psychiatric patients? J Emerg Med 2014. http://dx.doi.org/10.1016/j.jemermed.2013.12.003.

37. Shihabuddin BS, Hack CM, Sivitz AB. Role of urine drug screening in the medical clearance of pediatric psychiatric patients: is there one? Pediatr Emerg Care 2013;29(8):903–6. http://dx.doi.org/10.1097/PEC.0b013e31829e8050.

38. Tenenbein M. Do you really need that emergency drug screen? Clin Toxicol (Phila) 2009;47(4):286–91. http://dx.doi.org/10.1080/15563650902907798.

39. Hetrick SE, McKenzie JE, Cox GR, et al. Newer generation antidepressants for depressive disorders in children and adolescents. Cochrane Database Syst Rev 2012;(11):CD004851. http://dx.doi.org/10.1002/14651858.CD004851.pub3.

40. Spirito A, Plummer B, Gispert M, et al. Adolescent suicide attempts: outcomes at follow-up. Am J Orthopsychiatry 1992;62(3):464–8.

41. Prinstein MJ, Nock MK, Simon V, et al. Longitudinal trajectories and predictors of adolescent suicidal ideation and attempts following inpatient hospitalization. J Consult Clin Psychol 2008;76(1):92–103. http://dx.doi.org/10.1037/0022-006X.76.1.92.

42. Yen S, Weinstock LM, Andover MS, et al. Prospective predictors of adolescent suicidality: 6-month post-hospitalization follow-up. Psychol Med 2013;43(5):983–93. http://dx.doi.org/10.1017/S0033291712001912.

43. Cheung AH, Zuckerbrot RA, Jensen PS, et al. Guidelines for Adolescent Depression in Primary Care (GLAD-PC): II. Treatment and ongoing management. Pediatrics 2007;120(5):e1313–26. http://dx.doi.org/10.1542/peds.2006-1395.

44. American Academy of Child and Adolescent Psychiatry. Practice parameter for the assessment and treatment of children and adolescents with suicidal behavior. American Academy of Child and Adolescent Psychiatry. J Am Acad Child Adolesc Psychiatry 2001;40(Suppl 7):24S–51S.

45. Sher L, LaBode V. Teaching health care professionals about suicide safety planning. Psychiatr Danub 2011;23(4):396–7.

46. Simon OR, Swann AC, Powell KE, et al. Characteristics of impulsive suicide attempts and attempters. Suicide Life Threat Behav 2001;32(Suppl 1):49–59.

47. Plutchik R, van Praag HM, Picard S, et al. Is there a relation between the seriousness of suicidal intent and the lethality of the suicide attempt? Psychiatry Res 1989;27(1):71–9.

48. Vyrostek SB, Annest JL, Ryan GW. Surveillance for fatal and nonfatal injuries–United States, 2001. MMWR Surveill Summ 2004;53(7):1–57.

49. Baxley F, Miller M. Parental misperceptions about children and firearms. Arch Pediatr Adolesc Med 2006;160(5):542–7. http://dx.doi.org/10.1001/archpedi.160.5.542.

50. Brent DA, Perper JA, Allman CJ, et al. The presence and accessibility of firearms in the homes of adolescent suicides. A case-control study. JAMA 1991;266(21):2989–95.

51. McAneney CM, Shaw KN. Violence in the pediatric emergency department. Ann Emerg Med 1994;23(6):1248–51.

52. Knott JC, Bennett D, Rawet J, et al. Epidemiology of unarmed threats in the emergency department. Emerg Med Australas 2005;17(4):351–8. http://dx.doi.org/10.1111/j.1742-6723.2005.00756.x.

53. Felthous AR. The clinician's duty to protect third parties. Psychiatr Clin North Am 1999;22(1):49–60.

54. Busch AB, Shore MF. Seclusion and restraint: a review of recent literature. Harv Rev Psychiatry 2000;8(5):261–70.

55. Centers for Medicare & Medicaid Services (CMS), DHHS. Medicare and Medicaid programs; hospital conditions of participation: patients' rights. Final rule. Fed Regist 2006;71:71378–428.

56. Richmond JS, Berlin JS, Fishkind AB, et al. Verbal De-escalation of the Agitated Patient: Consensus Statement of the American Association for Emergency Psychiatry Project BETA De-escalation Workgroup. West J Emerg Med 2012; 13(1):17–25. http://dx.doi.org/10.5811/westjem.2011.9.6864.
57. Hilt RJ, Woodward TA. Agitation treatment for pediatric emergency patients. J Am Acad Child Adolesc Psychiatry 2008;47(2):132–8. http://dx.doi.org/10. 1097/chi.0b013e31815d95fd.
58. Christian R, Saavedra L, Gaynes BN, et al. Future research needs for first- and second-generation antipsychotics for children and young adults. Rockville (MD): AHRQ Comparative Effectiveness Reviews; 2012.
59. Chan EW, Taylor DM, Knott JC, et al. Intravenous droperidol or olanzapine as an adjunct to midazolam for the acutely agitated patient: a multicenter, random- ized, double-blind, placebo-controlled clinical trial. Ann Emerg Med 2013; 61(1):72–81. http://dx.doi.org/10.1016/j.annemergmed.2012.07.118.
60. Huf G, Coutinho ES, Adams CE. Rapid tranquillisation in psychiatric emergency settings in Brazil: pragmatic randomised controlled trial of intramuscular haloperidol versus intramuscular haloperidol plus promethazine. BMJ 2007; 335(7625):869. http://dx.doi.org/10.1136/bmj.39339.448819.AE.
61. Knott JC, Taylor DM, Castle DJ. Randomized clinical trial comparing intravenous midazolam and droperidol for sedation of the acutely agitated patient in the emergency department. Ann Emerg Med 2006;47(1):61–7. http://dx.doi.org/ 10.1016/j.annemergmed.2005.07.003.
62. Hsu WY, Huang SS, Lee BS, et al. Comparison of intramuscular olanzapine, orally disintegrating olanzapine tablets, oral risperidone solution, and intramus- cular haloperidol in the management of acute agitation in an acute care psychi- atric ward in Taiwan. J Clin Psychopharmacol 2010;30(3):230–4. http://dx.doi. org/10.1097/JCP.0b013e3181db8715.
63. Autism and Developmental Disabilities Monitoring Network Surveillance Year 2008, Centers for Disease Control and Prevention. Prevalence of autism spec- trum disorders–Autism and developmental disabilities monitoring network, 14 sites, United States, 2008. MMWR Surveill Summ 2012;61(3):1–19.
64. Mesibov GB, Shea V. Evidence-based practices and autism. Autism 2011;15(1): 114–33. http://dx.doi.org/10.1177/1362361309348070.
65. Adams C, Lockton E, Freed J, et al. The Social Communication Intervention Project: a randomized controlled trial of the effectiveness of speech and lan- guage therapy for school-age children who have pragmatic and social commu- nication problems with or without autism spectrum disorder. Int J Lang Commun Disord 2012;47(3):233–44. http://dx.doi.org/10.1111/j.1460-6984. 2011.00146.x.
66. Dawson G, Burner K. Behavioral interventions in children and adolescents with autism spectrum disorder: a review of recent findings. Curr Opin Pediatr 2011; 23(6):616–20. http://dx.doi.org/10.1097/MOP.0b013e32834cf082.
67. Gantman A, Kapp SK, Orenski K, et al. Social skills training for young adults with high-functioning autism spectrum disorders: a randomized controlled pilot study. J Autism Dev Disord 2012;42(6):1094–103. http://dx.doi.org/10.1007/ s10803-011-1350-6.
68. Gordon K, Pasco G, McElduff F, et al. A communication-based intervention for nonverbal children with autism: what changes? Who benefits? J Consult Clin Psychol 2011;79(4):447–57. http://dx.doi.org/10.1037/a0024379.
69. Ganz JB, Davis JL, Lund EM, et al. Meta-analysis of PECS with individuals with ASD: investigation of targeted versus non-targeted outcomes, participant

characteristics, and implementation phase. Res Dev Disabil 2012;33(2):406–18. http://dx.doi.org/10.1016/j.ridd.2011.09.023.

70. Howlin P, Gordon RK, Pasco G, et al. The effectiveness of Picture Exchange Communication System (PECS) training for teachers of children with autism: a pragmatic, group randomised controlled trial. J Child Psychol Psychiatry 2007;48(5):473–81. http://dx.doi.org/10.1111/j.1469-7610.2006.01707.x.

71. Yoder PJ, Lieberman RG. Brief Report: randomized test of the efficacy of picture exchange communication system on highly generalized picture exchanges in children with ASD. J Autism Dev Disord 2010;40(5):629–32. http://dx.doi.org/10.1007/s10803-009-0897-y.

Evaluation of Child Maltreatment in the Emergency Department Setting

An Overview for Behavioral Health Providers

Aaron N. Leetch, MD[a],*, John Leipsic, MD[b],
Dale P. Woolridge, MD, PhD[a]

KEYWORDS

- Nonaccidental trauma • Child abuse • Child maltreatment • Sexual abuse
- Emergency • Rib fractures • Shaken-baby syndrome • Retinal hemorrhage

KEY POINTS

- The key to diagnosing child abuse early is to keep a high clinical suspicion.
- High-risk chief complaints for child abuse include the Six B's: Bruises, Breaks, Bonks, Burns, Bites, and Baby blues.
- Medical evaluation and treatment should always supersede a forensic evaluation but should try to be as simultaneous as possible.
- All physical examination findings should be corroborated with a history and developmental level before it can be considered abusive.
- All emergency providers are mandatory reporters of a reasonable suspicion of abuse.

COMMENTARY

The evaluation of the abused or potentially abused child is a delicate matter that should be handled with the utmost precision, dignity, and care. Owing to the variable nature of the problem, the initial presentation often occurs in the Emergency Department (ED) wherein the child is evaluated by multiple providers from multiple agencies including medical, legal, and custodial groups. Evaluation usually includes screening for physical injury, collection of evidence for legal proceedings, and determination of guardianship.

This article is updated for *Child & Adolescent Psychiatric Clinics* from an article originally written for *Emergency Medicine Clinics of North America*; the article was entitled Emergency Department Evaluation of Child Abuse, by A.N. Leetch and D. Wooldridge, in the issue Pediatric Emergency Medicine, edited by L.N. Lu, D. Woolridge, and A.M. Dietrich; August 2013.

[a] Departments of Emergency Medicine and Pediatrics, University of Arizona, 1501 North Campbell Avenue, Tucson, AZ 85719, USA; [b] Department of Child and Adolescent Psychiatry, University of Arizona, 1501 North Campbell Avenue, Tucson, AZ 85719, USA
* Corresponding author.
E-mail address: aleetch@aemrc.arizona.edu

Abbreviations	
AAP	American Academy of Pediatrics
ALTE	Apparent life-threatening events
CPS	Child Protective Services
CT	Computed tomography
ED	Emergency department
EP	Emergency physician
ICH	Intracranial hemorrhage
MRI	Magnetic resonance imaging
NAT	Nonaccidental trauma
NIS-4	Fourth National Incidence Study of Child Abuse and Neglect
PECARN	Pediatric Emergency Care Applied Research Network
PPV	Positive predictive value
SIDS	Sudden infant death syndrome
SUIDS	Sudden infant unexplained death syndrome

The physical and legal implications are often dealt with immediately, but the emotional and psychological impact of the trauma and even the ED evaluation are usually managed later by a behavioral health provider who was not present at the time. For this reason, a foundational understanding of the initial ED evaluation is valuable for the behavioral health provider who will be managing the long-term sequelae of the initial trauma.

EMERGENCY DEPARTMENT EPIDEMIOLOGY

Child abuse or nonaccidental trauma (NAT) is a common occurrence in the United States. It is a diagnosis that many emergency physicians (EPs) find both clinically and personally challenging to diagnose. However, it is imperative that these diagnoses be made to prevent further physical, mental, and emotional harm to the affected children.

The most recently published data from the National Data Archive on Child Abuse and Neglect reported that nearly 1.25 million cases occurred annually.[1] Deeper evaluation of these data estimates that nearly 1 in 8 children are abused before the age of 18 years.[2] An estimated 12% of these cases presented to hospitals initially. Recent data also show that, in 2010, an estimated 1560 children died of abuse and neglect. Survivors of child abuse have a high propensity for mood disorders, anxiety disorders, and substance abuse. These individuals are 5 times more likely to attempt suicide.[3] Recent data from the Canadian Community Health Survey have shown results similar to the United States data.[4] Maltreatment has even been associated with increased risk of obesity and human immunodeficiency virus infection as well as an overall higher mortality rate than the general population. The cost of health care for abused children has been shown to be significantly more expensive than for nonabused children, and often continues to be incurred for years after the initial trauma.[5,6]

The ED is a common place for child abuse to present, whether overtly or latently. An estimated 2% to 10% of children visiting the ED are victims of either abuse or neglect. A study of 44 children who died of child abuse showed that 19% of them had been evaluated by a physician within a month of their death. Nearly 71% of those evaluations were in an ED for complaints ranging from fussiness to vomiting to poor feeding.[7] Many of these children have "sentinel injuries" such as bruising or intraoral injury, which are minor by medical standards but have a poor or implausible explanation.[8] A 2010 study showed that nearly one-fifth of abuse-related fractures had at least 1 previous physician visit during which the abuse was missed.[9] Without appropriate intervention, abuse may recur in nearly 35% to 50% of cases, and death may occur before the subsequent evaluation in nearly 25%.[10,11] The key to accurate diagnosis is a high level of clinical suspicion and a good understanding of the definitions.

DEFINITIONS IN CHILD ABUSE

There is no universally agreed definition for child abuse because it can range from blatant physical or sexual abuse to varying degrees of neglect or emotional abuse. However, a good understanding of the legal description of child abuse is imperative for EPs making the diagnosis and conducting appropriate referrals in the clinical setting. According the 2010 revised Child Abuse Prevention and Treatment Act, child abuse and neglect is defined as "at a minimum, any recent act or failure to act on the part of a parent or caretaker, which results in death, serious physical or emotional harm, sexual abuse or exploitation, or an act or failure to act which presents an imminent risk of serious harm" (Public Law 104-235, Section 111; 42 USC 5106g).

The Department of Health and Human Services defines the 4 main types of maltreatment in the Fourth National Incidence Study of Child Abuse and Neglect (NIS-4) Report to Congress as physical abuse, sexual abuse, neglect, and emotional abuse (**Table 1**).[1] Physical abuse is broadly defined as physical assault on a child. Sexual

Table 1		
Types of abuse, percentage of reports, and cited examples from NIS-4		
Physical abuse	58%	Beating, burning, choking, biting Shaking, pushing, restraining, kicking Any other mechanism that may have been meant to hurt or punish the child
Sexual abuse	24%	Intrusion: oral, anal, or genital penetration with any object Molestation: some form of genital contact without intrusion Other: cases of abuse without direct contact but includes exposure of a child or of a perpetrator to a child, lack of supervision of a child's sexual exposure, or touching areas other than the genitals with sexual intentions
Neglect	61%	Abandonment or other refusal to maintain custody, such as desertion, expulsion from home, refusal to accept custody of a returned runaway Permitting or encouraging chronic maladaptive behavior, such as truancy, delinquency, prostitution, serious drug/alcohol abuse Refusal to allow needed treatment for a professionally diagnosed physical, educational, emotional, or behavioral problem, or failure to follow the advice of a competent professional's recommendation thereof Failure to seek or unwarranted delay in seeking competent medical care for a serious injury, illness, or impairment Consistent or extreme inattention to the child's physical or emotional needs, including needs for food, clothing, supervision, safety, affection, and reasonably hygienic living conditions Failure to register or enroll the child in school, as required by state law
Emotional abuse	27%	Close confinement: binding a child to restrict movement or putting a child in a small space as a form of punishment Verbal abuse: threatening or demeaning words Other: allowing for unspecified acts that still have a profound effect on the child

Many different types of abuse are often inflicted on the same child, thus making the sum of percentages greater than 100%.

Data from Sedlak AJ, Mettenburg J, Basena M, et al. Fourth National Incidence Study of child abuse and neglect (NIS-4). Washington, DC: US Department of Health and Human Services; 2010. Available at: http://www.acf.hhs.gov/programs/opre/research/project/national-incidence-study-of-child-abuse-and-neglect-nis-4-2004-2009. Accessed July 9, 2010.

abuse is separated into intrusion, molestation, and other cases otherwise not described. Neglect entails failure to meet a child's basic needs of life, including physical, emotional, and educational neglect. Emotional abuse can include confinement, verbal abuse, or other unspecified forms.

For the purposes of research, the Harm Standard and Endangerment Standard were devised to better qualify abuse.[1] The Harm Standard is stricter, necessitating that the victim experienced some type of harm or injury that is then qualified as fatal, serious injury/condition, moderate injury/condition, probable, or impairment. The Endangerment Standard allows for more inclusion of potential child abuse with these criteria in addition to the category of Endangered (**Box 1**).[1]

Special mention should be paid to Munchausen syndrome by proxy, because it is a specialized form of abuse that is often associated with a medical setting. It is a factious disorder whereby caregivers derive an unknown (and hotly debated) benefit at the expense of the patient.[12,13] Allegations of abuse, whether physical or sexual, may be a type of Munchausen syndrome by proxy associated with repeated visits to EDs or primary care physicians claiming abuse. Unlike traditional abuse, victims of Munchausen syndrome by proxy often have a very close relationship with caregivers, receiving a lot of attention. Parents often appear very concerned and speak for the children. Although this should be considered, Munchausen is not a diagnosis easily made in the ED and is best determined using a multidisciplinary approach in an inpatient setting.[13]

Risk Factors in Patients

Patient characteristics most associated with increased rates of maltreatment include gender, age, race, disabilities, and school enrollment (**Table 2**). Historically and currently, there is no gender bias for physical abuse alone; however, girls are more often the victims of sexual abuse, which confers more overall abuse, compared with boys.[14] Children aged 6 to 8 years have the highest maltreatment rates, although there has been a recent increase in the youngest children, aged 0 to 2 years. The recent data show a significantly higher rate of maltreatment of African American children compared with white, Native American, and Hispanic children, which is a new

---

Box 1
Harm and endangerment standard definitions for abuse according to NIS-4

- Fatal: the abuse or neglect is suspected to have led to the child's death

- Serious injury/condition: injury or harm was significant enough to seriously impair the child's physical, mental, or emotional capacities long term or enough to require professional treatment to prevent such an outcome

- Moderate injury/condition: injury or harm was significant enough to seriously impair the child's physical, mental, or emotional capacities for at least longer than 48 hours

- Probable impairment: maltreatment so extreme or inherently traumatic in nature that significant emotional injury or impairment may reasonably be assumed to have occurred, even though the child may show no obvious physical or behavioral signs of injury

- Endangered: child's health or safety was or is seriously endangered, but child does not appear to have been harmed

Data from Sedlak AJ, Mettenburg J, Basena M, et al. Fourth National Incidence Study of child abuse and neglect (NIS-4). Washington, DC: US Department of Health and Human Services; 2010. Available at: http://www.acf.hhs.gov/programs/opre/research/project/national-incidence-study-of-child-abuse-and-neglect-nis-4-2004-2009. Accessed July 9, 2010.

Table 2 Risk factors for abuse		
Victims	**Perpetrators**	**Families**
Females (sexual abuse) Ages 0–1 and 6–8 African American race Not in school (sexual abuse, neglect)	Biological parents (physical abuse, neglect) Females (physical abuse) Males (sexual abuse) Unemployed Substance abuse Mental health issues	Low socioeconomic status Less than high school education of caregivers Single parents with live-in partners

trend from the previous data collection in 1996. Black children who are victims of NAT also carry a higher mortality than other races.[1]

Children with premature birth or children with disabilities/chronic medical illnesses traditionally were more often victims of abuse. However, the latest data show overall decreased rates of abuse, possibly owing to better recognition by medical providers and the widespread implementation of medical foster homes and respite care. However, when abused, these patients had higher morbidity and mortality.

Enrollment in school was evaluated for the first time in the most recent data collection. Children who were not enrolled in school were more likely than those who were in school to be sexually abused or neglected. By contrast, children who were enrolled in school had higher rates of physical abuse. The latter is not well explained, although there may be a component of selection bias caused by the presence of more caregivers (ie, teachers, coaches, principals), with those who attended school possibly being more apt to be identified. An important point for EPs is that the simple question of "How is school going?" can elicit important social history pertaining to latent abuse.

Risk Factors in Caregivers and Families

Risk factors such as gender, relationship to the child, age of the perpetrator, unemployment, and a history of the perpetrator being abusive in the past are all associated with higher rates of abuse (see **Table 2**).[1,14]

- Biological parents were most often the perpetrators (81%) in physical abuse or neglect, but were perpetrators in sexual abuse only a third of the time (36%).
- Female parents/caregivers are more likely to be perpetrators of physical abuse (75%), although NAT by men is more likely to result in the death of the child.
- Men are more often (87%) implicated in sexual abuse against children than are women.
- Rates of child maltreatment by unemployed parents are 2 to 3 times higher than by employed parents.
- Studies are inconclusive on whether caregivers who were themselves abused are more likely to abuse others, although there seems to be a trend toward this being true.[15]
- Substance abuse and mental illness in abusers were also more common.[1]

The Netherlands has recently instituted a protocol that screens adult ED patients with high-risk complaints for possible abuse of their children.[16] Adults presenting to the ED for substance abuse, suicide attempt, self-mutilation, or issues related to domestic violence were asked if they were responsible for the care of minors. Positive responses yielded a visit by a representative of the local child abuse center who screened the child for signs of abuse. The screening ultimately had a 91% positive predictive value (PPV) for maltreatment, indicating that such behavior in caretakers should heighten suspicion for abuse.

Low socioeconomic status, including income less than $15,000 annually, less than high school education for caregivers, and participation in public assistance programs contributed to increased maltreatment at 5 to 7 times the rates for those with higher socioeconomic status. Increasing rates of child maltreatment have been correlated with the socioeconomic inequality across the United States.[17] Children living with their married biological parents had the lowest rate of maltreatment, whereas children living with a single parent and a live-in partner had the highest rates of abuse.[1]

THE APPROACH TO AN ABUSED CHILD

The forensic or legal evaluation is best performed by a trained team of law enforcement and child abuse specialists. However, EPs are best suited to medically evaluate a child first, with the data gathered during this evaluation often being used for further investigation. Medical examination and treatment should always supersede legal evaluation for the good of the child. The following initial evaluation of abuse has been adapted from the previous *Clinics of North America* review and the most recent American Academy of Pediatrics recommendations.[18,19]

History

An appropriate history should be taken from all involved, including the child, parents, caregivers, and any witnesses. In a critically ill patient, history should be focused on information that can guide lifesaving intervention.

If possible, the child should be interviewed alone. Sit down at or below eye level and, in a gentle manner, ask questions in terms that the child can understand. Ask open-ended questions and document the child's exact responses. Involvement of social work or a child life specialist can be useful to make the child comfortable and to help document pertinent information. If available, video or audio recording may be used.

Caregivers should also be interviewed alone when possible. It is important to remain objective and nonjudgmental because the EP's role is a medical evaluation, not a legal evaluation. Without assigning blame, EPs can ask plainly, "Are you concerned someone is abusing your child?" Documentation on the injury or abuse should include timing, mechanism, preceding events, and witnesses to the injury. Responses concerning for NAT include lack of explanation, dramatic changes in important details, wide variability of explanation between caregivers, and explanations inconsistent with the injury or the physical/developmental capacity of the child.

A complete medical history should be obtained from the primary caregiver. Medical history should include birth history, chronic or congenital conditions, cognitive capacity of the child, and history of prior trauma or hospitalizations. Familial history of bleeding, bone, genetic, or metabolic disorders should be elicited. Current progress in developmental milestones should be documented. Important social history includes identification of primary and other caregivers, history of similar trauma to other siblings, history of substance abuse in the household, and prior Child Protective Services (CPS) involvement.

Physical Examination

A complete physical examination should be performed with exact documentation of findings. Older children are usually aware of the findings, and should be asked about the cause with their response documented. Their response, whether flat or tearful, should also be documented. Cardiovascular perfusion, work of breathing, and level of alertness can quickly identify a critically ill child. Lung auscultation can reveal a pneumothorax, and palpation of the chest and abdomen can uncover painful rib fractures or underlying solid organ injury. Symmetric and spontaneous movement of all extremities should be noted because failure to move one part can indicate a painful injury. The child should be completely undressed and the skin examined for patterned injuries such as bruising, burns, or bite marks. Children, especially young children, usually do not object to disrobing, although care should be taken with sexually abused children. Examination of the head for hematomas or step-offs can uncover a skull fracture. A fundoscopic examination can disclose retinal hemorrhages, although this can be difficult without dilatation in an uncooperative child. Oral cavity injuries such as a torn frenulum are often associated with forced feeding or forced oral sex. A full neurologic examination should be documented in cases of traumatic brain injury. Anogenital examination should be performed in cases of sexual abuse, but an external examination should also be performed in those with just physical abuse, and the two can be concurrent. General patterns of neglect can include cachexia, dental caries, severe diaper dermatitis, and poor wound care. Photography is useful to document injuries for legal purposes, and is often done in conjunction with law enforcement. Further description of specific findings and the evaluation of sexual abuse is discussed later in this article.

HIGH-RISK CHIEF COMPLAINTS

Abused children often present to EDs with chief complaints unrelated or latently related to the abuse. These children have a higher use of EDs compared with the general population.[20] Although it is unreasonable to treat every patient as if they are being abused, it is the role of EPs to keep a high index of suspicion. There have been numerous attempts at developing appropriate criteria for ED screening of abuse, including reminder systems, scheduled education, and automatic screening based on risk factors.[20,21] Although observational studies suggest that these may be useful, none have been shown to be sufficiently accurate or reproducible.[22–25] A brief introspection of whether the child is being abused is often enough of a consideration, but there are several chief complaints that deserve further investigation. There are "Six B's" that have high potentials for abuse and should heighten ED suspicion: bruises, breaks, bonks (head injury), burns, bites, and baby blues (**Box 2**).

THE SIX B'S
Bruises

Bruising is one of the most common findings of abuse but is often overlooked on initial evaluation. Nearly 44% of fatal or near-fatal cases of child abuse had previous medical

---

Box 2
The Six B's: high-risk chief complaints

- Bruises
- Breaks
- Bonks (head injuries)
- Burns
- Bites
- Baby blues (excessive crying, poor feeding)

evaluations in which bruising was noted.[26] Patient age and motor developmental stage should be carefully considered when bruising is found on young children. Most children progress from crawling at about 6 months to cruising (walking with assistance) between 6 and 12 months, to walking between 9 and 15 months, although some children show faster or slower gross motor development than others. The adage "those who don't cruise rarely bruise" was confirmed in a 1999 study by Sugar and colleagues.[27] In otherwise well children in whom abuse was not suspected, bruising was found over the bony prominences (ie, shins, forehead, scalp, or upper leg) in 54% of walkers and nearly 21% of cruisers, but in only 2% of precursors. Infants younger than 6 months with suspicious bruising carry nearly 50% risk of at least 1 additional underlying injury.[28]

Certain patterns of bruises also more strongly suggest abuse. A 2009 study by Pierce and colleagues[26] defined the TEN-4 (thorax, ears, neck) body region and age clinical decision rule, in which bruises on the torso (including genitals), ear, or neck on a child younger than 4 years or any bruising on a child less than 4 months old strongly suggested abuse, with a 97% sensitivity (**Box 3**, **Fig. 1**). However, specificity was only 84%, indicating that bruising in these areas or age groups is not necessarily diagnostic of abuse.

Any patterned bruising should also raise suspicion for abuse (**Fig. 2**). Sharp demarcation, uniform shape, or clusters of bruising often can indicate that the child was assailed with an object.[29] Types of patterned bruises may include linear bruises from a rod, looped bruises from a cord, band-like bruises from restraints around wrists or ankles, or mirror images of implements such as patterned belts or kitchen utensils.

In the past, dating bruises based on color was widely practiced to help distinguish accidental from nonaccidental trauma. However, recent literature suggests that dating of bruises by color has no scientific basis.[30,31] The accuracy of dating for fresh, intermediate, or old bruises was only 55% to 63%, and interobserver reliability regarding color was poor whether the bruise was photographed or in vivo.[30–32] However, multiple bruises in various stages of healing should prompt concern.

Bruising around the abdomen should raise specific concern for intra-abdominal injury, but bruising is often absent even with severe blows.[33] Inflicted abdominal trauma related to abuse is associated with a delayed presentation, higher rate of solid and hollow viscous injury, and overall higher morbidity and mortality.[34,35]

Pitfalls in evaluation of bruising

No bruise is diagnostic for abuse. It should prompt further investigation and should be correlated with a clinical history, development stage, and caregiver explanation. This information should ideally be confirmed by more than 1 source. Several normal childhood or medical conditions can cause or mimic bruising.

Box 3
TEN-4 rule for bruises suggestive of abuse

Bruises on the:

- T: thorax (including genitals)

- E: ears

- N: neck

Bruises on any child younger than 4 months

Data from Pierce MC, Kaczor K, Aldridge S, et al. Bruising characteristics discriminating physical child abuse from accidental trauma. Pediatrics 2010;125(1):67–74.

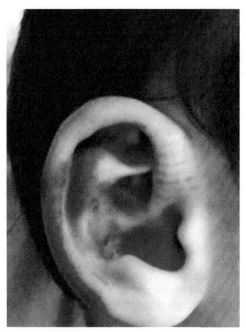

Fig. 1. Bruising on the ear of a child struck on the head.

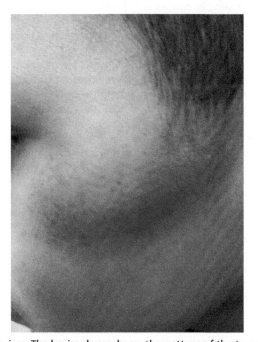

Fig. 2. Patterned bruises. The bruise shown bears the pattern of the tread on the bottom of the shoe the child was struck with.

Hemophilia, leukemia, postinfectious vasculitides, and idiopathic thrombocyto-penic purpura are well-described childhood illnesses that can cause easy bruising from poor clotting or platelet function. Minimal trauma can cause bruising similar to that described in abuse. A medical evaluation including a platelet count, platelet func-tion studies, prothrombin time, and partial thromboplastin time may be indicated for evaluation.[36]

Melanocytic nevus (previously called Mongolian spots) is a dark blue/green discol-oration in the low back and buttocks that is well described and can initially be seen at birth. These marks can be large, sometimes covering the buttocks and extending up to the mid or upper back, and are most common in African American, Hispanic, Native American, and Asian ethnicities. The natural course is to self-resolve in 2 to 3 years.

Several cultural practices that are not abusive can cause patterned bruises that can initially alarm EPs. Cao giao, or coining, is a Vietnamese folk remedy whereby a coin is vigorously rubbed against the skin to release sources of fever. The result is linear patterned bruises but no harm to the child. Cupping is similarly practiced by some Latin American cultures for relief of fever. Patterned circular bruises occur from a vac-uum effect after a heated glass bowl is applied to the skin and allowed to cool, thus creating a vacuum effect.

When documenting bruises, color, size, and shape should be documented, but al-ways objectively (ie, U-shaped bruise rather than belt buckle–shaped bruise). Bruises may also prompt radiographic imaging studies because they may be the only visible clue to a deeper fracture or injury.

Breaks

Skeletal fractures are common in the ED. Childhood fractures occur most commonly in boys and usually affect the upper extremity. The mechanism is usually related to falls, sports, or motor vehicle collisions.[37] Fractures of abuse are less common but are also often found incidentally and without rational explanation.[38] Important risk fac-tors of abusive fractures include age of the child, location of fracture, and number of fractures.

Toddlers and infants are most likely to have abusive fractures, with younger age be-ing more suggestive of abuse.[39,40] Again, development plays a key role in diagnosis because infants do not become mobile enough even to roll until about 4 months of age. In the premobile age group of 0 to 8 months, the most commonly fractured bones through accidental or iatrogenic trauma are the clavicle and skull.[39]

The specific bone fractured must fit with the given history, but some breaks more strongly suggest abuse than others. Rib fractures are frequently seen in abused chil-dren and are classically described as posteromedial, bilateral, and on contiguous ribs from a squeezing force as an infant is shaken (**Fig. 3**).[39] These signs can often be the only evidence of abuse. Rib fractures alone in children younger than 3 years are asso-ciated with 95% PPV for NAT. This value increased to 100% when clinical scenario and history were considered.[30] Cardiopulmonary resuscitation rarely causes rib frac-tures, and when it does they are anterior and may be multiple.[41,42]

Long bone fractures highly associated with abuse include midshaft and metaphy-seal fractures. Femoral fractures in the absence of a motor vehicle collision or other explained violent trauma conferred a significant probability that the inciting event was nonaccidental.[35] Humeral shaft fractures followed suit, especially when the child was younger than 15 months.[43] Fractures are typically midshaft, but neither spiral, transverse, nor oblique fractures correlated more with abuse.

In contrast to the direct force applied for midshaft fractures, metaphyseal fractures occur because of indirect forces. Shaking, pulling, or twisting mechanisms often

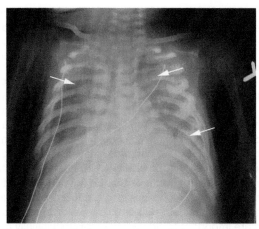

Fig. 3. Rib fractures. Multiple rib fractures (*arrows*) in various stages of healing in a 7-month-old abused child.

cause rapid acceleration and deceleration that shear the immature spongiosa of the growing bone. Metaphyseal fractures are the classic fractures described by Caffey[44] that are often associated with other abusive injuries such as rib fractures, retinal hemorrhages, or head trauma. These fractures, commonly referred to as bucket-handle or corner fractures, are highly specific for abusive injury and are almost never seen in accidental trauma.[45]

Appropriate imaging of fractures in the emergency department
If the fracture is suspicious for abuse, current recommendations by the American Academy of Pediatrics (AAP) are for a complete skeletal survey to be performed in the ED if the child is less than 24 months old.[37] The usefulness of skeletal survey in children older than 5 years is poor, and variable in children between 2 and 5 years old.[46] Skeletal surveys should be separate, high-quality radiographs of every bone. A "babygram" with multiple areas on the same image is not acceptable, and lowers the sensitivity of the survey. Skeletal survey alone does not identify all fractures, and can be performed in conjunction with bone scintigraphy to increase the sensitivity. However, this is not an imaging modality that is readily available in the ED and should be considered as part of the inpatient evaluation. Neither skeletal survey nor bone scintigraphy is sensitive enough to identify all fractures, and a repeat skeletal survey performed 2 weeks later will yield more findings. Repeat studies do not need to include the skull because it does not form calluses, as do cortical bones in the rest of the skeleton.[46]

The radiation exposure from a bone survey is estimated at 4 mSv and, although the concern of possible radiation effects is valid, the morbidity and mortality from missed abuse is well documented and high. The AAP recently published consensus guidelines on when a skeletal survey is necessary, and comments that it is always reasonable to obtain the films if suspicion is high.[47] Cases of confessed abuse, injury during domestic violence, delayed care, or injury attributed to impact from a toy or other object should prompt a skeletal survey on an age-dependent basis.

Skeletal survey is sensitive enough to be recommended for all suspected cases of abuse. A study of skeletal survey in children with burns concerning for abuse showed that 18% had concomitant fractures.[48] Finding these fractures not only helps identify further injuries in need of potential treatment but also helps build a case that the injuries sustained were nonaccidental. However, fractures cannot necessarily be correlated with exact injuries because dating of fractures is an inexact science reliant mostly on the radiologist's personal experience.[49]

Pitfalls in the evaluation of fractures

There are several medical conditions that confer bone fragility and a higher rate of fractures with minimal trauma.[50] Osteogenesis imperfecta is an autosomal dominant defect in collagen that causes fragility. Children may also have bluish sclera, short stature, a large fontanelle, and tooth discoloration, although several types exist with variable penetrance. Nutritional deficiencies such as rickets (vitamin D deficiency) and scurvy (vitamin C deficiency), and chronic kidney disease with persistent electrolyte loss can cause osteopenia that can be seen on imaging.[51] Pathologic fractures from childhood cancer can cause fractures that do not necessarily fit the mechanism of injury described. Identifying such physiologic causes of fracture often requires further medical evaluation, thus being linked to causation in retrospect.

Toddler fractures are important accidental fractures that initially appear suspicious. Fractures are associated with a twisting motion on a planted foot in children between 1 and 4 years old. At this age the cartilage is stronger than the bones, and resultant motion can cause a linear oblique fracture of the distal tibia (**Fig. 4**). Fractures of the midshaft tibia should be suspicious for abuse, as described earlier.[52] Similarly, distal radius or ulnar buckle fractures are thought to be plausibly accidental in ambulatory children. Other plausibly accidental injuries include unilateral, linear skull fractures with a significant fall (usually >3 ft) or trauma and clavicle fractures in infants younger than 30 days old that can be attributed to birth trauma.[47]

Bonks

Head trauma is the most common cause of death in cases of physical abuse.[53] Infants less than 1 year old are specifically at risk, and those who survive have significant morbidity related to neurologic sequelae. Children in this age group with intracranial injuries are frequently asymptomatic or have nonspecific symptoms, so a high clinical suspicion must lead EPs to the diagnosis.[54] Symptoms can be as vague as poor

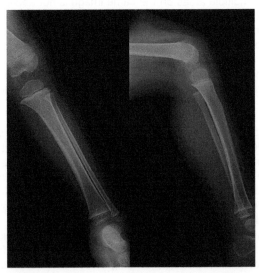

Fig. 4. Toddler fracture. Anteroposterior and lateral views of a tibia with thin lucency.

feeding, excessive crying, lethargy, or seizures. Abusive head trauma should be considered in any young child presenting in extremis or cardiac arrest.

Skull fractures and intracranial hemorrhage (ICH) are commonly encountered in abusive head trauma, but are also seen in accidental trauma. Skull fractures associated with accidental trauma are usually linear and parietal.[38] Fractures that are bilateral, complex as opposed to linear, depressed, or crossing suture lines should raise suspicion for abuse. History given by caregivers should always be evaluated in light of the patient's developmental level and the severity of trauma. The Pediatric Emergency Care Applied Research Network (PECARN) research group established an excellent decision rule to help identify those at low risk for clinically significant traumatic brain injury that can help in determining the plausibility of the caregiver's explanation.[55] Subdural hematomas are the most common type of ICH associated with abuse, whereas epidural hematomas are rarely associated with abuse (**Fig. 5**).[56] Of the subdural hematomas found, increasing number, location in the posterior fossa, and coincidence of cerebral edema were highly correlated with abuse.[57] A 2011 study showed 6 findings to be associated with abuse-related head trauma: rib fractures, retinal hemorrhages, long bone fractures, head/neck bruising, apnea, and seizures.[58] When 3 or more of these were present in children younger than 3 years, the PPV approached 100%. In addition, the combination of head injury and either retinal hemorrhages or rib fractures increased the PPV to nearly 100%.[59]

The triad of retinal hemorrhages, subdural hematomas, and posterior rib fractures is commonly known as shaken-baby syndrome. The injury to the retina is similar in mechanism to that of the subdural hematomas, and the rapid acceleration and deceleration causes a shearing injury to fragile vessels, resulting in hemorrhage. Although the term shaken-baby syndrome has been argued in the legal realm, the presence of retinal hemorrhages has a high specificity for abuse, especially when the hemorrhages are bilateral, extensive, and multilayered.[59,60] Because these cases often go to trial, detailed evaluation by an ophthalmologist is recommended for all suspected cases of abuse with evidence of traumatic brain injury on computed tomography

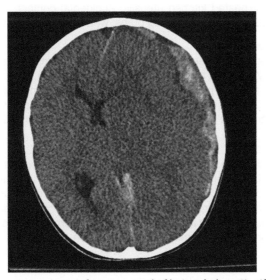

Fig. 5. Subdural hematomas in an infant suspected of being shaken. Significant midline shift is evident.

(CT). However, recent data suggest that retinal examination in infants with normal head CT scans is unlikely to reveal evidence of abuse.[61]

Appropriate imaging of head injuries in the emergency department

The standard modality for diagnosing intracranial hemorrhage in the ED is CT of the head. However, with increasing concerns for exposure of small children to radiation, there has been further investigation into the use of magnetic resonance imaging (MRI) as a primary alternative. However, the recommended sequence is head CT, followed by MRI and diffusion-weighted imaging of the brain to further evaluate findings.[62]

Pitfalls in evaluation of head injuries

Abusive head trauma can be difficult to diagnose, especially when a patient is asymptomatic. Several conditions can predispose children to hemorrhage more readily. Glutaric aciduria type 1 is an inborn error of metabolism associated with macrocranium, subdural hematomas, and retinal hemorrhages. Hemorrhagic disease of the newborn can cause severe ICH in cases where vitamin K prophylaxis is missed or refused. Simple birth trauma can cause ICH and retinal hemorrhage that persists up to 2 weeks of life and may be unrelated to the ED visit.[36]

Burns

Burn injuries are most commonly sustained as scalds from hot liquids or direct contact with hot objects. Although not usually deadly, burns are a permanent physical reminder of abuse. Much like with bruising, patterned burns, uniform burns, and burns with sharp demarcation should be concerning for abuse outside a rational history. Accidental scald burns tend to be on the head and back because toddlers pull hot water onto themselves. Splashing also causes satellite burns. By contrast, forced immersion burns are sharply demarcated and have uniform depth, indicating that the child was held still while being burned.[63] Spared areas of skin where flexion or extension prevented infiltration of hot liquids strongly suggest inflicted burns. Diapers provide excellent burn protection, so a history of a burn in the diaper area sustained while wearing a diaper should be suspicious for abuse. Contact burns often take the shape of the object used, such as cigarettes, irons, or heated kitchen utensils. Accidental contact burns often cause glancing injuries, as opposed to inflicted burns, which leave a more uniform mark.

Pitfalls in evaluating burns

Burns are common accidental injuries and must be explained by a rational history. Concerning history includes a supposedly unwitnessed burn, attribution of the burn to a sibling, and a delay in presentation.[64] Infectious or immunologic conditions such as staphylococcal scalded skin syndrome, Stevens-Johnson syndrome, or Kawasaki disease can cause sloughing of the skin and denuded areas similar to burns.

Bites

Bite marks on children are a disturbing sign of abuse. Often perpetrators lay blame on a sibling or animal, but careful history and measurement of the bite mark can help identify abuse. An intercanine distance of greater than 2.5 cm suggests an adult human bite rather than a bite from an animal or small child.[65] Photographs are helpful for documentation. Fresh bites are inoculated with the perpetrator's saliva, and should be swabbed by forensic personnel for DNA evaluation.

Baby Blues

Pediatricians spend considerable time with new parents preparing them for the challenges of parenthood.[66] Screening for postpartum depression and education in ways to avoid succumbing to stressors are done at each newborn visit. However, this role can often extend into the ED during off-business hours. ED visits for complaints of excessive crying, poor feeding, or apparent life-threatening events (ALTE) can sometimes be clues to abuse. Infants with excessive crying are more likely to be slapped, smothered, or shaken than are children who were not perceived to be excessive by caregivers.[67] The incidence curve of hospitalization for shaken-baby syndrome mirrors the incidence curve for crying in both the starting point and shape of the curve.[68] Parents who seem to be excessively concerned or frustrated about their infant's crying should be cautioned on ways to avoid abuse, including leaving the child with a responsible caregiver for a brief time and avoidance of substance use. Nonspecific signs of poor feeding or lethargy are often the only symptom of abuse, and children are often brought in by a caregiver other than the perpetrator. In cases of ALTE related to abuse, patients appeared well in the ED but were more likely to have focal findings, and had the highest mortality of any other causes of ALTE.[69]

Sudden infant unexplained death syndrome (SUIDS) is clinically difficult to distinguish in an ED setting. SUIDS is differentiated from sudden infant death syndrome (SIDS) because the latter is a diagnosis that can only be made by exclusion after full autopsy and forensic examination. Accidental causes, inborn causes, and nonaccidental causes are best determined by a medical examiner. AAP clinical policy states that the rate of SUIDS is higher than that of infanticide, and as such the family should be questioned in a nonjudgmental manner until a legal investigation can be completed.[70] Parents of SUIDS children demonstrate high levels of anxiety and depression after notification of death, with mothers typically having more symptoms than fathers.[71] As yet, however, no evidence exists to link parental response with either SUIDS or infanticide. Thorough objective documentation of history and physical examination findings and alerting law enforcement of a death is the appropriate role of the EP.

EMOTIONAL ABUSE AND NEGLECT

Often the most difficult type of abuse to diagnose in the ED is abuse that is not present on any examination, laboratory test, or imaging modality. Emotional abuse or neglect is often difficult to elicit or substantiate in an ED setting, but may be the subtle sign of latent physical abuse or further abuse to come. The EP's initial gestalt of the child's mood and interaction with the caregiver is pertinent to the evaluation of abuse. The internalization of abuse and subsequent progression to mental or behavioral disturbances is variable and age dependent.[72] Younger children may not internalize abuse in the same way as adolescents, and certainly have a different way of expressing their reaction to it. Toddlers may show a range of emotions from regression to aggression. School-aged children report anxiety, depression, feelings of guilt, or sleep disorders. Adolescents tend to act out the most, with problems as variable as eating disorders, personality disorders, suicidality, truancy, or self-mutilation, although some may become withdrawn instead. There is no clear connection between patient presentation and the type of abuse suffered, but some generalizations can be made for screening purposes. While in the ED, an abused child may show signs of emotional trauma such as inappropriate fear of caregivers and medical personnel, signs of attachment problems, or dissociation. Educational neglect is, again, more difficult to assess in the ED, but a basic knowledge of developmental milestones can help EPs determine whether a child is progressing appropriately. Parents may appear overconcerned, underconcerned, or intimidating to the child, other family members, or staff.

SEXUAL ASSAULT

Sexual assault of a child is a delicate scenario in the ED and deserves its own discussion. Victims should be prioritized in the ED. Prioritization is not always necessary for medical or forensic reasons, but is necessary for social and psychological reasons. These patients should be separated from the commotion of the waiting room into a quiet, nonthreatening area of the ED. An advocate should be assigned to the patient. This person is ideally a social worker trained as a sexual assault advocate. If not available, a social worker, nurse, or nurse assistant can remain with the patient. One must be conscious of gender issues. The victim may not respond well to being isolated in a room with a male staff member. The following initial evaluation of sexual abuse has been adapted from the most recent AAP recommendations and the US Department of Justice National Protocol.[73–75]

The Interview

Extensive training exists on how to appropriately conduct a forensic interview. This interview is ideally conducted before the medical evaluation because disclosure can often assist the clinician in focusing the examination and forensic collection. If the forensic interview has not been conducted, the goal is for a limited interview to gain the critical medical information needed while being cautious to avoid altering the disclosure. To minimize impact, allow patients to tell their stories using their own terms, at their own pace, and always ask open-ended questions as opposed to leading questions.

Understanding detailed events of an assault has the added benefit of directing your forensic collection. Listen without interruption, although occasional prompting with open-ended questions to encourage the victim through the disclosure may be warranted. As the victim divulges information, be meticulous to document exact words used so that these can be quoted in documentation. Exact phrases during the initial medical interview have been shown to be powerful in court proceedings. Key features of the event that should be documented include:

- Type of contact: genital-genital, oral-genital, and so forth
- Characteristics of the assailant: name if known, number of assailants, gender, ethnicity, identifying features, and so forth
- Presence of body fluids: wet areas that may imply saliva, sweat, ejaculate, and so forth
- Cleansing events since the assault: showering, bathing, urination, stooling

It is also necessary to know whether the victim had consensual intercourse before the assault (within the last week) and the date of the last menstrual period if the patient is postpubertal.

The Kit

The forensic collection kit (so-called rape kit) is regularly supplied by the law enforcement agency investigating the case. The contents of these kits are, for the most part, standardized but may vary slightly from region to region. Before use, inspect the kit to make sure it is sealed and intact. From this point forward, a clearly defined chain of custody must be maintained until it is completed and handed back to law enforcement personnel. The common elements of the forensic collection kit are summarized in **Box 4**.

The Examination

Make sure the patient is comfortable and explain everything that is going to happen. Unless they are suspects, have the parents involved as much as possible to keep the

---

Box 4
Inventory of a standard sexual assault forensics kit

- Paper bags to package clothing and underwear
- Folded paper mat to collect foreign materials such as dried blood, dried secretions, fibers, loose hairs, vegetation, soil/debris
- Envelope for collection of debris from pubic hair combings
- Swabs along with swab boxes for packaging of: vaginal/cervical swabs and smears; penile swabs and smears; anal/perianal swabs and smears; oral swabs and smears; body swabs
- Known victims' blood, saliva sample, or buccal swab for DNA analysis
- Bulb syringe and vial for vaginal washings
- Nail pick for fingernail scrapings
- Sealing tape and stickers

Additional equipment (if available) that can augment data collection

- Alternative light source (fluorescent light or Wood light)
- Colposcope or other photographic device
- Speculum and/or anoscope
- Toluidine blue
- 18F Foley catheter with Luer-lock syringe

---

child comfortable. If possible, have the victim assist during the examination. This involvement not only empowers the victim but also directs the collections (particularly combings and swabs) to regions of the body most likely to result in collection of biological evidence. Patients need to be fully disrobed and in a loose-fitting hospital gown. All regions of the body need to be inspected, including crevices, scalp, and fingernails (to check whether they are broken or retaining material). Positioning of the patient for the genital examination is critical not only for adequate visualization but for the comfort of the patient. For young girls, the knee-to-chest position is often comfortable when the child is in the parent's lap. The frog-legged and prone position can also help identify different aspects of the female genital examination for trauma or hymenal injury.

Keys to Processing and Packaging the Kit

Wear gloves at all times once the forensic kit is opened. Be cautious of what is touched. Work areas should be wiped clean with a disinfecting solution. Do not sneeze or cough onto the kit. Change gloves before and after each swab acquisition. Expect to change gloves more than 20 times throughout the examination. All evidence must be dried before storage. DNA within biological specimens is stable once desiccated. If specimens remain wet, fungus and bacteria can further degrade DNA in the collections. For this reason, material should never be packaged in plastic. Wet clothing can be laid out during the examination to dry but, if wet on packaging, law enforcement should be notified to expedite processing in the forensic laboratory. Commercial swab driers have a 1-hour timer with a swab compartment that gently circulates cool air over the swabs. An alternative can be a polystyrene cup turned upside down on the counter. Holes in the cup serve to hold and separate swabs while drying. Be careful to label the swabs in the swab rack or polystyrene cup.

Once dry, swabs and slides are packaged. Labeling should include the patient name, your name, body region of origin, and collection date/time on each package. Packages are then placed in separate envelopes once dry and tape sealed (it is important not to lick the envelope). Each envelope should be signed, with the signature extending across the tape. Once packaged, the outside of the kit has a region for the documentation of custody. On handing the completed kit to law enforcement, always witness their receipt and signature in the chain of custody section, thus documenting their receipt of the evidence.

Sexually Exploited Children

Sadly, the engagement of minors in prostitution is a consideration that must be made in the evaluation of suspected sexual abuse.[76] In 2001, a United States national study estimated that more than 200,000 children are at risk for sexual exploitation. Similarly to the statistics on physical abuse, many of these victims had contact with a health care provider who had a chance to intervene.[77] Risk factors for prostitution include runaway status, homelessness, truancy, recent immigration, substance abuse, and previous sexual abuse, which may then propagate the cycle. The child's affect will often be blunted, depressed, or guarded, and the caretaker may be inappropriately controlling or affectionate. The ED evaluation is an opportune time to isolate the child and screen for sexual exploitation with nonjudgmental and careful questioning. Involvement of social workers is highly recommended. Once identified, law enforcement should be notified and the child should be held in the ED or admitted until such a time as a safe disposition can be made.

MANAGEMENT AND DISPOSITION OF CHILD ABUSE IN THE EMERGENCY DEPARTMENT

When abused children present to the ED, identification and treatment of life-threatening injuries take precedence over any other part of the evaluation. A thorough history and complete examination, both visual and by palpation, are indicated in every child, much like in patients with trauma. Once the child has been appropriately stabilized, the legal evaluation can begin. Informing caregivers about the subsequent steps and need for mandatory reporting is vital and should be handled delicately, because some caregivers do not respond positively to being investigated. EPs can simply state, "I am concerned someone is abusing your child and I am legally obligated to report this."

EPs are required by law to report cases in which there is a reasonable suspicion of child abuse. However, in addition to there being no firm definition of child abuse, child abuse experts disagree on what constitutes reasonable suspicion as a threshold for mandatory reporting (**Box 5**).[74] Specific laws have minor variations from state to state, but all allow for immunity from criminal or civil prosecution for mandatory reporters who file reports in good faith (specific statutes can be found at the Web site for Administration for Children and Families, US Department of Health and Human Services, at https://www.childwelfare.gov/systemwide/laws_policies/state/). Despite this, many EPs choose not to report cases of abuse.[78] In an attempt to simplify a complex interaction, the role of EPs in child abuse is proposed to be 6-fold:

1. Identify abuse
2. Facilitate a thorough investigation
3. Treat medical needs
4. Protect the patient
5. Provide an unbiased medical consultation to law enforcement
6. Provide an ethical testimony if called to court

Box 5
Findings highly suspicious of abuse

- Aloof or inconsistent caregivers
- Young age
- Multiple injuries
- Patterned or sharply demarcated bruises or burns
- Bruises on the torso, ear, or neck
- Bruises in children younger than 4 months
- Rib fractures
- Midshaft or metaphyseal fractures
- Subdural hematomas
- Retinal hemorrhages
- Bite marks greater than 2.5 cm in diameter

The medical disposition of the child is determined by the EP. Even if the child does not medically meet inpatient criteria, an admission may still be warranted for the safety of the child until CPS can find another safe environment. This process is widely practiced and accepted by pediatricians, hospitals, and insurance companies.[79]

The ED is not the place to investigate suspects, accuse caregivers, or assign blame. Instead, it is important to stay focused on the medical evaluation of the child and allow law enforcement and CPS to investigate. Keeping objectivity allows an easier time testifying should the case go to court and the medical records and EP's testimony be subpoenaed.

Documentation

Documentation of abuse is carefully scrutinized in subsequent legal matters, so a meticulous record is critical. It is important to be objective and use quotes when possible. History should include where and when the injury occurred in addition to witnesses to the injury and explanations given for any delay in care. Events leading up to the event may elicit a cause for an abusive response. Physical examination should document color, size, and shape of any visible injuries. Developmental level of the child should be documented as what is given by history and what is observed in the ED encounter. The medical decision-making portion should give a concise opinion on whether the history and physical examination corroborate each other and whether the mechanism for injury is plausible or not.

For cases of sexual abuse each forensic collection kit has documentation forms included, and exact processing is vital. These forms are self-explanatory for the most part, with prompted fill-in sections and text areas for the examiner to complete. There is typically a signature line for consent from the victim's guardian. All pages need to be signed by the examiner, numbered, and have the victim's name and age along with the case number. Most paperwork is in triplicate (pressure-sensitive copy paper) for copies to law enforcement, crime laboratory, and medical facility. Examination portions of the documentation paperwork have body diagrams that can be marked to indicate location, with an associated page for the written description of each injury and finding. In general, the more verbose the better, because many of these cases take years to prosecute and no examiner can remember the examination over such a long period.

Table 3 Medical conditions that can mimic abuse	
Bruises	Hemophilia Leukemia Postinfectious vasculitides Idiopathic thrombocytopenic purpura Melanocytic nevus Cupping Coining
Breaks	Osteogenesis imperfecta Vitamin D deficiency (rickets) Vitamin C deficiency (scurvy) Chronic kidney disease Toddler fractures
Bonks	Bleeding diatheses Glutaric aciduria Vitamin K deficiency Birth trauma
Burns	Stevens-Johnson syndrome Staphylococcal scalded skin syndrome Kawasaki disease

Photographic Documentation

Photographic evidence has been beneficial in prosecution and in reminding examiners of their findings for testimony. An additional benefit is that images can be evaluated at a later date by outside medical specialists. Photography is best performed by a law enforcement agency with approved forensic cameras, which is typically facilitated by the law enforcement agent, and in small rural agencies can be as rudimentary as an officer (using an agency-approved camera) taking the photographs with the direction of the examiner. Smartphones or personal cameras should not be used.

SUMMARY

Child abuse is emotionally challenging and is a common problem in EDs globally. EPs are in a prime position to act on immediate threats to life and limb and to identify abuse before significant morbidity or mortality ensues. Early identification of abuse can also lead to early treatment of the psychological and emotional scars, which EPs cannot adequately treat in the emergency setting. Although no single finding is 100% specific for abuse, several findings are suspicious for abuse but can have medical reasons that first require evaluation (**Table 3**). Maintaining a high clinical suspicion for high-risk cases of abuse remains the most important skill an EP can have in helping to curb this serious social problem.

REFERENCES

1. Sedlak AJ, Mettenburg J, Basena M, et al. Fourth National Incidence Study of child abuse and neglect (NIS-4). Washington, DC: US Department of Health and Human Services; 2010. Available at: http://www.acf.hhs.gov/programs/opre/research/project/national-incidence-study-of-child-abuse-and-neglect-nis-4-2004-2009. Accessed July 9, 2010.
2. Wildeman C, Emanuel N, Leventhal JM, et al. The prevalence of confirmed maltreatment among US children, 2004 to 2011. JAMA Pediatr 2014;168(8):706–13.

3. Gilbert R, Widom CS, Browne K, et al. Burden and consequences of child maltreatment in high-income countries. Lancet 2009;373(9657):68–81.
4. Afifi TO, MacMillan HL, Boyle M, et al. Child abuse and mental disorders in Canada. Can Med Assoc J 2014;186(9):E324–32.
5. Florence C, Brown DS, Fang X, et al. Health care costs associated with child maltreatment: impact on Medicaid. Pediatrics 2013;132(2):312–8.
6. Peterson C, Xu L, Florence C, et al. The medical cost of abusive head trauma in the United States. Pediatrics 2014;134(1):91–9.
7. King WK, Kiesel EL, Simon HK. Child abuse fatalities: are we missing opportunities for intervention? Pediatr Emerg Care 2006;22(4):211.
8. Sheets LK, Leach ME, Koszewski IJ, et al. Sentinel injuries in infants evaluated for child physical abuse. Pediatrics 2013;131:701.
9. Ravichandiran N, Schuh S, Bejuk M, et al. Delayed identification of pediatric abuse-related fractures. Pediatrics 2010;125(1):60–6.
10. Skellern CY, Wood DO, Murphy A, et al. Non-accidental fractures in infants: risk of further abuse. J Paediatr Child Health 2000;36(6):590–2.
11. Deans KJ, Thackeray J, Askegard-Giesmann JR, et al. Mortality increases with recurrent episodes of nonaccidental trauma in children. J Trauma Acute Care Surg 2013;75(1):161–5.
12. Schreier H. Munchausen by proxy defined. Pediatrics 2002;110(5):985–8.
13. Stirling J. Beyond Munchausen syndrome by proxy: identification and treatment of child abuse in a medical setting. Pediatrics 2007;119(5):1026–30.
14. Barker LH, Howell RJ. Munchausen syndrome by proxy in false allegations of child sexual abuse: legal implications. J Am Acad Psychiatry Law 1994;22(4):499–510.
15. Mulpuri K, Tredwell SJ. The epidemiology of nonaccidental trauma in children. Clin Orthop Relat Res 2011;469:759–67.
16. Diderich HM, Fekkes M, Verkerk PH. A new protocol for screening adults presenting with their own medical problems at the emergency department to identify children at high risk for maltreatment. Child Abuse Negl 2013;37(12):1122–31.
17. Eckenrode J, Smith EG, McCarthy ME, et al. Income inequality and child maltreatment in the United States. Pediatrics 2014;133:454.
18. Jain AM. Emergency department evaluation of child abuse. Emerg Med Clin North Am 1999;17(3):575–93.
19. Kellogg ND. Evaluation of suspected child physical abuse. Pediatrics 2007;119(6):1232–41.
20. Guenther E, Knight S, Olson LM, et al. Prediction of child abuse risk from emergency department use. J Pediatr 2009;154(2):272–7.
21. Mikton C, Butchart A. Child maltreatment prevention: a systematic review of reviews. Bull World Health Organ 2009;87(5):353–61.
22. Teeuw AH, Derkx BH, Koster WA, et al. Detection of child abuse and neglect at the emergency room. Eur J Pediatr 2012;171(6):877–85.
23. Woodman J, Lecky F, Hodes D, et al. Screening injured children for physical abuse or neglect in emergency departments: a systematic review. Child Care Health Dev 2010;36(2):153–64.
24. Newton AS, Zou B, Hamm MP, et al. Improving child protection in the emergency department: a systematic review of professional interventions for health care providers. Acad Emerg Med 2010;17(2):117–25.
25. Louwers EC, Affourtit MJ, Moll HA, et al. Screening for child abuse at emergency departments: a systematic review. Arch Dis Child 2010;95(3):214–8.

26. Pierce MC, Kaczor K, Aldridge S, et al. Bruising characteristics discriminating physical child abuse from accidental trauma. Pediatrics 2010;125(1):67–74.
27. Sugar NF, Taylor JA, Feldman KW. Bruises in infants and toddlers: those who don't cruise rarely bruise. Arch Pediatr Adolesc Med 1999;153(4):399.
28. Harper NS, Feldman KW, Sugar NF, et al. Additional injuries in young infants with concern for abuse and apparently isolated bruises. J Pediatr 2014;165(2): 383–8.
29. Maguire S, Mann MK, Sibert J, et al. Are there patterns of bruising in childhood which are diagnostic or suggestive of abuse? A systematic review. Arch Dis Child 2005;90(2):182–6.
30. Maguire S, Mann MK, Sibert J, et al. Can you age bruises accurately in children? A systematic review. Arch Dis Child 2005;90(2):187–9.
31. Schwartz AJ, Ricci LR. How accurately can bruises be aged in abused children? Literature review and synthesis. Pediatrics 1996;97:254–7.
32. Munang LA, Leonard PA, Mok JY. Lack of agreement on colour description between clinicians examining childhood bruising. J Clin Forensic Med 2002;9(4): 171–4.
33. Thompson S. Accidental or inflicted? Evaluating cutaneous, skeletal, and abdominal trauma in children. Pediatr Ann 2005;34:372–81.
34. Canty TG Sr, Canty TG Jr, Brown C. Injuries of the gastrointestinal tract from blunt trauma in children: a 12-year experience at a designated pediatric trauma center. J Trauma 1999;46:234–40.
35. Wood J, Rubin DM, Nance ML, et al. Distinguishing inflicted versus accidental abdominal injuries in young children. J Trauma Acute Care Surg 2005;59(5): 1203–8.
36. Anderst JD, Carpenter SL, Abshire TC, et al. Evaluation for bleeding disorders in suspected child abuse. Pediatrics 2013;131(4):e1314–22.
37. Rennie L, Court-Brown CM, Mok JY, et al. The epidemiology of fractures in children. Injury 2007;38(8):913–22.
38. Kemp AM, Dunstan F, Harrison S, et al. Patterns of skeletal fractures in child abuse: systematic review. BMJ 2008;337:a1518.
39. Clarke NM, Shelton FR, Taylor C. The incidence of fractures in children under the age of 24 months—in relation to non-accidental injury. Injury 2012;43:762–5.
40. Leventhal JM, Thomas SA, Rosenfield NS, et al. Fractures in young children: distinguishing child abuse from unintentional injuries. Arch Pediatr Adolesc Med 1993;147(1):87.
41. Bulloch B, Schubert CJ, Brophy PD, et al. Cause and clinical characteristics of rib fractures in infants. Pediatrics 2000;105(4):e48.
42. Barsness KA, Cha ES, Bensard DD, et al. The positive predictive value of rib fractures as an indicator of nonaccidental trauma in children. J Trauma Acute Care Surg 2003;54(6):1107–10.
43. Williams R, Hardcastle N. Humeral fractures and non-accidental injury in children. Emerg Med J 2005;22(2):124–5.
44. Caffey J. Some traumatic lesions in growing bones other than fractures and dislocations: clinical and radiological features. Br J Radiol 1957;30:225–38.
45. Kleinman PK, Perez-Rossello JM, Newton AW, et al. Prevalence of the classic metaphyseal lesion in infants at low versus high risk for abuse. AJR Am J Roentgenol 2011;197(4):1005–8.
46. Kemp AM, Butler A, Morris S, et al. Which radiological investigations should be performed to identify fractures in suspected child abuse? Clin Radiol 2006; 61(9):723–36.

47. Wood JN, Fakeye O, Feudtner C, et al. Development of guidelines for skeletal survey in young children with fractures. Pediatrics 2014;134(1):45–53.
48. DeGraw M, Hicks RA, Lindberg D. Incidence of fractures among children with burns with concern regarding abuse. Pediatrics 2010;125(2):e295–9.
49. Prosser I, Maguire S, Harrison SK, et al. How old is this fracture? Radiologic dating of fractures in children: a systematic review. AJR Am J Roentgenol 2005;184(4):1282–6.
50. Flaherty EG, Perez-Rossello JM, Levine MA, et al. Evaluating children with fractures for child physical abuse. Pediatrics 2014;133(2):e477–89.
51. Ayoub DM, Hyman C, Cohen M, et al. A critical review of the classic metaphyseal lesion: traumatic or metabolic? AJR Am J Roentgenol 2014;202(1):185–96.
52. Tenenbein M, Reed MH, Black GB. The toddler's fracture revisited. Am J Emerg Med 1990;8(3):208–11.
53. Duhaime AC, Christian CW, Rorke LB, et al. Nonaccidental head injury in infants—the "shaken-baby syndrome". N Engl J Med 1998;338(25):1822–9.
54. Laskey AL, Holsti M, Runyan DK, et al. Occult head trauma in young suspected victims of physical abuse. J Pediatr 2004;144(6):719–22.
55. Kupperman N, Holmes JF, Dayan PS, et al. Identification of children at very low risk of clinically-important brain injuries after head trauma: a prospective cohort study. Lancet 2009;374:1160–70, 20.
56. Piteau SJ, Ward MG, Barrowman NJ, et al. Clinical and radiographic characteristics associated with abusive and nonabusive head trauma: a systematic review. Pediatrics 2012;130(2):315–23.
57. Kemp AM, Jaspan T, Griffiths J, et al. Neuroimaging: what neuroradiological features distinguish abusive from non-abusive head trauma? A systematic review. Arch Dis Child 2011;96(12):1103–12.
58. Maguire SA, Kemp AM, Lumb RC, et al. Estimating the probability of abusive head trauma: a pooled analysis. Pediatrics 2011;128(3):e550–64.
59. Togioka BM, Arnold MA, Bathurst MA, et al. Retinal hemorrhages and shaken baby syndrome: an evidence-based review. J Emerg Med 2009;37(1):98–106.
60. Bhardwaj G, Chowdhury V, Jacobs MB, et al. A systematic review of the diagnostic accuracy of ocular signs in pediatric abusive head trauma. Ophthalmology 2010;117(5):983–92.
61. Greiner MV, Berger RP, Thackeray JD, et al. Dedicated retinal examination in children evaluated for physical abuse without radiographically identified traumatic brain injury. J Pediatr 2013;163(2):527–31.
62. Kemp AM, Rajaram S, Mann M, et al. What neuroimaging should be performed in children in whom inflicted brain injury (iBI) is suspected? A systematic review. Clin Radiol 2009;64(5):473–83.
63. Greenbaum AR, Donne J, Wilson D, et al. Intentional burn injury: an evidence-based, clinical and forensic review. Burns 2004;30(7):628–42.
64. Stone NH, Rinaldo L, Humphrey CR, et al. Child abuse by burning. Surg Clin North Am 1970;50(6):1419.
65. Wagner GN. Bitemark identification in child abuse cases. Pediatr Dent 1986;8(1):96–100.
66. Flaherty EG, Stirling J Jr. The pediatrician's role in child maltreatment prevention. Pediatrics 2010;126(4):833–41.
67. Reijneveld SA, van der Wal MF, Brugman E, et al. Infant crying and abuse. Lancet 2004;364(9442):1340–2.

68. Barr RG, Trent RB, Cross J. Age-related incidence curve of hospitalized shaken baby syndrome cases: convergent evidence for crying as a trigger to shaking. Child Abuse Negl 2006;30(1):7–16.
69. Parker K, Pitetti R. Mortality and child abuse in children presenting with apparent life-threatening events. Pediatr Emerg Care 2011;27(7):591–5.
70. Hymel KP. Distinguishing sudden infant death syndrome from child abuse fatalities. Pediatrics 2006;118(1):421–7.
71. Vance JC, Foster WJ, Najman JM, et al. Early parental responses to sudden infant death, stillbirth or neonatal death. Med J Aust 1991;155(5):292–7.
72. Schwarz ED, Perry BD. The post-traumatic response in children and adolescents. Psychiatr Clin North Am 1994;17(2):311–26.
73. Kellogg N. The evaluation of sexual abuse in children. Pediatrics 2005;116(2):506–12.
74. A national protocol for sexual assault medical forensic examinations 2004. The United States Department of Justice website: office on violence against women: selected publications. Available at: http://www.ovw.usdoj.gov/publications.html. Accessed December 18, 2012.
75. Levi BH, Crowell K. Child abuse experts disagree about the threshold for mandated reporting. Clin Pediatr 2011;50(4):321–9.
76. Estes RJ, Weiner NA. The commercial sexual exploitation of children in the U.S., Canada and Mexico. Full Report of the U.S. National Study. 2001. Revised February 20, 2002. Available at: http://www.hawaii.edu/hivandaids/Commercial%20Sexual%20Exploitation%20of%20Children%20in%20the%20US,%20Canada%20and%20Mexico.pdf. Accessed August 25, 2014.
77. Ijadi-Maghsoodi R, Todd EJ, Bath EP. Commercial sexual exploitation of children and the role of the child psychiatrist. J Am Acad Child Adolesc Psychiatry 2014;53(8):825–9.
78. Van Haeringen AR, Dadds M, Armstrong KL. The child abuse lottery—will the doctor suspect and report? Physician attitudes towards and reporting of suspected child abuse and neglect. Child Abuse Negl 1998;22(3):159.
79. Medical necessity for the hospitalization of the abused and neglected child. American Academy of Pediatrics, Committee on Hospital Care and Committee on Child Abuse and Neglect. Pediatrics 1998;101:715–6.

Playing Violent Video Games and Desensitization to Violence

Jeanne Funk Brockmyer, PhD

KEYWORDS

- Video games • Violence • Desensitization • Media violence • Aggression • Empathy
- Moral evaluation • fMRI

KEY POINTS

- Desensitization, the reduction of cognitive, emotional and/or behavioral responses to a stimulus, is an automatic and unconscious phenomenon often experienced in everyday life.
- Exposure to media violence has been identified as potentially desensitizing for children and adolescents.
- This study reviewed data from questionnaire, behavioral, and psychophysiologic research to examine links between exposure to violent video games and desensitization to violence in children and adolescents.
- It was concluded that exposure to violent video games increases the relative risk of desensitization to violence, which in turn may increase aggression and decrease prosocial behavior.
- Parents should be counseled to discuss the differences between real and screen violence, to encourage non-violent problem-solving, and to provide empathy-building experiences.

THE PHENOMENON OF DESENSITIZATION

Desensitization, the reduction of cognitive, emotional, and/or behavioral responses to a stimulus, is an automatic and unconscious phenomenon often experienced in typical, everyday life experiences. This can be best demonstrated through the following exercise: Recall a difficult experience. Remember your thoughts and emotional reactions. Now consider your current response to this recollection. Most likely this response is not as intense as your original reaction. This change reflects normal desensitization. Human beings are simply incapable of long-term maintenance

Funding Source: University of Toledo.

Conflict of Interest: None.

Emeritus, Department of Psychology, University of Toledo, MS 948, 2800 West Bancroft, Toledo, OH 43606-3390, USA

E-mail address: jeanne.brockmyer@gmail.com

1056-4993/15/$ – see front matter © 2015 Elsevier Inc. All rights reserved.

of an acute level of distress. Those whose reactions do not habituate are likely to develop various forms of psychopathology. However, unconscious desensitization can also be maladaptive. For example, researchers have found that children who are exposed to high levels of community violence often view violence as an ordinary part of life and may act accordingly.[1,2] This perspective reflects desensitization to violence. Similarly, exposure to media violence has been identified as potentially desensitizing for children and adolescents.[3,4] This article summarizes research that examines exposure to video game violence as a risk factor for desensitization to violence.

THE PREVALENCE OF VIDEO GAME PLAY

The popularity of video games with players of all ages continues to grow. According to the Entertainment Software Association, in 2013 US consumers spent approximately $21.53 billion on games, equipment, and accessories.[5] Children and adolescents make up a sizable proportion of these consumers: according to a 2008 to 2009 study by the Kaiser Family Foundation, 8 to 18 year olds spent, on average, 73 minutes every day playing video games on a variety of platforms.[6] A telephone survey conducted in 2003 conveys the emerging importance of media in the lives of very young children (birth to 6 years): among those who play, the average daily playing time was 61 minutes per day.[7] Given the trend for increasing time spent with media, including video games, these figures probably underrepresent current play.[6–8]

Research suggests that many games that are popular with children and adolescents have violent content.[9] In the 2008 to 2009 Kaiser survey, more than half of 8 to 18 year olds reported having played a game from the violent Grand Theft Auto series, and almost half reported playing Halo, another violent game.[6] More recent research, including cross-cultural studies, suggests that violent video games remain popular among adolescents.[10,11] Updated data are needed regarding the video game preferences of young and very young children, given the increasing involvement of this group in video game play. However, it seems clear that video games with violent content continue to be a popular leisure choice for children and youth. Such games represent a large portion of total exposure to media violence for children and youth.

MEDIA VIOLENCE EFFECTS: A RELATIVE-RISK MODEL

Video games are only one of several sources of potential exposure to media violence. Concern about the prevalence and influence of exposure to media violence has been raised by several organizations concerned with the welfare of children and youth. For example, the American Academy of Pediatrics' policy statement on media violence includes the following: "Although exposure to media violence is not the sole factor contributing to aggression, antisocial attitudes, and violence among children and adolescents, it is an important health risk factor."[12(p1498)]

Media violence effects have been given considerable research attention. The evidence is conclusive, despite minority views: for many, exposure to media violence can increase aggressive thought, behavior, and emotion.[13–15] Anderson and colleagues'[16] General Aggression Model provides a relevant theoretic framework for understanding these effects. The General Aggression Model integrates several theoretic perspectives including social learning, social cognition, affective aggression, and excitation transfer. Predictions based on the General Aggression Model suggest that repeated exposure to media violence can lead to the development of aggressive beliefs and attitudes, aggressive behavioral scripts, and desensitization to violence. Relevant stimuli are considered to be either short- or long-term influences.

Long-term influences may be most important for the process of desensitization to violence.[17] In early childhood, media violence is first encountered through cartoon characters who present violent actions as entertaining and fun. This leads to positive emotional reactions that are incompatible with any negative reaction to violence and may reflect what has been termed "sensitization."[18] Older children and adults are exposed to more realistic violence with more obvious negative characteristics, but the increases are gradual and guided by the industry's views of the preferences of the target audience. However, violence often continues to be presented as fun and justified. This developmental progression of exposure to media violence represents an effective form of long-term systematic desensitization.[19]

Obviously not all consumers of media violence act out aggressively. Protective factors, such as a family that models and teaches nonviolent problem-solving, may balance risk factors, such as exposure to violent media. The relative risk model suggests that the more risk factors, the more likely it is that there will be a negative outcome as a result of exposure to media violence.[20] Recent work by Gentile and Bushman supports this conceptualization.[21] These researchers surveyed 430 third and fourth graders (51% male), and the students' teachers and peers, twice in a school year. Six factors (considered either risk or protective, depending on the specific experience) for aggression were measured: media violence exposure (television, movies, video games), physical victimization, participant sex, hostile attribution bias, parental monitoring, and prior aggression. Every risk factor (eg, high media violence exposure) was associated with an increased risk of physical aggression at the second survey time, whereas protective factors (eg, low media violence exposure) were associated with decreased risk. In addition, the combination of risk factors was a better predictor of aggression than individual factors considered separately or added together. Multiple risk factors were not simply additive but also multiplicative.

Because of their interactive nature, and the carefully graded reinforcement cycle when aggressive actions are chosen, the impact of exposure to violent video games may be proportionately greater than the impact of exposure to passive experiences of media violence.[16,22] In violent video games, violence is presented as being necessary, justified, and fun. In addition, the antisocial behavior demonstrated and required to win rarely generates realistic consequences, and the true impact of violent actions is disguised.[22,23] Popular first-person shooter games actually require players to actively identify with the aggressor.[24] In violent video games, the unremitting exposure to violence and the concomitant reward (game success) for continuously choosing violent actions may desensitize the player to the actual consequences of real-life violence. Desensitization to violence is a matter of concern because such desensitization prevents initiation of the process of moral reasoning that would inhibit inappropriate aggression or initiate a helping response.[25] Desensitization to violence may result in increased aggression, including bullying, or in a failure to recognize the true plight of victims and subsequent failure to help those in need.[3]

MEASURING DESENSITIZATION

Measurement issues impeded early research on violent video game–related desensitization in part because, by definition, desensitization is the absence of an expected response.[26] Long- and short-term studies of video game–related desensitization are now available using multiple research modalities. In addition to survey and behavioral studies, current research takes advantage of the fact that cognitive and emotional desensitization may result, at least in part, from diminished physiologic arousal. The following is guided by this principle: in research on real-world phenomena, such as media effects, a convergence of evidence from a variety of research approaches is the gold standard for drawing conclusions about whether or not the evidence supports an effects model.[16] One logical way to organize this evidence is to separately consider research using questionnaire, behavioral, and physiologic measures, recognizing that some studies may use a combination of indices.

QUESTIONNAIRE DATA

Questionnaires are typically used to collect large amounts of information from cross-sectional samples, often based on self-report. In the case of violent video games, comparisons are made between self-reported exposure to such games and responses to questions related to indices of cognitive and emotional desensitization. Desensitization to violence involves changes in emotional and cognitive responsivity.[3] Changes in emotional responsivity are seen in the blunting or absence of emotional reactions to violent events that would commonly elicit a strong response. Cognitive changes are demonstrated when the customary view that violence is uncommon and unlikely is transformed to the belief that violence is mundane and inevitable.

One way to evaluate desensitization to violence is to examine indicators of moral evaluation. Moral evaluation is an automatic psychological process that is triggered when the individual encounters a situation where ethical issues are relevant and behavioral choices must be made. The process of moral evaluation is disrupted by desensitization to violence when the desensitized individual does not either perceive or respond to the cues that typically would initiate evaluative processes. The moral evaluation process is determined in part by the individual's affective repertoire, especially empathy, and by their attitudes toward violence.[26,27] Empathy and attitudes toward violence are components of the process of moral evaluation that may reflect emotional and cognitive desensitization, with empathy decreasing and proviolence attitudes being strengthened. Therefore, lower empathy and stronger attitudes toward violence may reflect desensitization to violence.

Contemporary definitions of empathy include cognitive (perspective-taking) and affective (experiencing the emotional state of another) elements.[27] Although the substrate of empathy is innate, the development of mature empathy requires certain experiences. These include, for example, opportunities to view empathic models, to interact with others in certain kinds of stressful situations, and to experience feedback about behavioral choices.[4] Success at violent video games requires the choice of violent actions that are often presented as normal, acceptable, and fun, with realistic consequences typically nonexistent. Victims are frequently dehumanized, a strategy that is also used in real-life situations, particularly by the military, to minimize the activation of moral reasoning. These experiences, repeated incessantly, could affect empathic capacity in susceptible individuals.

One early study examined empathy in relation to video game preference. Sixty-six children ages 5 through 12 (27 female) responded to vignettes about everyday occurrences after playing either a violent or nonviolent video game. They also reported video game preferences and length of play. Long-term exposure to violent video games contributed to lower empathy vignette scores, which could be consistent with desensitization.[26]

Attitudes are a type of knowledge structure that results from complex and selective evaluation processes. These processes are based on an individual's experience, cognitions, and affective reactions to a situation or object. Although useful in organizing information, established attitudes may interfere with accurate perception in new situations. Attitudes can exert a direct, cognitively unmediated impact on judgment and behavior. The development of positive or neutral attitudes toward violence is influenced by many factors including exposure to violence in real life either directly or indirectly, and in entertainment media. Proviolence attitudes may play an important role in the translation of negative cognitions and affect into behavior.[4]

Several survey-based studies have examined empathy and attitudes toward violence in relation to exposure to violent video games. For example, fourth and fifth graders (N = 150; 68 girls) completed measures of a variety of forms of real-life and media violence exposure, empathy, and attitudes toward violence. Only exposure to video game violence was associated with (lower) empathy. Both video game and movie violence exposure were associated with stronger proviolence attitudes.[25] In a survey of 312 Chinese adolescents (35% female) Wei[28] found that a higher level of exposure to violent video games online was associated with lower empathy and stronger proviolence attitudes, with stronger effects for males than for females. The author concluded that these results are consistent with desensitization theory. Moller and Krahe[29] surveyed 143 German adolescents (71 females) twice over a 30-month period, assessing exposure to violent video games, attitudes toward violence, and aggressive behavior. Exposure to violent video games at Time 1 influenced physical aggression at Time 2 through a strengthening of proviolence attitudes. A large sample of seventh and eighth graders (N = 1237; 51.5% female) in Germany was surveyed by Krahe and Moller[30] twice over a 12-month period. Self-reports of habitual violent media usage at Time 1 were related to self-reports of lower empathy and higher physical aggression at Time 2. Additional analyses suggested that higher aggressive and lower prosocial behavior resulted from the acceptance of aggression as normative following exposure to media violence, which could imply desensitization to violence.

Indirect evidence for the impact of playing violent video games is provided by research on prosocial media. Prot and colleagues[31] examined relationships among prosocial media and helping behavior through two studies conducted with a large cross-cultural sample. Results from one survey with participants from seven countries (ranging from about 200 to 400; 60% female) indicate that helping was positively related to exposure to positive video games, and this effect was mediated by empathy. In the second study, longitudinal relations among prosocial and violent video game use, empathy, and helping (N = about 3000 children and adolescents; 27% female) were examined. Students from Singapore were surveyed three times across a 2-year period. Violent video game use was negatively associated with empathy and prosocial behavior. Use of prosocial video games was positively associated with prosocial behavior in real life, and empathy was a key mediator of prosocial media effects.

The possible consequences of desensitization to the needs of others is also demonstrated in research reported by Anderson.[32] He analyzed telephone survey data from the Pew Internet & American Life Project[33] to examine how exposure to violent, as opposed to nonviolent games, would be associated with differences in attitudes toward civic engagement and actual behavior. He also assessed how those effects may be influenced by parental involvement. Information from 821 youth (ages 12–17; 43% female) was available for teenage gaming habits, civic engagement attitudes and behaviors, and family characteristics. Parents reported on their monitoring of and involvement in their teenager's gaming (teenagers answered the same questions about parent involvement). Parents also reported on their own civic engagement. Path analysis indicated that more violent gaming was negatively associated with attitudes toward civic engagement and with civic engagement behavior. However, more prosocial and nonviolent gaming was positively associated with civic attitudes and behavior. High levels of parent involvement reduced the negative effects of violent gaming on youth civic attitudes and engagement, confirming a moderation effect. Other researchers have found similar relationships between prosocial game-playing and prosocial behavior in children and adolescents.[34] That playing prosocial games influences prosocial behavior provides support for the possibility of an opposite effect for antisocial games.

BEHAVIORAL INDICATORS

Behavioral studies are used to more directly examine the impact of current experience. In an early study examining the relationship between video game violence exposure and desensitization, 92 college students (46 females) played either a more violent or a less violent video game and then assigned prison sentences to hypothetical violent criminals. The experimental procedure was repeated 1 hour later. Men who had played the more violent game endorsed lower sanctions for criminals immediately and again at the second experimental session. Females, however, showed sensitization to criminal behavior (assigned more severe sentences) after the second playing session. The researchers concluded that females and males may be affected differently by exposure to violent video games.[35] This finding is particularly important because, if researchers do not separately examine the responses of males and females, a true desensitization effect for one gender could be masked. This research did not, however, measure prior exposure to game-playing, which could have provided additional insight into the apparent male desensitization effect.

Using even more realistic paradigms, two studies were conducted by Bushman and Anderson to examine how exposure to violent media affected helping responses in college students and adults. One studied violent and nonviolent video games, the other studied violent and nonviolent movies.

Violent and Nonviolent Video Game

In the first study, participants played either a violent or nonviolent video game. After play they were exposed to a simulated altercation: participants heard what seemed to be a loud fight just outside the door. Those who played the violent video game took longer to help the apparently injured victim than nonviolent game players. Violent game players also rated the fight as being less serious and were less likely to even acknowledge the altercation. There were also differences related to gender and past gaming experience: men rated the fight as less serious than women and those who reported a preference for violent video games were less likely to help than those whose favorite game was nonviolent (suggesting possible long-term desensitization).

Violent and Nonviolent Movie

In the second study, adults who attended either a nonviolent or a violent movie observed a young woman struggling with crutches either before or after viewing the movie. Those who had just watched the violent movie took longer to help the young woman than those who were not exposed to the violent movie. The researchers concluded that these results suggest that short-term exposure to violent media can be desensitizing.[36]

Association Between Violent Video Games and Real-World Behaviors

Researchers have also examined associations between exposure to violent video games and documented negative real-world behaviors. For example, DeLisi and colleagues[37] examined associations between violent video game play and measures of delinquent behavior in a sample of institutionalized juveniles (N = 227; 45% female) ages 14 to 18. Using interview and survey methods, the researchers found that frequency of violent video game play and a measure of liking for violent games were significantly associated with general and violent delinquency after controlling for the effects of screen time, years playing video games, age, gender, race, delinquency history, and psychopathic personality traits. Although desensitization to violence was not measured directly, the juveniles all had histories of extreme criminality, often including violent behavior, which could reflect desensitization.

Canadian researchers surveyed about 800 parents and their children (ages 10–17; about half female). The online survey assessed bullying behavior (reported by both children and parents) and the child's three favorite games, which were coded by the researchers for level of violence. For male and female children, general bullying and cyberbullying were related to preferences for playing violent video games, based the parents' and children's responses. This may reflect desensitization to the suffering of others.[38]

The Role of Empathy

In research combining questionnaire and behavioral methods, Bartholow and colleagues[39] examined, among other variables, the possible mediating role of empathy in the relationship between exposure to violent video games and aggressive behavior. Male college students (N = 92) completed questionnaires and played a violent or nonviolent video game. Participants who played the violent video game delivered louder and longer noise blasts to presumed opponents than participants who played the nonviolent game, suggesting a short-term effect caused by violent video game play. Regarding desensitization, those high in prior exposure to violent video games had higher levels of aggression than those low in such exposure. Empathy was one mediator of this effect, and the researchers concluded that repeated exposure to video game violence increases aggressive behavior in part through changes in cognitive and personality factors that are associated with desensitization.

PSYCHOPHYSIOLOGIC MEASURES

Neurodevelopment is a continuous, dynamic process that is sequential and use-dependent. When an individual repeatedly engages in repetitive, structured, patterned activities, permanent changes in brain reactivity may occur.[40] There is emerging evidence that exposure to violent media may be linked to decreases in the activity of brain structures needed for the regulation of aggressive behavior, and to increases in the activity of structures needed to carry out aggressive plans.[19] In the case of exposure to violent video games, if the process of moral reasoning is chronically subverted, then disuse-related extinction of the emotional reactivity substrate of moral reasoning could result. In that case, the distress response to violence would not be triggered, indicating desensitization.

A variety of psychophysiologic measures have been used to examine short- and long-term effects of exposure to violent video games on brain function.

Heart and Respiratory Rate

Early research typically used peripheral psychophysiologic indicators, such as heart and respiratory rate, and galvanic skin response to examine short-term violent video game exposure effects. For example, in a study with 257 undergraduates (133 female), Carnagey and colleagues[41] found that playing a violent video game resulted in lower arousal (heart rate and galvanic skin response) to actual videos of people being physically assaulted, compared with those who played a nonviolent game. No significant gender differences or differences for those with a preference for violent video games were identified in this sample. The authors concluded that short-term exposure to violent video games desensitized the players to filmed scenes of real-life violence. Researchers in Germany compared the physiologic responses (heart rate and respiration) of 42 adult males who played either high-or low-violence video games.[42] They also examined postgame physiologic (skin conductance) and self-report responses to pictures selected from the International Affective Picture System.[43] Participants who played games with high video game violence had weaker responses (desensitization) to aversive picture stimuli (eg, mutilated corpses) and reacted significantly more strongly (sensitization) to aggressive cues (pictures of weapons). These researchers also considered past game experience, noting that highly experienced participants reacted less strongly than participants with lower experience, which may reflect a long-term desensitization process. Similar results, again with college students (N = 38; 14 females), were reported more recently by Lang and colleagues.[44] They found that physiologic arousal (heart rate and skin conductance) in response to violent activity decreased over time during game play. Various measure-specific differences related to prior game experience and gender were also found, reinforcing the importance of considering these characteristics. These researchers also considered the phenomenon of game engagement (in the Lang and colleagues study termed "presence"). Described by Brockmyer and colleagues,[45] game engagement is considered to be an individual difference in propensity to become involved in media experience. The theoretic assumption is that deeper involvement could increase the impact of media violence exposure.[25,45] Lang and colleagues[44] found a link between game engagement and physiologic arousal. They reported that, as players felt more engaged, their physiologic arousal data suggested that the scenarios encountered by their character were engaging the players' sympathetic nervous system, suggesting that the violence felt "real." The researchers suggested that, over time, engagement in media violence with unrealistic consequences could lead to desensitization to the real-life consequences of violence.

Functional Magnetic Resonance Imaging: Function of Specific Neural Structures

Advances in neuroimaging techniques have begun to demonstrate how exposure to violent video games and other violent media may affect the functioning of specific neural structures. Using functional magnetic resonance imaging (fMRI), Weber and coworkers[46] measured 13 adult males' (age range, 18–26) brain activity during violent video game play. Reduced neural activity in areas of the brain responsible for emotion (affective areas of the anterior cingulate cortex, and the amygdala) occurred when participants performed aggressive acts in the game. Involvement in virtual violence also led to decreased activity in the rostral anterior cingulate cortex and increased activity in the dorsal anterior cingulate cortex, suggesting suppression of affective information processing. Although this was a study only of short-term effects, repeated activation of this suppression of affective information processing could ultimately lead to desensitization to violence. It is worth noting that chronic consumption of violent media in general has also been linked to suppression of the anterior cingulate cortex.[47]

Functional Magnetic Resonance Imaging: Cortical Networks

Kelly and colleagues[48] also used fMRI to examine how short-term exposure to media violence affects neural functioning, specifically cortical networks that regulate behavior. Their results indicated that laboratory exposure to media violence (film clips) led to diminished response in the right lateral orbitofrontal cortex and a decrease in right lateral orbitofrontal cortex–amygdala interaction. Reduced function in this network has been previously associated with decreased control over a variety of be-haviors, including reactive aggression. The lateral orbitofrontal cortex is generally active during situations in which external cues demand that behaviors be changed or suppressed. The precise mechanism of the Kelly study's effect of exposure to film violence is unclear, but desensitization seems a reasonable possibility.

Functional Magnetic Resonance Imaging: Altered Emotional Processing

Montag and colleagues[49] investigated the possible association between long-term frequent violent video gaming and altered emotional processing. They identified adult males who played first-person shooters regularly, and a control group who had never played such games. During fMRI scanning, the 40 participants were presented with a series of pictures that included pleasant, unpleasant, neutral, and first-person shooter game images. A significantly higher activation of the left lateral frontal cortex was seen in the control group, compared with the gamers, when viewing violent images. The re-searchers suggested that this may indicate that gamers had developed some habitu-ation to such stimuli (indicating desensitization) because of their frequent exposure to violent images through regular violent game-playing. They also suggested that this lower activity in the lateral prefrontal cortex could be interpreted as a dulling of the experience of empathy. Using a similar design, one fMRI study with 22 adult males (age range, 21–33) did not identify a difference in neural response related to violent video game exposure.[50] In this study, however, it is possible that there was not suffi-cient statistical power for the analyses conducted to identify the small to medium effects that are characteristic of media research.

Functional Magnetic Resonance Imaging: Event-Related Brain Potential

Several psychophysiologic studies have examined the long- and short-term effects of exposure to violent video games. For example, a 2006 event-related brain potential study was conducted by Bartholow and colleagues[51] with 39 adult male participants. The researchers found that viewing violent images produced reduced P300 ampli-tudes among players with an extensive history of playing violent video games, compared with players who preferred nonviolent games. The reduced brain response also predicted increased aggressive behavior later in a competitive reaction time task where participants delivered noise blasts to a supposed competitor. The researchers concluded that the reduced cortical response to violent images in players with high exposure to violent video games demonstrates desensitization to violence, that desensitization limits emotional arousal to violent stimuli, and that this could remove normal inhibitions for aggressive behavior. Englehardt and colleagues[52] randomly assigned 70 low and high violent video game exposure young adult participants (46% female) to play a violent or nonviolent video game. Similar to Bartholow and col-leagues' findings, high-exposure participants had a smaller P300 response to violent images than those with low exposure, suggesting long-term desensitization. Those with low exposure who played a violent video game in the laboratory had a smaller P300 response than low-exposure participants who played a violent video game, sug-gesting short-term desensitization. This brain response mediated the effect of video game content on subsequent aggressive behavior in a competitive reaction time task.

Functional Magnetic Resonance Imaging: Short- and Long-Term Effects of Violent Video Game Exposure

Most recently, Gentile and colleagues[53] used fMRI to study short- and long-term ef-fects of exposure to violent video games. Their participants were 22 young adult males with a preference for violent games and a similar group with a stated preference for nonviolent games. Each participant played two versions of a popular video game, one violent and one nonviolent. Play of each version occurred for short blocks, followed by rest, followed by play of the alternate version. fMRI scanning was conducted throughout the session. Contrary to expectations, no signal differences were observed in the amygdala or other emotion-related brain regions for violent compared with nonviolent game play across all participants. Significant differences were found based on long-term exposure: when playing the violent game, players with a preference for nonviolent games demonstrated an increase in activity in emotional response regions, whereas those with a preference for violent games showed active suppression of the same regions during violent game play. The researchers concluded that this may be an indication of a long-term desensitization effect, as a cumulative result of prior violent video game exposure.

Summary

The preponderance of evidence from questionnaire, behavioral, and psychophysiologic approaches demonstrates a relationship between exposure to violent video games and desensitization to violence; in some research paradigms, a causal relationship has been demonstrated. This is not a simple one-to-one relationship: other risk and protective factors likely moderate or mediate the relationship. It is evident, however, that exposure to violent video games increases the relative risk of desensitization to violence, which in turn may increase aggression and decrease prosocial behavior.

CLINICAL IMPLICATIONS

Both increased aggression and a decrease in empathy and prosocial behavior may result when a child or adolescent is desensitized to violence as a result of exposure to media, and specifically video game, violence. It is important for the clinician to evaluate the media experience, including video game playing habits, of any child or adolescent with aggressive or other antisocial behavior issues. Particularly in a high-risk individual, exposure to violent media can increase the relative risk of such behavior. Parents should be encouraged to limit exposure to violent video games as much as possible, although it must be acknowledged that this is increasingly difficult as children grow older and more independent. Monitoring children's media exposure has been shown to have a protective effect on a variety of child outcomes including decreased aggression and increased prosocial behavior.[54] Emerging research suggests that exposure to prosocial video games and other media may be accompanied by increased prosocial behavior. Providing prosocial media choices as part of the media diet is a parent's prerogative, although some may need to be reminded and empowered. Parents should also be counseled to discuss the differences between real and screen violence, to model and encourage nonviolent ways to solve problems, and to provide empathy-building experiences (eg, early exposure to volunteering).

REFERENCES

1. Guerra NG, Huesmann LR, Spindler A. Community violence exposure, social cognition, and aggression among urban elementary school children. Child Dev 2003;75:1561–76.
2. Orue I, Bushman BJ, Calvete E, et al. Monkey see, monkey do, monkey hurt: longitudinal effects of exposure to violence on children's aggressive behavior. Soc Psychol Personal Sci 2011;2:432–7.

3. Brockmyer JB. Media violence, desensitization, and psychological engagement. In: Dill K, editor. Handbook of media psychology. New York: Oxford; 2013. p. 212–22.
4. Funk JB. Children's exposure to violent video games and desensitization to violence. Child Adolesc Psychiatr Clin N Am 2005;14:387–404.
5. Entertainment Software Association. 2013 sales, demographic, and usage data: essential facts about the video game industry. Available at: http://www.theesa.com/facts/. Accessed May 2, 2014.
6. Rideout VJ, Foehr UG, Roberts DF. Generation M2: media in the lives of 8- to 18-year-olds. Menlo Park (CA): Kaiser Family Foundation; 2010.
7. Rideout VJ, Hamel E. Zero to six: electronic media in the lives of infants, toddlers, and preschoolers. Menlo Park (CA): Kaiser Family Foundation; 2003.
8. Kaiser Family Foundation. Children and video games. Menlo Park (CA): Kaiser Family Foundation; 2002.
9. Brockmyer JB. Video games. In: Strasburger V, Wilson B, Jordan A, editors. Children, adolescents, and the media. 3rd edition. Thousand Oaks (CA): Sage; 2014. p. 457–86.
10. Bijvank MN, Konijn EA, Bushman BJ. We don't need no education: video game preferences, video game motivations, and aggressiveness among adolescent boys of different educational ability levels. J Adolesc 2012;35:153–62.
11. Chory RM, Goodboy AK. Is basic personality related to violent and non-violent video game play and preferences? Cyberpsychol Behav Soc Netw 2011;14: 191–8.
12. American Academy of Pediatrics. Policy statement–media violence. Pediatrics 2009;124:1495–503.
13. Anderson CA, Shibuya A, Ihori N, et al. Violent video game effects on aggression, empathy, and prosocial behavior in Eastern and Western countries: a meta-analytic review. Psychol Bull 2010;136:151–73.
14. Gentile DA, Li D, Khoo A, et al. Mediators and moderators of long-term effects of violent video games on aggressive behavior. JAMA Pediatr 2014;168(5):450–7.
15. Strasburger VC, Wilson BJ, Jordan AB, editors. Children, adolescents and the media. 3rd edition. Thousand Oaks (CA): Sage; 2014.
16. Anderson CA, Gentile DA, Buckley KE. Violent video game effects on children and adolescents: theory, research, and public policy. New York: Oxford; 2007.
17. Huesmann LR, Kirwil L. Why observing violence increases the risk of violent behavior by the observer. In: Flannery DJ, Vazsonyi AT, Waldman I, editors. The Cambridge handbook of violent behavior and aggression. Cambridge (England): Cambridge University Press; 2007. p. 545–70.
18. Krahe B. Violent video games and aggression. In: Dill K, editor. Handbook of media psychology. New York: Oxford; 2013. p. 352–73.
19. Carnagey NL, Anderson CA, Bartholow BD. Media violence and social neuroscience. Curr Dir Psychol Sci 2007;16:178–82.
20. Funk JB. Violent video games: who's at risk? In: Ravitch D, Viteritti J, editors. Kid stuff: marketing violence and vulgarity in the popular culture. Baltimore (MD): Johns Hopkins University Press; 2003. p. 168–92.
21. Gentile DG, Bushman BJ. Reassessing media violence effects using a risk and resilience approach to understanding aggression. Psychol Pop Media Cult 2012;1:138–51.
22. Funk JB, Buchman DD. Playing violent video and computer games and adolescent self-concept. J Commun 1996;46:19–32.
23. Funk JB. Video games: benign or malignant? J Dev Behav Pediatr 1992;13:53–4.

24. Gentile DA, Anderson CA. Violent video games: the newest media hazard. In: Gentile DA, editor. Media violence and children: a complete guide for parents and professionals. Westport (CT): Praeger Publishers; 2003. p. 131–52.
25. Funk JB, Bechtoldt H, Pasold T, et al. Violence exposure in real-life, video games, television, movies, and the Internet: Is there desensitization? J Adolesc 2004;27:23–39.
26. Funk JB, Buchman DD, Jenks J, et al. Playing violent video games, desensitization, and moral evaluation in children. J Appl Dev Psychol 2003;24:413–36.
27. Funk JB, Fox C, Chan M, et al. The development of the children's empathic attitudes questionnaire using classical and Rasch analyses. J Appl Dev Psychol 2008;29:187–96.
28. Wei R. Effects of playing violent videogames on Chinese adolescents' pro-violence attitudes, attitudes toward others, and aggressive behavior. CyberPsychol Behav 2007;10:371–80.
29. Moller I, Krahe B. Exposure to violent video games and aggression in German adolescents: a longitudinal analysis. Aggress Behav 2009;35:75–89.
30. Krahe B, Moller I. Longitudinal effects of media violence on aggression and empathy among German adolescents. J Appl Dev Psychol 2010;31:401–9.
31. Prot S, Gentile DA, Anderson CA, et al. Long-term relationships between prosocial media use, empathy, and prosocial behavior. Psychol Sci 2014;25(2):358–68.
32. Anderson CA. Violent, nonviolent, and prosocial gaming effects on teens' civic engagement. Oxford handbooks online. New York: Oxford; 2014.
33. Lenhart A, Kahne J, Middaugh E, et al. Teens' video games and civics. Washington, DC: Pew Internet & American Life Project; 2008. Available at: http://www.pewinternet.org/Reports/2008/Teens-Video-Games-and-Civics.aspx. Accessed May 5, 2014.
34. Gentile DA, Anderson CA, Yukaw S, et al. The effects of prosocial video games on prosocial behaviors: international evidence from correlational, longitudinal, and experimental studies. Pers Soc Psychol Bull 2009;35:752–63.
35. Deselms JL, Altman JD. Immediate and prolonged effects of videogame violence. J Appl Soc Psychol 2003;33:1553–63.
36. Bushman BJ, Anderson CA. Comfortably numb: desensitizing effects of violent media on helping others. Psychol Sci 2009;20:273–7.
37. DeLisi M, Vaughn MG, Gentile DA, et al. Violent video games, delinquency, and youth violence: new evidence. Youth Violence Juv Justice 2012;11:132–42.
38. Dittrick CJ, Beran TN, Mishna F, et al. Do children who bully their peers also play violent video games? A Canadian national study. J Sch Violence 2013;12:297–318.
39. Bartholow BD, Sestir MA, Davis EB. Correlates and consequences, of exposure to video game violence: hostile personality, empathy, and aggressive behavior. Pers Soc Psychol Bull 2005;31:1573–86.
40. Perry B. Using a neurodevelopmental lens when working with children who have experienced maltreatment. Parramatta NSW (Australia): Uniting Care Children, Young People and Families; 2011. brochure.
41. Carnagey NL, Anderson CA, Bushman BJ. The effect of video game violence on physiological desensitization to real-life violence. J Exp Soc Psychol 2007;43:489–96.
42. Staude-Müller F, Bliesener T, Luthman S. Hostile and hardened? an experimental study on (de-)sensitization to violence and suffering through playing video games. Swiss J Psychol 2008;67:41–50.

43. Lang PJ, Bradley MM, Cuthbert BN. International affective picture system (IAPS): Instruction manual and affective ratings. Gainesville (FL): The Center for Research in Psychophysiology, University of Florida; 1999.
44. Lang A, Bradley SD, Schneider EF, et al. Killing is positive! Intra-game responses meet the necessary (but not sufficient) theoretical conditions for influencing aggressive behavior. J Media Psychol 2012;24:154–65.
45. Brockmyer JB, Fox C, Mc Broom E, et al. The development of the game experience questionnaire: a measure of levels of engagement in video game-playing. J Exp Soc Psychol 2009;49:624–34.
46. Weber R, Ritterfeld U, Mathiak K. Does playing violent video games induce aggression? Empirical evidence of a functional magnetic resonance imaging study. Media Psychol 2006;8:39–60.
47. Matthews VP, Kronenberger WG, et al. Media violence exposure and frontal lobe activation measure by functional magnetic resonance imaging in aggressive and nonaggressive adolescents. J Comput Assist Tomogr 2005;29:287–92.
48. Kelly CR, Grinband J, Hirsch J. Repeated exposure to media violence is associated with diminished response in an inhibitory frontolimbic network. PLoS One 2007;2:e1268.
49. Montag C, Weber B, Trautner P, et al. Does excessive play of violent first-person-shooter-video-games dampen brain activity in response to emotional stimuli? Biol Psychol 2012;89:107–11.
50. Regenbogen C, Herrmann M, Fehr T. The neural processing of voluntary completed, real and virtual violent and nonviolent computer game scenarios displaying predefined actions in gamers and nongamers. Soc Neurosci 2010;5: 221–40.
51. Bartholow BD, Bushman BJ, Sestir MA. Chronic violent video game exposure and desensitization to violence. J Exp Soc Psychol 2006;42:532–9.
52. Englehardt CR, Bartholow BD, Kerr GT, et al. This is your brain on violent video games: neural desensitization to violence predicts increased aggression following violent video game exposure. J Exp Soc Psychol 2011;47:1033–6.
53. Gentile DA, Swing, EL, Anderson CA, et al. Differential neural recruitment during violent video game play in violent and nonviolent game players. Psychol Pop Media Cult, in press.
54. Gentile DA, Reimer RA, Nathanson AI, et al. Protective effects of parental monitoring of children's media use: a prospective study. JAMA Pediatr 2014;168: 479–84.

Psychosocial Interventions in Attention-Deficit/Hyperactivity Disorder: Update

Kevin M. Antshel, PhD

KEYWORDS

- ADHD • Psychosocial • Behavioral • Treatment • Child • Adolescent

KEY POINTS

- Medications are useful for managing the symptoms of attention-deficit/hyperactivity disorder (ADHD), but are less effective for improving functioning.
- Psychosocial interventions for child/adolescent ADHD target functional impairments as the intervention goal, and rely heavily on behavioral therapy techniques and operant conditioning principles.
- Behavioral parent training, elementary school–based interventions that rely on behavioral modification, intensive multimodal middle- and high-school interventions that rely on teaching skills and operant conditioning principles, in addition to an intensive summer treatment program are the most evidence-based psychosocial interventions for managing pediatric ADHD.
- While showing some promise, more research is needed on nontraditional social skills training for children and cognitive-behavioral treatment interventions for adolescents before recommendations can be made.
- Psychosocial interventions should be used in conjunction with medication management.

INTRODUCTION

Attention-deficit/hyperactivity disorder (ADHD) is the most common reason for referral to child and adolescent psychiatry clinics, and affects approximately 5% to 10% of youth worldwide.[1,2] The defining features of ADHD include developmentally inappropriate and impairing levels of inattention and/or hyperactivity-impulsivity that begin before age 12 years and cannot be better explained by other factors (eg, anxiety, defiance).[3] The academic,[4] social,[5] and family[6,7] domains are generally the most impaired in children with ADHD. Once considered to be a condition that children outgrew in adolescence,[8] there is now compelling evidence that ADHD often continues into adolescence and adulthood.[9,10] Though sometimes portrayed as a benign condition

The author does not have any financial disclosures or conflicts of interest to report.
Department of Psychology, Syracuse University, 802 University Avenue, Syracuse, NY 13244, USA
E-mail address: kmantshe@syr.edu

Abbreviations	
ADHD	Attention-deficit/hyperactivity disorder
BPT	Behavioral parent training
CBT	Cognitive-behavioral treatment
CHP	Challenging Horizons Program
DRC	Daily report card
HOPS	Homework, Organization, and Planning Skills program
IEP	Individualized education plan
MTA	Multimodal Treatment of ADHD study
SST	Social skills training
STP	Summer treatment program

in the popular media,[11] ADHD is an impairing psychiatric disorder that imparts considerable lifetime economic costs (medical, education, legal, and so forth) that rival the costs for major depressive disorder and stroke.[12]

FRONT-LINE INTERVENTIONS FOR ATTENTION-DEFICIT/HYPERACTIVITY DISORDER

Given the chronic nature of ADHD, both pharmacologic and psychosocial interventions are used to manage the disorder. A front-line intervention is stimulant medications, which are effective in approximately 80% of youth with ADHD.[13] Stimulant side effects can include decreased appetite and increased sleep-onset latencies and, while positively affecting the core ADHD symptoms (eg, inattention, impulsivity), stimulants generally do not normalize peer relationships,[14] lessen family dysfunction,[15] or improve academic achievement.[16] The use of conjoint psychosocial treatments with ADHD medications can result in the need for lower doses of each form of treatment.[17] Parents are also more accepting of and interested in treatments that include psychosocial components.[18] For all these reasons, psychosocial interventions have continued to play a prominent role in the management of youth with ADHD.

For the purposes of this article, psychosocial interventions are defined as any intervention that stresses psychological or social factors rather than biological variables. This is not to say that biological treatments (eg, medication, dietary modifications) do not have a place in ADHD management; most treatment guidelines recommend medication as a front-line intervention.[19] Several stimulant (eg, methylphenidate, amphetamine salts) and nonstimulant medications (eg, guanfacine, atomoxetine) are approved by the US Food and Drug Administration for ADHD management, with large effect sizes (Cohen $d = 0.9$) reported for stimulant medications.[20] Likewise, although with smaller effect sizes (Cohen $d = 0.3$), dietary interventions, including single nutrient supplements,[21] multinutrient supplements,[22,23] and supplementation with omega-3 fatty acids,[24–27] have received more empirical attention in the past 10 years and are now used more in ADHD management. Nonetheless, these biological interventions are not be considered in this review.

Biological treatments such as stimulant medications explicitly target ADHD symptoms, not functional impairments. However, it is functional impairments, not symptoms, which compel parents to seek treatment for ADHD.[28] As a group, the psychosocial interventions reviewed herein target functional impairments as the intervention goal.

In addition to this common factor, the psychosocial interventions for ADHD management considered in this article all share another common factor: the heavy reliance on behavioral therapy techniques and operant conditioning principles. Research demonstrating that children with ADHD are less responsive to inconsistent, delayed, or weak reinforcement, and are less responsive to punishment cues,[29,30] supports the usefulness of behavioral therapy techniques and operant conditioning principles in ADHD. Barkley's[31] theory of ADHD as a problem in response inhibition and self-regulation, with the secondary consequences this may create for their poor self-motivation to persist at assigned tasks, provides a theoretically based rationale for the use of behaviorally based interventions with ADHD. Barkley's theoretic stance is that these psychosocial interventions are not being done primarily to increase skills that children with ADHD may appear to lack, but are being used to enhance the deficient self-motivation and working memory of these children to help them demonstrate what they already know. From this perspective, ADHD is a disorder of performance, not of knowledge of skills. Thus, psychosocial interventions are used to cue the use of such skills at key points of performance in natural settings, and to motivate their display through the use of artificial consequences that ordinarily do not exist at those points of performance in natural settings.

Parent Training in Behavioral Management

Behavioral parent training (BPT) programs (also referred to as parent management training or parent training) are effective for children with disruptive behaviors whether or not the children have co-occurring inattention/hyperactive-impulsive symptoms.[32,33] Although nonspecific to ADHD, BPT programs also seem to be efficacious for children with ADHD[34–44] yet are somewhat less effective for adolescents with ADHD.[45] Three separate reviews in the past 15 years[46–48] have concluded that BPT is a well-established evidence-based treatment for managing ADHD in children.

There is a variety of BPT programs that have been studied with ADHD children, including Cunningham's COPE program (Community Parent Education Program[49]), Webster-Stratton's *The Incredible Years*,[50] and Barkley's *Defiant Children*.[51] Other programs used with oppositional or noncompliant children, some of whom undoubtedly also have ADHD, are Eyberg's *Parent-Child Interaction Therapy*[52] and Sanders' *Triple P* (positive parenting program),[53] which have demonstrated efficacy according to a meta-analysis of the literature.[54] All of these programs are founded on a social learning model of disruptive child behavior (disrupted parenting and social coercion), and all have demonstrated efficacy for disruptive children, including those with ADHD.[34]

BPT programs generally consist of weekly training sessions, either in groups of parents or with individuals, each focusing on a discrete operant conditioning technique. These methods can be grouped into 3 basic types of procedure:

1. Those that manipulate the environmental events that may precede or surround a child's tasks/activities so as to increase positive or negative behavior (ie, parental commands, task demands, teacher instructions, and so forth)
2. Those that may restructure the tasks to be done (reduce work quotas, insert more interesting task materials, and so forth)
3. Those that manipulate the nature of the consequences for child behavior in that setting (ie, attention, praise, token reinforcement, punishment, and so forth)

For example, Webster-Stratton's *Incredible Years*[50] curriculum for school-aged children consists of a minimum of twelve 2-hour weekly group sessions that focuses on such topics as:

a. Providing positive parental attention and special time
b. Engaging in social, emotion, and persistence coaching
c. Utilizing effective praise and encouragement
d. Using tangible reward programs to motivate your child

e. How to effectively implement rules, responsibility, and routines
f. Using predictable learning routines and delivering clear limit-setting messages
g. Ignoring misbehavior
h. Using time-outs to calm down

In most BPTs, the initial focus is on the implementation of reinforcement techniques (eg, positive attention, praise), for 3 primary reasons:

1. The use of reinforcement may result in less disruptive behaviors, thus lessening the need for punishment techniques
2. The coercive cycle is disrupted by the use of reinforcement
3. It is easier to implement reinforcement than punishment programs consistently and effectively.

Functional impairments as targets

BPTs such as *The Incredible Years* do not target ADHD symptoms but rather are directed at functional impairments.[46] For children and adolescents with ADHD, these functional targets often include improving adherence to parental requests (eg, do homework at the prescribed time), reducing dependence on parents to manage daily routines (eg, getting ready for school in the morning) and lessening defiance toward parental requests. In addition to targeting child functional impairments, BPTs also aim to address coercive or dysfunctional parenting practices.[55] For example, parents of children with ADHD often demonstrate more negative and less consistent parenting practices in addition to less positive parenting behaviors.[15,56] These coercive parent-child interaction cycles predict a variety of functional impairments outside of the home environment.[57,58]

BPTs are generally efficacious across different races and ethnicities.[59] More favorable BPT treatment outcomes, however, are associated with parents who attend BPT sessions regularly and report consistently using the interventions,[60,61] as well as those families in which the parents are optimistic about the child's ability to improve.[62] Intact families and those with lower levels of parental psychopathology and stress also generally improve more with BPT.[48] Finally, when present, maternal ADHD seems to significantly limit the outcomes of BPT.[63]

In addition to the general BPT programs already listed, BPTs have also been developed that are specific to ADHD areas of impairment. For example, a BPT called Parental Friendship Coaching has been developed to target social problems. In this intervention, parents are taught strategies to help promote and reinforce their children in the engagement of successful peer interactions.[64] Likewise, another BPT involves training parents and teachers to reinforce children contingently for meeting improvement goals for organizational, homework, and school performance.[65] This program also includes the use of a daily report card (DRC) that goes home with the children, a home-based point system for achieving goals, and the implementation of a homework routine. Thus, in addition to the use of general BPTs, several ADHD-specific BPTs have been developed.

Inadequacies of therapy

Despite the aforementioned benefits of BPTs, several inadequacies exist. First, despite improvements in ADHD symptoms and increased adherence to parental requests, BPTs do not normalize child functioning. Second, most studies of BPTs have only assessed outcomes in the months following the BPT, not across years.[66] Thus, the maintenance of these effects remains an open question. Finally, the positive outcomes are generally only observed in the environment where the BPT is focused.

Interventions used at home therefore typically do not generalize to other settings (eg, school).[67,68]

School-Based Interventions

In addition to BPTs, several evidence-based management approaches for ADHD occur in the school setting. This fact is not surprising, given that school functional impairments are often listed as one of the most impaired domains for children with ADHD.[69,70] For the sake of simplicity, the interventions are organized by target population.

Elementary school

Many of the school-based behavioral interventions seek to improve positive behaviors by understanding the context (antecedents and consequences) of the negative behaviors. Negative or off-task behaviors are hypothesized to serve 1 of 4 primary functions[71]:

1. Escape or avoidance of a nonpreferred activity or setting
2. Gain access to materials or preferred settings
3. Gain attention
4. Sensory stimulation

Behavioral interventions can be either proactive or reactive. Proactive interventions (eg, reviewing cafeteria rules, use of cues and prompts) are directed at disruptive behavior antecedents, thereby making the child with ADHD less likely to engage in these behaviors. On the other hand, reactive interventions target behavior consequences, reinforcing positive behavior (eg, token economy) and ignoring or punishing negative behaviors (eg, time-out for aggression).

Concurrently implementing one of more of the reactive and proactive strategies can lead to more positive outcomes.[17,72] Contingent application of reinforcers for reduced level of activity or increased sustained attention can rapidly alter the levels of these ADHD symptoms.[73] These programs generally incorporate token rewards, as praise may not be sufficient to increase or maintain normal levels of on-task behavior in children with ADHD.[74,75] The role of punishment in the management of classroom behavior in ADHD children has been less well studied. What data exist suggest that response cost is the most effective punishment technique.[74,76] A recent meta-analysis concluded that behavioral interventions in the school setting are effective, with overall mean effect sizes in the large range for dependent measures of behavior.[77]

DRCs are designed to improve communication between the school and home, and allow the use of both proactive and reactive strategies.[78–80] Typically consisting of a list of well-defined behavioral targets, a DRC provides a vehicle to assess the target behavior throughout the day. The DRC is then taken home to the parents, who can administer a predetermined incentive. A recent meta-analysis suggests that the DRC is an evidence-based intervention for ADHD, with overall mean effect sizes in the medium range for dependent measures of behavior.[81]

Similarly to BPT, few studies have assessed for maintenance of these improvements after treatment withdrawal. In addition, none of these studies examined whether generalization of behavioral control occurred in other school settings where no treatment procedures were in effect.

Middle school and high school

Educational impairment persists into middle and high school in students with ADHD.[82] The most common service provided to adolescents with ADHD is academic accommodations (eg, testing accommodations, preferential seating, copies of class notes) as a function of an individualized education plan (IEP) or Section 504 plan. These accommodations, however, are not predicated on the notion that the adolescent will develop or improve skills but rather that the expectations are being lowered to permit the student a better chance at advancement. A recent review reported that these services are only minimally beneficial to the students.[83]

Although accommodations are the most common service provided to adolescents with ADHD, accommodations are not the most effective intervention for middle and high school students with ADHD. Relative to the literature on interventions for elementary school–aged children with ADHD, the extant literature on interventions for adolescents with ADHD is less vast and has only really begun to develop in the last 15 years.[84]

One of the better researched interventions for middle and high school students with ADHD is the Challenging Horizons Program (CHP), a comprehensive school-based treatment program that includes interventions targeting social, academic, and family impairment. Two CHP versions have been evaluated, an after-school model and a mentoring model.

After-school model The after-school model of CHP is an intensive program provided over an entire academic year for 150 minutes per session up to 3 days per week. In a typical CHP intervention, undergraduate students from a local university serve as counselors, with graduate students or faculty serving as supervisors.

Interventions that are included in the after-school CHP include academic skills training (eg, organizational training, note-taking instruction, study strategies), an interpersonal skills group (eg, aim to teach adolescents to understand relationships between their behavior and their own personal identity, assist students to learn to monitor and revise interpersonal behavior so that their behavior aligns with their identity goals), sports skills (eg, provide an opportunity to practice interpersonal skills), mentoring (eg, brief meetings with CHP counselors that occur at each CHP session), and monthly parent meetings (eg, parents are provided with information about ADHD and adolescence, parents receive instruction on effective parenting practices).

Mentoring model In an attempt to improve the feasibility of the CHP, the CHP mentoring model was designed to provide a subset of the after-school model CHP interventions during the standard academic day. School mental health professionals (eg, social workers, school psychologists) and teachers meet weekly with the adolescents to provide the academic skills training interventions. Extant data from 3 randomized trials support the efficacy of the CHP, especially the after-school model for middle school students.[85–89]

Homework, Organization, and Planning Skills Program Another relatively well-researched intervention for adolescents with ADHD is the Homework, Organization, and Planning Skills (HOPS) program, originally developed as an extension of the CHP. As the name implies, the HOPS program focuses exclusively on teaching organization, time management, and planning skills to middle and high school students with ADHD. The HOPS intervention is administered by a school-based mental health professional in sixteen 20-minute sessions that occur during the standard academic day. The entire HOPS intervention is delivered over the course of one semester, beginning with twice-weekly meetings and tapering to weekly meetings approximately halfway through the intervention. The HOPS intervention also includes two 1-hour "family" meetings that the adolescent and his/her parents/guardians attend with the school-based mental health professional. The primary purpose of these meetings is to discuss and refine the home-based reinforcement system that all HOPS participants have in place at the beginning of the intervention.

Several randomized intervention trials have supported the efficacy of the HOPS intervention, especially with regard to parent ratings of adolescent organization and time-management/planning skills.[90–92] In both the CHP and HOPS studies, approximately 70% of participants were taking ADHD medications while receiving the interventions, yet none of the studies reported an association between medication use and outcome.[85,91]

Summer Treatment Program

An evidence-based multimodality intervention program for managing ADHD is the summer treatment program (STP) developed by Pelham and Hoza.[93] Markedly different to the clinic-based or school-based interventions already described, an STP is a package of intensive interventions that engage the child in a camp-like setting. This program includes 5 major components of treatment:

1. Parent training in child behavior management
2. Classroom implementation of behavior modification techniques
3. Academic and sports skills practice and tutoring
4. Social skills training (typically involving sports)
5. Stimulant medication

Most of these interventions rely on operant conditioning and social learning principles that are delivered by adults (eg, camp counselors, teachers, parents) in the child's natural environment.

Most STPs are a 6- to 8-week program for school-aged children and adolescents. The children are placed into age-matched groups of approximately 12, and the groups remain together for the duration of the STP. Contingency management interventions are used continuously throughout the camp day, and a DRC accompanies every child/adolescent when they leave for the day. In addition to the child-focused interventions, weekly BPT sessions are provided for the parents.

STP participants who are prescribed medication receive their customary doses. A feature of the STP is that if parents desire, a child may have an ecologically valid, controlled evaluation of the stimulant effectiveness as part of the STP. Several studies have indicated that STP participants require lower doses of stimulant medication when participating in the STP, even when delivered in a modified, less intensive fashion.[17,94]

STPs have a substantial research base; more than 15 randomized controlled trials (either between-group or crossover design) have been completed, which support the efficacy of STPs.[47] The STP was included in the largest previous intervention study of ADHD, the Multimodal Treatment of ADHD (MTA) Study.[79] Most of these previous STP intervention studies were directed at academic (eg, work completion, adherence to rules, improved note taking) and social functional outcomes (peer and adult interactions).

PSYCHOSOCIAL INTERVENTIONS REQUIRING FURTHER STUDY BEFORE RECOMMENDATIONS CAN BE MADE
Clinic-Based Cognitive-Behavioral Treatment for Adolescents

Although once believed to be effective for children with ADHD,[95] neither cognitive-behavioral treatment (CBT) nor cognitive therapy has much research support in pediatric ADHD.[73,96–99] Meta-analyses of CBT have typically reported the effect sizes to be less than one-third of a standard deviation.[98] Because of its limited efficacy, CBT was not included in the MTA treatment protocols.

There is a growing body of literature suggesting that CBT can be effective for managing adult ADHD.[100–111] Adult ADHD CBT interventions are focused on skill building and teaching specific skills,[112] and are more heavily skewed toward teaching behavioral techniques than changing cognitions. While behavioral therapy has been well researched for adolescents with ADHD,[113] far less empirical attention has been devoted to CBT in adolescents with ADHD, possibly because of previous findings indicating that children and adolescents with ADHD are "treatment refractory" to any "cognitive" intervention.[114]

Within the past few years, one clinic-based adolescent ADHD CBT intervention trial that concurrently incorporated principles of contingency management reported modestly positive outcomes on several functional domains.[115] Other recent clinic-based (not school-based) intervention studies with adolescents with ADHD have included CBT components, and have reported positive results on several functional domains.[116–118] In addition, secondary analyses in the clinic-based Treatment of Adolescent Depression Study[119] examined the role of comorbid ADHD as a moderator of treatment outcomes in adolescent depression. Data from these analyses suggested that comorbid ADHD did not negatively affect CBT response in adolescents with depression.[120] Likewise, in a clinic-based study of adolescent anxiety disorders, co-morbid ADHD did not affect CBT treatment outcomes.[121] Thus, there is some reason to suggest that larger clinic-based trials for CBT in adolescent ADHD may be worthy of consideration.

Social Skills Training

Social impairments are a prominent feature of ADHD[3] and are likely to manifest as being a sore loser and/or interrupting ongoing conversations.[122] Social skills training (SST) has been traditionally conducted in groups held in a clinic setting, and is predicated on the belief that children with ADHD lack the core skills to demonstrate prosocial behaviors.[123] Social skills taught in SST for children with ADHD include topics such as taking turns, initiating and maintaining conversation, and emotion awareness and regulation.[124] The extant literature suggests that traditional clinic-based SST for ADHD can improve social functioning in the group setting,[125,126] but with poor generalization to the home and school environments.[127–130] In fact, 2 recent reviews of psychosocial treatments for children with ADHD have concluded that traditional clinic-based SST is ineffective for ADHD.[46,47]

Barkley's[31] theoretic model of ADHD posits that ADHD is not a knowledge deficit as much as the disorder is a performance disorder. Thus, teaching additional skills to children with ADHD is not so much the issue as is assisting them to perform the skills they have when it would be useful to do so. Rather than in a clinic setting, this instruction should likely also occur at the point of performance (the place and time in the natural setting) where such skills are most likely to prove useful to the long-term social acceptance of the individual.

Although traditional clinic-based SST has not been proved to be effective for improving the social impairments that often accompany ADHD, several alternative SST interventions have been developed in the past 10 years that emphasize instruction at the point of performance. Rather than focusing on the children, training parents, STP counselors, and/or teachers to provide in vivo reminders and incentives to children with ADHD to carry out socially skilled behaviors with real peers has been a focus of these alternative approaches.[64,93,126,130–134] Several of these alternative SST approaches involve no child treatment component, instead focusing exclusively on training parents[64] or teachers[135] to administer the social skills knowledge instruction and provide the contingencies necessary to permit skill generalization. In addition to working with teachers, one of the more novel SST approaches, MOSAIC (Making Socially Accepting Inclusive Classrooms), includes training for teachers on how to encourage non-ADHD peers to be accepting of children with ADHD.[135]

At this point further research is needed before considering if these alternative SST approaches should be recommended as a front-line psychosocial intervention. However, compared with traditional, clinic-based SST programs, these alternative approaches appear to be more promising.

SUMMARY AND FUTURE DIRECTIONS

ADHD is conceptualized now as a largely chronic disorder for most, but not all children, similar in some respects to chronic medical disorders such as diabetes or phenylketonuria. Stimulant medications are a front-line intervention for managing ADHD in children and adolescents. In addition to the use of medication, psychosocial interventions that seem most promising, and thus should be included in a combined treatment program, include contingency management methods applied in classrooms and elsewhere (STPs), training of parents (BPT) in these same methods to be used in the home and community settings, and comprehensive school-based treatment programs (CHP, HOPS). Evidence for CBT for adolescents and alternative child SST programs focused more on parents and teachers appears promising, but requires further research before stronger recommendations can be made.

Role of Psychosocial Therapies

Future research should continue to consider the role that psychosocial therapies will play in the treatment of ADHD in children and adolescents. A primary and fundamental research goal for future psychosocial interventions is to specifically target generalization and maintenance of treatment gains. Psychosocial treatments, especially behavioral ones, are comparable with medication management in that they produce solid benefits as long as they are in place. However, most psychosocial treatments for ADHD yield little evidence of maintenance or generalization once withdrawn.

Barkley refers to many ADHD psychosocial treatments, especially those with significant behavioral approaches, as "designing prosthetic environments."[136] In Barkley's view, behavioral treatments, like hearing aids, wheelchairs, ramps into public facilities, lower bathroom fixtures, glasses, large print books, and prosthetic limbs for amputees, are artificial means of altering environments so as to reduce the adverse impact of a biological handicap on the performance of major life activities.[136] Behavioral methods are prostheses: a means of rearranging environments by artificial means so as to yield improved participation in major life activities. Once the prostheses are withdrawn, however, the child is once again impaired. Future research should continue to consider how best to address this prosthetic dilemma and better promote maintenance and generalization of treatment effects.

Whereas psychosocial interventions work for many youths with ADHD, not all children and adolescents with ADHD respond positively. Future psychosocial research should continue to consider the mechanisms of change (using treatment-dismantling approaches) and mediators/moderators of outcomes.

Psychosocial Treatment Accessibility and Portability

There is a crucial need to improve psychosocial treatment portability and accessibility. The children who need the interventions the most are often from high-risk families that lack resources.[137] In addition to the CHP and HOPS (which are delivered directly in schools), some recent interventions have moved in this direction.[138,139] Likewise, the

STP model, not feasible for many families, is being piloted in a less intensive version in after-school, school, and community settings.[94] Nonetheless, future research should continue to focus on improving psychosocial treatment portability and accessibility. These efforts will likely use various existing technologies (eg, interactive Internet-based treatment and/or training) applied in a more novel fashion to high-risk groups.

Stigma Effect on Psychosocial Interventions

Normalization of functioning for children and adolescents with ADHD is difficult to achieve with medications[140,141] and psychosocial interventions.[10] Nearly all of the psychosocial interventions have been focused on the child/adolescent and/or training the parents/teachers. Very few psychosocial interventions have included non-ADHD peers in an intervention package. Future psychosocial interventions should also consider the role that stigma plays in affecting psychosocial treatment outcomes and maintenance. For example, there are many data to suggest that children with ADHD are stigmatized by typically developing peers,[142–145] parents,[146–148] and teachers.[149] Given the pervasiveness of the stigma that ADHD seems to engender, it is surprising that more interventions have not considered the role that stigma may play in negatively affecting outcomes (eg, the child with ADHD improves skills, yet others continue to have negative perceptions of the child). Some work[135,150] has begun recently to explore this domain, although more research should focus on the role of stigma as a possible moderator of treatment outcomes.

Adolescent Versus Child Treatment Guidelines

Finally, the American Academy of Child and Adolescent Psychiatry practice parameters outline practice guidelines for managing adolescents that are substantively different to child guidelines.[151] Despite this, there have been far fewer psychosocial research studies that have focused on treating adolescents with ADHD relative to children with ADHD[152] (and more recently, even adults with ADHD). ADHD and the associated functional impairments often persist into adolescence, so there remains a clear need for effective psychosocial treatments for adolescents with ADHD.

REFERENCES

1. Ceneters for Disease Control and Prevention. Increasing prevalence of parent-reported attention-deficit/hyperactivity disorder among children—United States, 2003 and 2007. MMWR Morb Mortal Wkly Rep 2010;59(44):1439–43.
2. Polanczyk G, de Lima MS, Horta BL, et al. The worldwide prevalence of ADHD: a systematic review and metaregression analysis. Am J Psychiatry 2007;164(6):942–8.
3. American Psychiatric Association. Diagnostic and statistical manual of mental disorders. 5th edition. Arlington (VA): American Psychiatric Publishing; 2013.
4. Kent KM, Pelham WE Jr, Molina BS, et al. The academic experience of male high school students with ADHD. J Abnorm Child Psychol 2011;39(3):451–62.
5. Danckaerts M, Sonuga-Barke EJ, Banaschewski T, et al. The quality of life of children with attention deficit/hyperactivity disorder: a systematic review. Eur Child Adolesc Psychiatry 2010;19(2):83–105.
6. Bussing R, Gary FA, Mason DM, et al. Child temperament, ADHD, and caregiver strain: exploring relationships in an epidemiological sample. J Am Acad Child Adolesc Psychiatry 2003;42(2):184–92.
7. Wymbs BT, Pelham WE Jr, Molina BS, et al. Rate and predictors of divorce among parents of youths with ADHD. J Consult Clin Psychol 2008;76(5):735–44.

8. Hill JC, Schoener EP. Age-dependent decline of attention deficit hyperactivity disorder. Am J Psychiatry 1996;153(9):1143–6.

9. Barkley RA, Murphy K, Fischer M. ADHD in adults: what the science says. New York: Guilford Press; 2008.

10. Molina BS, Hinshaw SP, Swanson JM, et al. The MTA at 8 years: prospective follow-up of children treated for combined-type ADHD in a multisite study. J Am Acad Child Adolesc Psychiatry 2009;48(5):484–500.

11. Schwarz A. Drowned in a sea of prescriptions. New York Times 2013.

12. Pelham W, Foster EM, Robb JA. The economic impact of attention-deficit/hyperactivity disorder in children and adolescents. J Pediatr Psychol 2007; 32(6):711–27.

13. Faraone SV, Biederman J, Spencer TJ, et al. Comparing the efficacy of medications for ADHD using meta-analysis. MedGenMed 2006;8(4):4.

14. Hoza B, Gerdes AC, Mrug S, et al. Peer-assessed outcomes in the multimodal treatment study of children with attention deficit hyperactivity disorder. J Clin Child Adolesc Psychol 2005;34(1):74–86.

15. Johnston C, Mash EJ. Families of children with attention-deficit/hyperactivity disorder: review and recommendations for future research. Clin Child Fam Psychol Rev 2001;4(3):183–207.

16. Raggi VL, Chronis AM. Interventions to address the academic impairment of children and adolescents with ADHD. Clin Child Fam Psychol Rev 2006;9(2):85–111.

17. Fabiano GA, Pelham WE Jr, Gnagy EM, et al. The single and combined effects of multiple intensities of behavior modification and methylphenidate for children with attention deficit hyperactivity disorder in a classroom setting. Sch Psychol Rev 2007;36:195–216.

18. Pelham W, Fabiano GA, Gnagy EM, et al. ADHD. In: Hibbs ED, Jensen PS, editors. Psychosocial treatments for child and adolescent disorders: empirically based strategies for clinical practice. 2nd edition. Washington, DC: American Psychological Association; 2005. p. 377–410.

19. Wolraich M, Brown L, Brown RT, et al, Subcommittee on Attention-Deficit/Hyperactivity Disorder, Steering committee on quality improvement and management. ADHD: clinical practice guideline for the diagnosis, evaluation and treatment of attention deficit/hyperactivity disorder in children and adolescents. Pediatrics 2011;128(5):1007–22.

20. Faraone SV, Buitelaar J. Comparing the efficacy of stimulants for ADHD in children and adolescents using meta-analysis. Eur Child Adolesc Psychiatry 2010; 19(4):353–64.

21. Hurt EA, Arnold LE, Lofthouse N. Dietary and nutritional treatments for attention-deficit/hyperactivity disorder: current research support and recommendations for practitioners. Curr Psychiatry Rep 2011;13(5):323–32.

22. Rucklidge JJ, Johnstone J, Kaplan BJ. Nutrient supplementation approaches in the treatment of ADHD. Expert Rev Neurother 2009;9(4):461–76.

23. Rucklidge JJ, Frampton CM, Gorman B, et al. Vitamin-mineral treatment of attention-deficit hyperactivity disorder in adults: double-blind randomised placebo-controlled trial. Br J Psychiatry 2014;204:306–15.

24. Bloch MH, Qawasmi A. Omega-3 fatty acid supplementation for the treatment of children with attention-deficit/hyperactivity disorder symptomatology: systematic review and meta-analysis. J Am Acad Child Adolesc Psychiatry 2011;50(10):991–1000.

25. Gillies D, Sinn J, Lad SS, et al. Polyunsaturated fatty acids (PUFA) for attention deficit hyperactivity disorder (ADHD) in children and adolescents. Cochrane Database Syst Rev 2012;(7):CD007986.

26. Sonuga-Barke EJ, Brandeis D, Cortese S, et al. Nonpharmacological interventions for ADHD: systematic review and meta-analyses of randomized controlled trials of dietary and psychological treatments. Am J Psychiatry 2013;170(3):275–89.
27. Hawkey E, Nigg JT. Omega-3 fatty acid and ADHD: blood level analysis and meta-analytic extension of supplementation trials. Clin Psychol Rev 2014; 34(6):496–505.
28. Angold A, Costello EJ, Farmer EM, et al. Impaired but undiagnosed. J Am Acad Child Adolesc Psychiatry 1999;38(2):129–37.
29. Pfiffner LJ. More rewards or more punishment?. In: Pfiffner LM, editor. Attention deficit/hyperactivity disorder: concepts, controversies, new directions. New York: Informa Health Care; 2008. p. 291–300.
30. Sonuga-Barke EJ. Causal models of attention-deficit/hyperactivity disorder: from common simple deficits to multiple developmental pathways. Biol Psychiatry 2005;57(11):1231–8.
31. Barkley RA. Behavioral inhibition, sustained attention, and executive functions: constructing a unifying theory of ADHD. Psychol Bull 1997;121(1):65–94.
32. Hartman RR, Stage SA, Webster-Stratton C. A growth curve analysis of parent training outcomes: examining the influence of child risk factors (inattention, impulsivity, and hyperactivity problems), parental and family risk factors. J Child Psychol Psychiatry 2003;44(3):388–98.
33. Bor W, Sanders MR, Markie-Dadds C. The effects of the triple P-Positive parenting program on preschool children with co-occurring disruptive behavior and attentional/hyperactive difficulties. J Abnorm Child Psychol 2002;30(6): 571–87.
34. Chronis AM, Chacko A, Fabiano GA, et al. Enhancements to the behavioral parent training paradigm for families of children with ADHD: review and future directions. Clin Child Fam Psychol Rev 2004;7(1):1–27.
35. Chronis AM, Jones HA, Raggi VL. Evidence-based psychosocial treatments for children and adolescents with attention-deficit/hyperactivity disorder. Clin Psychol Rev 2006;26(4):486–502.
36. Chronis AM, Lahey BB, Pelham WE Jr, et al. Maternal depression and early positive parenting predict future conduct problems in young children with attention-deficit/hyperactivity disorder. Dev Psychol 2007;43(1):70–82.
37. Anastopoulos AD, DuPaul GJ, Barkley RA. Stimulant medication and parent training therapies for attention deficit-hyperactivity disorder. J Learn Disabil 1991;24(4):210–8.
38. Sonuga-Barke EJ, Daley D, Thompson M, et al. Parent-based therapies for preschool attention-deficit/hyperactivity disorder: a randomized, controlled trial with a community sample. J Am Acad Child Adolesc Psychiatry 2001;40(4):402–8.
39. Sonuga-Barke EJ, Thompson M, Daley D, et al. Parent training for attention deficit/hyperactivity disorder: is it as effective when delivered as routine rather than as specialist care? Br J Clin Psychol 2004;43(Pt 4):449–57.
40. Strayhorn JM, Weidman CS. Reduction of attention deficit and internalizing symptoms in preschoolers through parent-child interaction training. J Am Acad Child Adolesc Psychiatry 1989;28(6):888–96.
41. Pisterman S, McGrath P, Firestone P, et al. Outcome of parent-mediated treatment of preschoolers with attention deficit disorder with hyperactivity. J Consult Clin Psychol 1989;57(5):628–35.
42. Anastopoulos AD, Shelton TL, DuPaul GJ, et al. Parent training for attention-deficit hyperactivity disorder: its impact on parent functioning. J Abnorm Child Psychol 1993;21(5):581–96.

43. Chronis-Tuscano A, Clarke TL, O'Brien KA, et al. Development and preliminary evaluation of an integrated treatment targeting parenting and depressive symptoms in mothers of children with attention-deficit/hyperactivity disorder. J Consult Clin Psychol 2013;81(5):918–25.
44. Fabiano GA, Pelham WE, Cunningham CE, et al. A waitlist-controlled trial of behavioral parent training for fathers of children with ADHD. J Clin Child Adolesc Psychol 2012;41(3):337–45.
45. Barkley RA, Guevremont DC, Anastopoulos AD, et al. A comparison of three family therapy programs for treating family conflicts in adolescents with attention-deficit hyperactivity disorder. J Consult Clin Psychol 1992;60(3):450–62.
46. Pelham WE Jr, Fabiano GA. Evidence-based psychosocial treatments for attention-deficit/hyperactivity disorder. J Clin Child Adolesc Psychol 2008;37(1):184–214.
47. Evans SW, Owens JS, Bunford N. Evidence-based psychosocial treatments for children and adolescents with attention-deficit/hyperactivity disorder. J Clin Child Adolesc Psychol 2014;43(4):527–51.
48. Nonpharmacological treatments for childhood ADHD and their combination with medication. In: Nathan PE, Gordon JM, editors. A guide to treatments that work. 4th edition. New York: Oxford University Press; 2014.
49. Cunningham CE, Bremner R, Secord M. COPE: the community parent education program: a school-based family systems oriented workshop for parents of children with disruptive behavior disorders. Hamilton (Canada): COPE Works; 1997.
50. Webster-Stratton C. The incredible years. Toronto (Canada): Umbrella Press; 1992.
51. Barkley RA. Defiant children: a clinician's manual for assessment and parent training. New York: Guilford Press; 1997.
52. Eyberg SM, Robinson EA. Parent-child interaction training: effects on family functioning. J Clin Child Psychol 1982;11:130–7.
53. Sanders MR, Markie-Dadds C, Tully LA, et al. The triple P-positive parenting program: a comparison of enhanced, standard, and self-directed behavioral family intervention for parents of children with early onset conduct problems. J Consult Clin Psychol 2000;68(4):624–40.
54. Thomas R, Zimmer-Gembeck MJ. Behavioral outcomes of parent-child interaction therapy and triple p-positive parenting program: a review and meta-analysis. J Abnorm Child Psychol 2007;35(3):475–95.
55. Patterson GR. Coercive family process. Eugene (OR): Castalia Publishing Company; 1982.
56. Gerdes AC, Hoza B, Pelham WE. Attention-deficit/hyperactivity disordered boys' relationships with their mothers and fathers: child, mother, and father perceptions. Dev Psychopathol 2003;15(02):363–82.
57. Hinshaw SP, Owens EB, Wells KC, et al. Family processes and treatment outcome in the MTA: negative/ineffective parenting practices in relation to multimodal treatment. J Abnorm Child Psychol 2000;28(6):555–68.
58. Kaiser NM, McBurnett K, Pfiffner LJ. Child ADHD severity and positive and negative parenting as predictors of child social functioning: evaluation of three theoretical models. J Atten Disord 2011;15(3):193–203.
59. Jones HA, Epstein JN, Hinshaw SP, et al. Ethnicity as a moderator of treatment effects on parent—child interaction for children with ADHD. J Atten Disord 2010;13(6):592–600.

60. Clarke AT, Marshall SA, Mautone JA, et al. Parent attendance and homework adherence predict response to a family–school intervention for children with ADHD. J Clin Child Adolesc Psychol 2013;1–10 [Epub ahead of print].

61. Villodas MT, McBurnett K, Kaiser N, et al. Additive effects of parent adherence on social and behavioral outcomes of a collaborative school–home behavioral intervention for ADHD. Child Psychiatry Hum Dev 2014;45(3):348–60.

62. Kaiser NM, Hinshaw SP, Pfiffner LJ. Parent cognitions and behavioral parent training: engagement and outcomes. The ADHD Report 2010;18(1):6–12.

63. Sonuga-Barke EJ, Daley D, Thompson M. Does maternal ADHD reduce the effectiveness of parent training for preschool children's ADHD? J Am Acad Child Adolesc Psychiatry 2002;41(6):696–702.

64. Mikami AY, Lerner MD, Griggs MS, et al. Parental influence on children with attention-deficit/hyperactivity disorder: II. Results of a pilot intervention training parents as friendship coaches for children. J Abnorm Child Psychol 2010; 38(6):737–49.

65. Abikoff H, Gallagher R, Wells KC, et al. Remediating organizational functioning in children with ADHD: immediate and long-term effects from a randomized controlled trial. J Consult Clin Psychol 2013;81(1):113–28.

66. Kazdin AE. Parent management training: evidence, outcomes, and issues. J Am Acad Child Adolesc Psychiatry 1997;36(10):1349–56.

67. Owens JS, Murphy CE, Richerson L, et al. Science to practice in underserved communities: the effectiveness of school mental health programming. J Clin Child Adolesc Psychol 2008;37(2):434–47.

68. Pfiffner LJ, Hinshaw S, Owens E, et al. A two-site randomized clinical trial of integrated psychosocial treatment for ADHD-inattentive type. J Consult Clin Psychol 2014. [Epub ahead of print].

69. Dupaul G, Stoner G. ADHD in the schools: assessment and intervention strategies. 2nd edition. New York: Guilford Press; 2003.

70. DuPaul GJ, Weyandt LL. School-based interventions for children and adolescents with attention-deficit/hyperactivity disorder: enhancing academic and behavioral outcomes. Educ Treat Children 2006;29:341–58.

71. Cooper JO, Heron TE, Hewards L. Applied behavior analysis. 2nd edition. Upper Saddle River (NJ): Pearson; 2007.

72. Jurbergs N, Palcic J, Kelley ML. School-home notes with and without response cost: increasing attention and academic performance in low-income children with attention-deficit/hyperactivity disorder. Sch Psychol Q 2007;22:358–79.

73. DuPaul GJ, Eckert TL. The effects of school-based interventions for attention deficit hyperactivity disorder: a meta-analysis. Sch Psychol Dig 1997; 26:5–27.

74. Pfiffner LJ, Rosen LA, O'Leary SG. The efficacy of an all-positive approach to classroom management. J Appl Behav Anal 1985;18(3):257–61.

75. Pfiffner LJ, Barkley RA, DuPaul GJ. Treatment of ADHD in school settings. In: Barkley RA, editor. Attention deficit hyperactivity disorder: A handbook for diagnosis and treatment. 3rd Edition. New York: Guilford Press; 2006. p. 547–89.

76. Pfiffner LJ, O'Leary SG, Rosen LA, et al. A comparison of the effects of continuous and intermittent response cost and reprimands in the classroom. J Clin Child Psychol 1985;14:348–52.

77. DuPaul GJ, Eckert TL, Vilardo B. The effects of school-based interventions for attention deficit hyperactivity disorder: a meta-analysis 1996-2010. Sch Psychol Rev 2012;41(4):387–412.

78. Volpe RJ, Fabiano GA. Daily behavior report cards: an evidence-based system of assessment and intervention. New York: Guilford; 2013.

79. MTA Collaborative Group. A 14-month randomized clinical trial of treatment strategies for attention-deficit/hyperactivity disorder. The MTA Cooperative Group. Multimodal treatment study of children with ADHD. Arch Gen Psychiatry 1999; 56(12):1073–86.

80. Atkinson BM, Forehand R. Home-based reinforcement programs designed to modify classroom behavior: a review and methodological evaluation. Psychol Bull 1979;86:1298–308.

81. Vannest KJ, Davis JL, Davis CR. Effective intervention for behavior with a daily behavior report card: a meta-analysis. Sch Psychol Rev 2010;39:654–72.

82. Langberg JM, Molina BS, Arnold LE, et al. Patterns and predictors of adolescent academic achievement and performance in a sample of children with attention-deficit/hyperactivity disorder. J Clin Child Adolesc Psychol 2011;40(4):519–31.

83. Harrison J, Bunford N, Evans SW. Educational accommodations for students with behavioral challenges: a systematic review of the literature. Rev Educ Res 2013;83:551–97.

84. DuPaul GJ, Evans SW. School-based interventions for adolescents with attention-deficit/hyperactivity disorder. Adolesc Med State Art Rev 2008;19(2): 300–12, x.

85. Evans SW, Schultz BK, DeMars CE, et al. Effectiveness of the challenging horizons after-school program for young adolescents with ADHD. Behav Ther 2011; 42(3):462–74.

86. Schultz BK, Storer J, Watabe Y, et al. School-based treatment of attention-deficit/hyperactivity disorder. Psychol Schools 2011;48(3):254–62.

87. Molina BS, Flory K, Bukstein OG, et al. Feasibility and preliminary efficacy of an after-school program for middle schoolers with ADHD a randomized trial in a large public middle school. J Atten Disord 2008;12(3):207–17.

88. Evans SW, Serpell ZN, Schultz BK, et al. Cumulative benefits of secondary school-based treatment of students with attention deficit hyperactivity disorder. Sch Psychol Rev 2007;36(2):256–73.

89. Evans SW, Axelrod J, Langberg JM. Efficacy of a school-based treatment program for middle school youth with ADHD—pilot data. Behav Modif 2004;28(4): 528–47.

90. Langberg JM, Becker SP, Epstein JN, et al. Predictors of response and mechanisms of change in an organizational skills intervention for students with ADHD. J Child Fam Stud 2013;22(7):1000–12.

91. Langberg JM, Epstein JN, Becker SP, et al. Evaluation of the homework, organization, and planning skills (HOPS) intervention for middle school students with attention deficit hyperactivity disorder as implemented by school mental health providers. Sch Psychol Rev 2012;41(3):342–64.

92. Langberg JM, Epstein JN, Urbanowicz CM, et al. Efficacy of an organization skills intervention to improve the academic functioning of students with attention-deficit/hyperactivity disorder. Sch Psychol Q 2008;23(3):407–17.

93. Pelham W, Hoza B. Intensive treatment: a summer treatment program for children with ADHD. In: Hibbs E, Jensen EH, editors. Psychosocial treatments for child and adolescent disorders: empirically based strategies for clinical practice. New York: APA Press; 1996. p. 311–40.

94. Pelham WE, Burrows-Maclean L, Gnagy EM, et al. A dose-ranging study of behavioral and pharmacological treatment in social settings for children with ADHD. J Abnorm Child Psychol 2014;42(6):1019–31.

95. Kendall PC, Braswell L. Cognitive-behavioral therapy for impulsive children. New York: Guilford Press; 1985.

96. Abikoff H, Gittelman R. Hyperactive children treated with stimulants. Is cognitive training a useful adjunct? Arch Gen Psychiatry 1985;42(10):953–61.

97. Dush DM, Hirt ML, Schroeder HE. Self-statement modification in the treatment of child behavior disorders: a meta-analysis. Psychol Bull 1989;106(1):97–106.

98. Baer RA, Nietzel MT. Cognitive and behavioral treatment of impulsivity in children: a meta-analytic review of the outcome literature. J Clin Child Psychol 1991;20:400–12.

99. Bloomquist ML, August GJ, Ostrander R. Effects of a school-based cognitive-behavioral intervention for ADHD children. J Abnorm Child Psychol 1991;19: 591–605.

100. Weiss M, Murray C, Wasdell M, et al. A randomized controlled trial of CBT therapy for adults with ADHD with and without medication. BMC Psychiatry 2012;12:30.

101. Emilsson B, Gudjonsson G, Sigurdsson JF, et al. Cognitive behaviour therapy in medication-treated adults with ADHD and persistent symptoms: a randomized controlled trial. BMC Psychiatry 2011;11:116.

102. Virta M, Salakari A, Antila M, et al. Short cognitive behavioral therapy and cognitive training for adults with ADHD - a randomized controlled pilot study. Neuropsychiatr Dis Treat 2010;6:443–53.

103. Bramham J, Young S, Bickerdike A, et al. Evaluation of group cognitive behavioral therapy for adults with ADHD. J Atten Disord 2009;12(5):434–41.

104. Safren SA, Otto MW, Sprich S, et al. Cognitive-behavioral therapy for ADHD in medication-treated adults with continued symptoms. Behav Res Ther 2005; 43(7):831–42.

105. Rostain AL, Ramsay JR. A combined treatment approach for adults with ADHD—results of an open study of 43 patients. J Atten Disord 2006;10(2):150–9.

106. Stevenson CS, Stevenson RJ, Whitmont S. A self-directed psychosocial intervention with minimal therapist contact for adults with attention deficit hyperactivity disorder. Clin Psychol Psychother 2003;10:93–101.

107. Stevenson CS, Whitmont S, Bornholt L, et al. A cognitive remediation programme for adults with attention deficit hyperactivity disorder. Aust N Z J Psychiatry 2002;36(5):610–6.

108. Safren SA, Sprich S, Mimiaga MJ, et al. Cognitive behavioral therapy vs relaxation with educational support for medication-treated adults with ADHD and persistent symptoms: a randomized controlled trial. JAMA 2010;304(8):875–80.

109. Solanto MV, Marks DJ, Wasserstein J, et al. Efficacy of meta-cognitive therapy for adult ADHD. Am J Psychiatry 2010;167(8):958–68.

110. Hesslinger B, Tebartz van Elst L, Nyberg E, et al. Psychotherapy of attention deficit hyperactivity disorder in adults—a pilot study using a structured skills training program. Eur Arch Psychiatry Clin Neurosci 2002;252(4):177–84.

111. Philipsen A, Richter H, Peters J, et al. Structured group psychotherapy in adults with attention deficit hyperactivity disorder: results of an open multicentre study. J Nerv Ment Dis 2007;195(12):1013–9.

112. Knouse LE, Safren SA. Current status of cognitive behavioral therapy for adult attention-deficit hyperactivity disorder. Psychiatr Clin North Am 2010;33(3): 497–509.

113. Sibley MH, Kuriyan AB, Evans SW, et al. Pharmacological and psychosocial treatments for adolescents with ADHD: an updated systematic review of the literature. Clin Psychol Rev 2014;34(3):218–32.

114. Miller M, Hinshaw SP. Treatment for children and adolescents with ADHD. In: Kendall PC, editor. Child and adolescent therapy: cognitive-behavioral procedures. 4th edition. New York: Guilford Press; 2012. p. 61–91.

115. Antshel KM, Faraone SV, Gordon M. Cognitive behavioral treatment outcomes in adolescent ADHD. J Atten Disord 2012;18(6):483–95.

116. van de Weijer-Bergsma E, Formsma AR, de Bruin EI, et al. The effectiveness of mindfulness training on behavioral problems and attentional functioning in adolescents with ADHD. J Child Fam Stud 2012;21(5):775–87.

117. Sibley MH, Pelham WE, Derefinko KJ, et al. A pilot trial of supporting teens' academic needs daily (STAND): a parent-adolescent collaborative intervention for ADHD. J Psychopathol Behav Assess 2013;35:436–49.

118. Fabiano GA, Hulme K, Linke S, et al. The supporting a teen's effective entry to the roadway (STEER) program: feasibility and preliminary support for a psychosocial intervention for teenage drivers with ADHD. Cogn Behav Pract 2011;18:267–80.

119. March J, Silva S, Curry J, et al. The treatment for adolescents with depression study (TADS): outcomes over 1 year of naturalistic follow-up. Am J Psychiatry 2009;166(10):1141–9.

120. Kratochvil CJ, May DE, Silva SG, et al. Treatment response in depressed adolescents with and without co-morbid attention-deficit/hyperactivity disorder in the treatment for adolescents with depression study. J Child Adolesc Psychopharmacol 2009;19(5):519–27.

121. Flannery-Schroeder E, Suveg C, Safford S, et al. Comorbid externalising disorders and child anxiety treatment outcomes. Behav Change 2004;21(1):14–25.

122. Landau S, Milich R, Diener MB. Peer relations of children with attention-deficit hyperactivity disorder. Read Writ Q 1998;14(1):83–105.

123. de Boo GM, Prins PJ. Social incompetence in children with ADHD: possible moderators and mediators in social-skills training. Clin Psychol Rev 2007; 27(1):78–97.

124. Pfiffner LJ. Social skills training. In: McBurnett K, Pfiffner LJ, editors. Attention-deficit/hyperactivity disorder: concepts, controversies, new directions. New York: Informa Healthcare; 2008. p. 179–90.

125. Fenstermacher K, Olympia D, Sheridan SM. Effectiveness of a computer-facilitated interactive social skills training program for boys with attention deficit hyperactivity disorder. Sch Psychol Q 2006;21(2):197–224.

126. Pfiffner LJ, McBurnett K. Social skills training with parent generalization: treatment effects for children with attention deficit disorder. J Consult Clin Psychol 1997;65(5):749–57.

127. Abikoff HB, Hechtman L, Klein RG, et al. Social functioning in children with ADHD treated with long-term methylphenidate and multimodal psychosocial treatment. J Am Acad Child Adolesc Psychiatry 2004;43(7):820–9.

128. Antshel KM, Remer R. Social skills training in children with attention deficit hyperactivity disorder: a randomized-controlled clinical trial. J Clin Child Adolesc Psychol 2003;32(1):153–65.

129. Abikoff HB. Efficacy of cognitive training interventions in hyperactive children: a critical review. Clin Psychol Rev 1985;5(5):479–512.

130. Pelham WE, Wheeler T, Chronis A. Empirically supported psychosocial treatments for attention deficit hyperactivity disorder. J Clin Child Psychol 1998; 27(2):190–205.

131. Frankel F, Myatt R, Cantwell DP, et al. Parent-assisted transfer of children's social skills training: effects on children with and without attention-deficit hyperactivity disorder. J Am Acad Child Adolesc Psychiatry 1997;36(8):1056–64.

132. Pfiffner LJ, Mikami AY, Huang-Pollock C, et al. A randomized, controlled trial of integrated home-school behavioral treatment for ADHD, predominantly inattentive type. J Am Acad Child Adolesc Psychiatry 2007;46(8):1041–50.

133. Frankel F, Myatt R, Cantwell DP. Training outpatient boys to conform with the social ecology of popular peers: effects on parent and teacher ratings. J Clin Child Psychol 1995;24(3):300–10.

134. Pelham WE, Bender ME. Peer relationships in hyperactive children: description and treatment. In: Gadow KD, Bailer I, editors. Advances in learning and behavioral disabilities, vol. 1. Greenwich (CT): JAI Press; 1982. p. 365–436.

135. Mikami AY, Griggs MS, Lerner MD, et al. A randomized trial of a classroom intervention to increase peers' social inclusion of children with attention-deficit/hyperactivity disorder. J Consult Clin Psychol 2013;81(1):100–12.

136. Barkley RA. ADHD and the nature of self-control. New York: Guilford; 1997.

137. Hoagwood K, Kelleher KJ, Feil M, et al. Treatment services for children with ADHD: a national perspective. J Am Acad Child Adolesc Psychiatry 2000; 39(2):198–206.

138. McGrath PJ, Lingley-Pottie P, Thurston C, et al. Telephone-based mental health interventions for child disruptive behavior or anxiety disorders: randomized trials and overall analysis. J Am Acad Child Adolesc Psychiatry 2011;50(11):1162–72.

139. Pfiffner LJ, Villodas M, Kaiser N, et al. Educational outcomes of a collaborative school–home behavioral intervention for ADHD. Sch Psychol Q 2013;28(1):25.

140. Rostain A, Jensen PS, Connor DF, et al. Toward quality care in ADHD: defining the goals of treatment. J Atten Disord 2013. [Epub ahead of print].

141. Ramos-Quiroga JA, Casas M. Achieving remission as a routine goal of pharmacotherapy in attention-deficit hyperactivity disorder. CNS Drugs 2011;25(1): 17–36.

142. O'Driscoll C, Heary C, Hennessy E, et al. Explicit and implicit stigma towards peers with mental health problems in childhood and adolescence. J Child Psychol Psychiatry 2012;53(10):1054–62.

143. Bussing R, Koro-Ljungberg M, Noguchi K, et al. Willingness to use ADHD treatments: a mixed methods study of perceptions by adolescents, parents, health professionals and teachers. Soc Sci Med 2012;74(1):92–100.

144. Walker JS, Coleman D, Lee J, et al. Children's stigmatization of childhood depression and ADHD: magnitude and demographic variation in a national sample. J Am Acad Child Adolesc Psychiatry 2008;47(8):912–20.

145. Law GU, Sinclair S, Fraser N. Children's attitudes and behavioural intentions towards a peer with symptoms of ADHD: does the addition of a diagnostic label make a difference? J Child Health Care 2007;11(2):98–111.

146. DosReis S, Barksdale CL, Sherman A, et al. Stigmatizing experiences of parents of children with a new diagnosis of ADHD. Psychiatr Serv 2010;61(8):811–6.

147. Pescosolido BA, Jensen PS, Martin JK, et al. Public knowledge and assessment of child mental health problems: findings from the national stigma study-children. J Am Acad Child Adolesc Psychiatry 2008;47(3):339–49.

148. Martin JK, Pescosolido BA, Olafsdottir S, et al. The construction of fear: Americans' preferences for social distance from children and adolescents with mental health problems. J Health Soc Behav 2007;48(1):50–67.

149. Bell L, Long S, Garvan C, et al. The impact of teacher credentials on ADHD stigma perceptions. Psychol Schools 2011;48(2):184–97.

150. Mikami AY, Reuland MM, Griggs MS, et al. Collateral effects of a peer relationship intervention for children with ADHD on typically developing classmates. Sch Psychol Rev 2013;42(4):458–76.

151. Pliszka S, AACAP Work Group on Quality Issues. Practice parameter for the assessment and treatment of children and adolescents with attention-deficit/hyperactivity disorder. J Am Acad Child Adolesc Psychiatry 2007;46:894–921.
152. Smith BH, Waschbusch DA, Willoughby MT, et al. The efficacy, safety, and practicality of treatments for adolescents with attention-deficit/hyperactivity disorder (ADHD). Clin Child Fam Psychol Rev 2000;3(4):243–67.

Social Skills Training for Youth with Autism Spectrum Disorders: A Follow-Up

Tiffany L. Otero, MSEd[a],*, Rochelle B. Schatz, MSEd[a],
Anna C. Merrill, BA[a], Scott Bellini, PhD[b]

KEYWORDS

• Autism • Social skills • Youth • Interventions • Evidence-based practice

KEY POINTS

• Social communication remains one of the core deficits associated with autism spectrum disorders.
• Several interventions with strong empirical support are available for practitioners to choose from and information on them is readily available.
• Strategies are most successful when they are implemented with fidelity and match the individual's skill deficit.
• Assessment measures have been updated to identify social deficits and to align more closely with DSM-5 diagnostic criteria.

INTRODUCTION

The substantial increase in prevalence rates for autism spectrum disorders (ASD) over the last 10 years has sparked debate regarding cause and critical need for effective services. The most recent reports released by the Centers for Disease Control and Prevention (CDC) estimate that as many as 1 in every 68 children are affected by ASD, a 78% increase from 2002 to 2010.[1] It affects more boys than girls with prevalence estimates being as high as 1 in 42 boys being diagnosed with ASD compared with 1 in 189 girls. The increase in prevalence rates has been referred to as an "epidemic" by some autism organizations and news organizations. However, the

Funding: There are no known funding sources to disclose.
Conflicts of Interest: There are no known conflicts of interest.
[a] School Psychology Program, Department of Counseling and Educational Psychology, Indiana University, W.W. Wright School of Education, 201 North Rose Avenue, Bloomington, IN 47405, USA; [b] Department of Counseling and Educational Psychology and Social Skills Research Clinic, Indiana University, W.W. Wright School of Education, 201 North Rose Avenue, Bloomington, IN 47405, USA
* Corresponding author. Department of Curriculum and Instruction, Indiana University School of Education, 201 North Rose Avenue, Bloomington, IN 47405-1006.
E-mail address: tlotero@umail.iu.edu

Child Adolesc Psychiatric Clin N Am 24 (2015) 99–115
http://dx.doi.org/10.1016/j.chc.2014.09.002
1056-4993/15/$ – see front matter © 2015 Elsevier Inc. All rights reserved.

childpsych.theclinics.com

Abbreviations	
ASD	Autism spectrum disorders
CBI	Cognitive behavioral intervention
CDC	Centers for Disease Control and Prevention
DSM	Diagnostic and Statistical Manual of Mental Disorder
EBP	Evidence-based practices
ESDM	Early Start Denver Model
NAC	National Autism Center
NPDC	National Professional Development Center on Autism Spectrum Disorders
PRT	Pivotal response training
SCD	Social (pragmatic) communication disorder
SRS-2	Social Responsiveness Scale-2
SSIS	Social Skills Improvement System
SSRS	Social Skills Rating System
SST	Social skills training
VSM	Video self-modeling

CDC has pointedly chosen to avoid using the term "epidemic," opting instead to refer to the increase as an "important public health concern." Irrespective of the terms used to describe the increase in prevalence, the demand for effective intervention modalities for youth with ASD has never been greater. Educators, therapists, and physicians have been inundated with an increase in the number of students and patients with ASD in their classrooms and clinics.

Definition of Autism

The definition of autism has changed several times since first described by Leo Kanner[2] in 1943. However, one characteristic has remained consistent: a marked impairment in social relatedness. In fact, "social communication" remains 1 of the 2 core deficits of ASD in the most recent edition of the Diagnostic and Statistical Manual of Mental Disorder (DSM-5).[3] According to the manual, characteristic deficits in social communication and social interaction occur across multiple contexts. Specifically, they include the following:

1. Deficits in social emotional reciprocity
2. Deficits in nonverbal communicative behaviors used for social interaction
3. Deficits in developing, maintaining, and understanding relationships.

Historically, the impairment in social relatedness presents itself in several ways, including limited eye contact, limited engagement with others, a tendency to be alone, impaired Theory of Mind, deficits in social reciprocity, and the inability to infer sociocultural constructs of interaction.[4–8]

Asperger Syndrome

The 1994 release of the DSM-IV introduced Asperger syndrome as one of the diagnoses to fall under the umbrella of Autism Spectrum Disorders. Individuals diagnosed with Asperger syndrome have characteristic deficits in social skills and display specific interests or preferences or may have repetitive or stereotypical behaviors. However, they lack impairment in language development and have an IQ ranging from low average to highly gifted. The recent issue of the DSM-5 has removed the diagnosis of Asperger syndrome, offering only a diagnosis of ASD with the notation of mild, moderate, or severe. In addition, a separate diagnosis of Social (Pragmatic)

Communication Disorder (SCD) has been added. Although it is too early to tell how the change to the definition will impact the identification rate of ASD, there remains a growing population of individuals impacted by social communication deficits. Given the common deficits associated with ASD and SCD, this prevalence has tremendous implications for future work as educators and clinicians, primarily because these skills are critical to successful social, emotional, and cognitive outcomes.[9]

Lack of Social Skills in Autism Spectrum Disorders

Some researchers argue that of the core deficits associated with ASD, perhaps the most debilitating, is the lack of social skills.[7] For those youth who fall along the high-functioning end of the spectrum, significant deficits in social skills combined with a level of intelligence that falls within the normal to gifted range minimize the cultural understanding and empathy typically received by those with a more profound and obvious disability. As a result, these children are often targets of bullying and social rejection, which further increase their social isolation and take a tremendous toll on their emotional and cognitive well-being.[10] In fact, Tantam[11(p367)] stated, "It has been said that the 'mildness' of the handicap in Asperger Disorder is what makes its emotional and social impact so severe." For an adolescent, impairments in social communication skills can lead to a variety of negative outcomes, including poor academic achievement,[12] social anxiety,[13] and poor self-esteem and depression.[11] Given the magnitude of difficulty encountered with even mild forms of the disability, it is imperative to consider treatment options for this vulnerable population.

Fortunately, there is an extensive body of research that has been done to address the social skill deficits commonly associated with ASD. In 2008, Bellini and Peters[14] provided an overview of child-specific practices used to build social skills in youth with ASD. Because child-specific approaches continue to be used most often by practitioners in clinical settings, this article focuses on those types of interventions. Child-specific approaches are those that include the following[15(p361)]:

a. General instructional interventions to increase knowledge and social problem-solving (including social stories)
b. High-density reinforcement to "prime" social responding
c. Social skills training
d. Adult-mediated prompting and reinforcement
e. Various generalization promotion techniques (particularly self-monitoring).

In recent years, there has been significant attention to developing and disseminating information regarding social skill interventions that have consistently demonstrated positive outcomes for those with ASD. In the past decade, several empirically supported child-specific social skill interventions have been established through systematic reviews of the literature.[16–18] Reichow and Volkmar[18] examined the empirical evidence of recently studied social skill interventions within the framework of a best evidence synthesis. The findings suggest there is much empirical evidence supporting many different treatments for the social deficits of individuals with ASD. The effectiveness of social skill groups and video modeling has accumulated the evidence necessary for the classifications of established evidence-based practices (EBP) and "promising" EBP, respectively.

Evidence-based Practices for Youth with Autism Spectrum Disorder

Committee work devoted to the identification and dissemination of EBPs for youth with ASD has further elucidated effective practices. The National Professional

Development Center on Autism Spectrum Disorders (NPDC) is a multiuniversity center that functions to review literature, provide professional development and assistance, and further evaluate the use of EBPs in schools across the United States. Using rigorous evaluation criteria, the center has identified 27 EBPs as of their most recent report.[19] Also, in 2005, the National Autism Center (NAC) initiated the National Standards Project in hopes of providing resources to parents and practitioners that allow them to make well-informed decisions regarding the interventions they choose for a child with ASD.[20] After an exhaustive review of the literature, they have categorized interventions based on the level of support they have received in the research. Established interventions are those that have consistently demonstrated positive outcomes and are determined to be effective interventions for youth with ASD. Emerging interventions are those that show promise but have a research base that is either still developing or has inconsistent outcomes. The remaining category lists those interventions that are unestablished, or those interventions for which there is little or no evidence to demonstrate that they are effective.

To follow up the report by Bellini and Peters,[14] research on social skill interventions published from 2008 to the present has been reviewed. In the following sections, an overview of social skills training (SST) is provided as well as the research on social skill interventions by describing the findings of recent meta-analyses that have examined more than one social skills intervention strategy. Then, a descriptive synthesis of child-specific social skills intervention programs that have emerged or have continued to develop as EBP (as considered by the NAC and NPDC on ASD) is provided. Finally, advancements in the assessment of social skills are reviewed.

OVERVIEW OF SOCIAL SKILLS TRAINING

SST procedures involve the application of techniques to enhance the social behaviors of individuals who experience social deficits. Specifically, SST "refers to instruction that facilitates the acquisition or performance of social skills."[14(p858)] The NPDC on ASD defines SST as:

Group or individual instruction designed to teach learners with autism spectrum disorders (ASD) ways to appropriately interact with peers, adults, and other individuals. Most social skill meetings include instruction on basic concepts, role-playing or practice, and feedback to help learners with ASD acquire and practice communication, play, or social skills to promote positive interactions with peers.[19(p21)]

SST is considered an EBP by the NPDC on ASD. The NAC has this categorized as a Social Skills Package and has it ranked as an emerging practice. This discrepancy is not unexpected. First, the NAC standards were published in 2009, whereas the NPDC report was released early this year, allowing for more research to be included in the NPDC report. In addition, although there are several strategies that have shown success in increasing social skills for youth having ASD, given the variation among the delivery of SST programs and small sample sizes, the assessment of quality of an intervention is difficult to determine.[17,21]

Typically, social skills are taught in small group settings with 5 to 8 participants with a teacher or adult facilitator.[22] Within social skills groups, a variety of evidence-based techniques can be used to teach several social interaction skills, including, but not limited to, emotional regulation, basic conversation skills, nonverbal communication skills, perspective taking, initiating, responding, and maintaining a social interaction. Given the evidence, as long as interventions used in combination are administered with fidelity, they can be used in a group or with individual children and can yield positive results.

META-ANALYTIC REVIEWS OF SOCIAL SKILLS INTERVENTIONS

Since 2008, meta-analytic reviews have been conducted to examine the collective outcomes of SST and to establish the efficacy of various social intervention strategies. Wang and Spillane[23] reviewed the literature on social skills interventions published between 1997 and 2008. They identified 5 categories of social skill interventions including social stories, peer-mediated interventions, video modeling, cognitive behavioral training, and other. Using a percentage of nonoverlapping data scores, the authors concluded that of the 5 categories, only video modeling met the criteria for being evidence-based and demonstrating high-effectiveness as an intervention strategy. The remaining strategies showed promise, but had moderate effectiveness. The authors concluded that more research is needed to establish these strategies as evidence-based. These findings are consistent with those of previous meta-analyses, which found low to questionable effectiveness and generalization of social skills interventions.[9]

In addition, de Bruin and colleagues[24] evaluated 4 categories of interventions for youth with ASD implemented in a public-school setting. Dependent variables for the studies included academic, functional, and social skills. Antecedent interventions were those strategies that were implemented before the targeting behavior or setting and included social stories, chaining, modeling, task sequencing, strategy training, prompting, and time delay. Consequence interventions were those that were generally applied after the targeted skill or behavior occurred and included praise, contingency mapping, error correction, differential reinforcement, and embedded instruction. Self-management interventions were those that required youth to observe, record, and evaluate their own behavior. These strategies included self-monitoring, self-reinforcement, self-recording, and self-management. Finally, video interventions used some sort of video component with feedback and included video modeling, video scheduling, and video prompting. Based on the number of quality investigations for each category, the authors determined that antecedent, consequence, and video interventions were considered evidence-based. Using percentage of all non-overlapping data, the authors determined that video interventions demonstrated the most consistently favorable outcomes. Consequence and antecedent interventions resulted in moderate outcomes. Self-management procedures also had positive outcomes, but there were not enough studies to establish a meaningful average effect size.

In another meta-analysis, the authors used hierarchical linear modeling to evaluate the effectiveness of social skill interventions examined via a single case design.[25] They found that, in general, social skill interventions are effective at improving the social functioning of youth with ASD. However, their findings differ from other previous analyses[26] in that intervention length, gender and age of participants, and the quality of the research methods did not significantly impact the efficacy of the interventions. The only variable that significantly affected the intervention effectiveness was the single-case design chosen, with multiple-baseline and reversal methods demonstrating the most dramatic outcomes.

SOCIAL SKILLS INTERVENTION STRATEGIES

Eight strategies have been identified, including cognitive behavioral intervention (CBI), modeling, naturalistic intervention, pivotal response training (PRT), self-management, social narratives, technology-aided instruction, and video-modeling. Four strategies that appeared in the article by Bellini and Peters (2008)[14] will not be described. Social problem-solving has not met sufficient criteria to be evidence-based on its own; however, it may still be used within other EBPs such as cognitive-behavioral intervention.

Prompting, priming, and scripting have also been excluded from this synthesis because recent research has typically evaluated these strategies as components of "treatment packages" and not as the primary intervention strategy for social skills. For more information regarding these interventions, please refer to the NPDC Evidence Based Practices Report[19] and the findings of the NAC's National Standards Project.[20]

Cognitive Behavioral Intervention

CBI, or cognitive behavioral therapy, is a therapeutic method that focuses on targeting positive and negative thought processes to change behavior. It is used primarily with those who experience anxiety or difficulty controlling expressions of anger and aggressive behavior. Individuals using CBI are taught to identify their feelings and the thoughts associated with those feelings and then use strategies to express their behavior in a more appropriate manner. According to the literature, it is effective with youth from elementary school age to high school.[27] Although CBI has been used to address living skills, anger and anxiety management, and communication skills, it has also been used to address social skill deficits for youth with ASD. Social problem-solving may also be targeted in some CBI, as participants are required to assess a social situation and decide on an appropriate plan of action. Some researchers have posited that social skill deficits occur as a function of avoidance due to increased social anxiety.[13] Therefore, by addressing the thoughts and feelings associated with social anxiety, one may learn to function in a more socially appropriate manner.

Research shows that CBI is typically administered in a group setting and in combination with other social skill intervention strategies. In a review of the literature on SST groups, Cappadocia and Weiss[28] found that groups that used some form of CBI demonstrated gains in skills using premeasures and postmeasures, more so than those that used traditional training (instruction and feedback only) and those with a parent component. However, on closer review of the techniques used in the different types of groups, the authors noted that the primary difference among the group of CBI social skill groups was the amount of intervention hours provided, and not the CBI techniques. CBI features such as identifying feelings and self-evaluation were used in some form even in the traditional groups and the parent groups. However, the CBI groups offered between 50 and 180 hours of intervention, whereas the traditional and parent groups offered no more than 18 and 30 hours of intervention, respectively. Therefore, longer or more intense interventions may result in greater outcomes.

Cotugno[29] created 4 social skill groups. Using a combination of group therapy, CBI, and skills instruction techniques within a developmental framework, participants met weekly with a lead facilitator for 1 hour for 30 weeks. Each session was structured to address a developmental stage through targeted activities. For example, in a group session, participants may choose from activities focused on group cohesion and then have an evaluative discussion following the activity to address skills learned and problem solved. Using pretest and posttest measures, teacher and parent ratings demonstrated a significant improvement in skills in the areas of anxiety management, joint attention, and flexibility/transitions. White and colleagues[30] described the development of a program that used CBI to alleviate anxiety experienced by youth with ASD and increase social competence. They completed an initial study to test the feasibility of the program and found it to be promising in that it is acceptable to their participants and can be implemented with fidelity. Research to determine treatment outcomes are currently underway. Other studies reported that the use of CBI in group settings was effective in increasing executive functioning skills, facial recognition, problem-solving,

Theory of Mind, reading nonverbal cues, and accurately describing how to respond in a social situation.[31,32]

Modeling

Modeling involves the demonstration of a skill in order for a learner to imitate the skill. Typically, when modeling is used as an intervention strategy, it occurs within an intervention package and not in isolation. When used in conjunction with repetition, praise, and reinforcement, skill acquisition can take place. In the first randomized control trial study of a social intervention for 2-year-olds with ASD, Landa and colleagues[33] found that intervention groups that used modeling procedures among other strategies benefitted participants. Participants made gains in socially engaged imitation, expressive language, and cognitive and social functioning abilities. Similarly, modeling, prompting, and reinforcement were used to teach empathy responses to 4 children with ASD. Researchers used dolls and puppets to express affect, such as sadness, pain, or fear, and participants were taught to respond empathetically. In addition, generalization of the empathy responses was observed, but decreased as time passed.[34] When compared with a video-modeling intervention, the most recent research has shown that video-modeling and in vivo modeling have similar effectiveness in terms of gains in social skills; however, the participants were more visually attentive to video models, and practitioners found the video-modeling condition to be slightly more preferred than in vivo modeling.[35]

Naturalistic Intervention

Naturalistic intervention is a behavior therapy technique that uses manipulations of the natural environment, and interaction strategies to develop social communication skills in youth with ASD. The primary difference between naturalistic intervention and more formalized behavioral therapy is that naturalistic interventions typically occur in the child's natural environment and is embedded within the child's routines that may be naturally reinforcing. For example, a practitioner may layout the child's favorite toys and elicit requests from the child based on the toys they most prefer. By using already established reinforcement routines, teachers, parents, and other practitioners can build more skills that are appropriate to the context.

In a study demonstrating the effectiveness of this type of intervention on the neural activity of participants, the investigators implemented the Early Start Denver Model (ESDM) with children ranging in ages from 18 to 30 months old for 2 years.[36] The ESDM is a naturalistic teaching strategy that uses a variety of agents (ie, teachers, parents, clinicians) to encourage children to engage socially within their own preferred tasks. Applied behavioral analysis strategies, such as reinforcement and prompting, are used systematically throughout the session to encourage communication, joint attention, and socialization. For comparison, the investigators had a neurotypical comparison group and another control group of children with ASD who received therapies typically offered in the community.

After 2 years of using this intervention, samples from the 3 groups of children participated in an EEG while images of faces and images of objects were flashed in front of them. Children who received the ESDM intervention showed a shorter latency in the attention-related event-related potential and increased cortical activation when faces were shown and opposite when objects were shown. This pattern is the same as was observed in neurotypical children. However, children with ASD who solely received community interventions had the reverse pattern. They had more cortical activation and shorter event-related potential latency in response to objects than in response to faces. Another study compared a naturalistic intervention strategy with a developmental social pragmatic intervention in which adults increased their responsiveness to the child. Remaining consistent with previous findings, the authors found that the naturalistic intervention condition and a combined condition resulted in greater gains in social communication skills for 4 young children with ASD.[37]

Pivotal Response Training

PRT is a naturalistic intervention strategy based on the principles of applied behavior analysis. Similar to naturalistic interventions, it uses the child's existing interests, settings, and routines to target desired skill acquisition.[38] Specifically, PRT allows the child to choose the activity and provides the child with systematic reinforcement for every correct response and appropriate attempt to respond that the child makes.[39] What makes this approach unique is that it is designed to enhance specific learning variables, or pivotal skills, that are thought to underlie other more complex skills. These pivotal skills are motivation, responding to multiple cues, self-management, and self-initiation.[38] More recently, PRT has been found to be extremely effective in teaching symbolic, manipulative, and sociodramatic play skills to youth with ASD. The newly acquired skills have also been generalized to new toys and new adults.[39]

Developed as an alternative to interventions focused on single target behaviors,[40] PRT has a long history of success and has been considered an evidence-based practice by both the NPDC and an established practice by the NAC. Most published PRT intervention studies are implemented with individuals, as opposed to a group, yet the implementers have ranged from researchers/clinicians to parents, primary care takers, peers, and teachers. An analysis of many studies targeting social skills functioning through the use of PRT was conducted, and the results indicate that having different intervention implementers aided with the generalizability of the skills being taught.[41]

Many PRT interventions emphasize a focus on parent involvement to support the goal of producing naturalized behavioral improvements.[42,43] As there is an ever-increasing demand for access to effective interventions for families who have children with ASD, more evidence-based resources are being developed for this purpose. Nefdt and colleagues[44] created a self-directed learning program using an interactive DVD to provide parents of children with ASD with introductory PRT. The findings indicate that most parents who completed the program demonstrated learning of specified procedures, higher confidence levels during parent-child interactions, high satisfaction ratings, and an increase in the functional verbal sounds made by their children with ASD. Minjarez and colleagues[43] found that, in addition to individual training, a group training model for parents is also beneficial in targeting specific language-based and communication-based deficits in youth with ASD. In an effort to further extend knowledge on PRT implementation, Robinson[45] examined a modeling and video-based feedback training package to enable paraprofessionals to implement PRT in the school environment. Because children spend most of their days in school settings, schools are another key naturalistic location for them to receive intervention. The paraprofessionals who were taught using this technique demonstrated maintenance of the PRT implementation several weeks afterward, and each of the youth who participated in the study demonstrated positive improvements in each of their social communication target behaviors.

Self-Management

Self-management refers to strategies that are used to teach children how to identify, record, assess, and manage their behavior. According to Rafferty,[46] there are 5 types of self-management interventions that are frequently used to help foster self-regulated performance:

1. Self-monitoring
2. Goal setting
3. Self-evaluation
4. Self-instruction
5. Strategy instruction.

Self-monitoring is a strategy commonly used to develop self-regulation skills and involves the observation and recording of one's own behavior. Typically, children are taught to record their behavior following a specific prompt, such as a tone from an interval timer. Goals are set based on the occurrence or nonoccurrence of the target behavior, and children may evaluate their performance in relation to their goals. It has been shown to be effective with a wide range of individuals from preschoolers to adults with and without disabilities on both academic and behavioral skills.[47,48] In addition, self-monitoring contributes to the development of self-management, which is a pivotal skill[40] that, when mastered, provides a catalyst to the mastery of several other related skills. This strategy is effective for youth with ASD because they commonly lack self-awareness and self-regulation skills.

Although research supports the utilization of this method as an EBP, "self-management" intervention packages in general vary widely in terms of the specific implementation strategies, making it difficult to determine the true effectiveness of this intervention.[49] In the most recent review of the literature on the use of self-management procedures to address core deficits of ASD, Southall and Gast[50] found that most studies using a self-management package use self-monitoring, self-recording, and self-reinforcement. Also, studies often used additional technologies such as tokens, videos, and pictures to make the intervention more attainable for those with more severe forms of ASD. Deitchman and colleagues[51] used self-management training during a video feedback session to increase the use of social initiations for 3 children with ASD. The children were video-taped entering the general education setting and interacting with their peers. Then, in daily feedback sessions, they reviewed the footage with the interventionist and were asked to observe and record their social initiations. The researchers found that the rate of social initiations increased for all participants. In addition, 2 of the participants increased their use of social initiations to novel settings and the behavior was maintained following the intervention.

Social Narratives

Social narratives encompass a variety of interventions that function to introduce and teach appropriate behavior via written story form, such as Social Stories, Power Cards, and other written story-based prompts. They may also include illustrations, pictures, and songs.[52] The most common of these are Social Stories, developed by Carol Gray. According to The Gray Center Web site, "A Social Story describes a situation, skill, or concept in terms of relevant social cues, perspectives, and common responses in a specifically defined style and format."[53] To be considered a Social Story, the written passage must contain the following statements[54]:

a. Descriptive: objective statements that describes the situation and the people in it
b. Perspective: statements that describe the reactions, feelings, and responses of others
c. Directive: statements that describe the appropriate action
d. Cooperative: statements that describe what others will do to help

e. Affirmative: statements that validate the common values of a given culture
f. Control: statements written or developed by the child that provide strategies for using the appropriate behaviors.

In general, Social Stories are read to the child before they enter the difficult situation being described in the story.

Power Cards are another intervention strategy that uses short written prompts to elicit desired behavior. The primary differentiation between Social Stories and Power Cards is that Power Cards incorporate the child's special interest area.[55] Special interests are common for youth with ASD and can be highly motivating in eliciting desired behaviors.[56] By using special interests, such as a favorite hero or character as the "person" describing the behavior to be changed, the child may be more inclined to attend to the Power Card and perform the desired skills.

A recent meta-analysis on the effectiveness of Social Stories[52] found that they resulted in low to questionable effects. This low to questionable effect is surprising given the strong attention that Social Stories have received in the past few years. However, on further examination of the scores, the authors found that the most of the studies reviewed either resulted in a high degree of effectiveness or were not effective at all, suggesting that not all youth may benefit equally from this intervention. Intervention effects were greater when the child was their own agent of the intervention, as opposed to having the story read by a parent, teacher, or researcher, and when it was read just before the situation described. In addition, simple stories presented within a brief time frame resulted in better outcomes for the child. Power Cards have demonstrated effectiveness in developing social behaviors, such as increasing the percentage of time that adolescents engaged in conversation outside of their preferred topic[57] and increasing pro-social playground behaviors of a 5-year-old boy with ASD.[56]

Technology-aided Instruction

Technology-aided instruction refers to any intervention in which technology (such as a computer, DVD/video, timer, or virtual environment) is used as the principal component of the intervention.[58] It is used to address a variety of behaviors including academic, social, and problem behaviors. Given the availability of technology to practitioners and families of those with disabilities, it may come as no surprise that technology-assisted interventions have become a popular and effective practice. In addition, many youth with ASD are more prone to interact with technology and, therefore, interventions using technology may be reinforcing in their design, further increasing their potential efficacy. Although the technology-aided interventions of video-modeling and self-monitoring (when a timer is used) are EBP on their own, there are other ways of using technology to address the unique characteristics of individuals with ASD.

DiGennaro Reed and colleagues[59] reviewed the literature on technology-aided interventions to teach social skills to youth with ASD. They found that the most interventions used video or DVDs and that most of the studies were aimed at initiation of conversations. Other types of technology commonly used were computer programs, tactile prompts (such as a vibrating timer or MotivAider), or audio scripts. Ramdoss and colleagues[60] reviewed computer-assisted interventions and found that these interventions were generally effective in producing positive outcomes in social skills, but there was great variability among the outcomes of the studies. However, those interventions in which the technology interventions and measurement tool was developed by the researcher showed the most positive outcomes.

Video Modeling

Video modeling and video self-modeling (VSM) are 2 of the most consistently success-ful methods of providing SST to youth with ASD. Video modeling refers to an individual watching a video that demonstrates a target behavior and then reproducing the same modeled behavior. VSM is a form of video modeling that enables the individual to perform specific, targeted behavior by watching himself or herself perform a positive behavior effectively.[14,61] Research suggests that VSM can generalize across multiple settings and that the learned skills throughout this process are sustained for months after the intervention.[62] The success of VSM has been demonstrated in a variety of areas when teaching youth with ASD.[35,63,64] Some of these areas include language, play, self-help, and social skills[65] and are particularly significant for youth with ASD, who have difficulty applying skills to multiple settings.[14] The VSM technique has shown to be especially effective for those with high-functioning ASD.

Wang and colleagues[66] conducted a meta-analysis to determine the effectiveness of peer-mediated and video-modeling techniques. Both peer-mediated interventions and video modeling were effective in improving the children's social behavior. How-ever, it seems that age functioned as a significant moderator between the effective-ness of the 2 types of intervention. Specifically, the results indicate that younger children may benefit more from both interventions than older children. This study pro-vides valuable evidence indicating that when children are younger, they receive the most positive outcomes from video-modeling interventions.

One study aimed at teaching vocational skills to adolescents with ASD in social set-tings.[67] In this study, using direct instruction and a multiple baseline design, 4 adoles-cents with ASD were taught how to dress as a mascot and entertain customers in a retail setting via VSM. The participants learned how to interact with customers in socially appropriate ways that both the managers and the customers appreciated. Kleeberger and Mirenda[68] also extended the application of VSM by measuring the effectiveness of interventions designed to address the generalized imitation deficit that is commonly seen in young youth with ASD. The results indicated that imitative behaviors could be significantly improved by providing video-modeling instructional techniques. Despite all of the evidence of the effectiveness of VSM, there was one study that did not find VSM to be effective for making gains in the frequency of social initiations.[69] As such, continued research is still needed in this area to determine best practices for the use of this technique across youth of different ages and setting.

ASSESSMENT OF SOCIAL FUNCTIONING

Since 2008, the development of social skill assessments has continued to grow. Re-visions have been made to old assessments and new assessments continue to be developed to measure social functioning in individuals with ASD. As reviewed by Bellini and Peters,[14] there are 3 different methods of measuring social functioning according to Gresham and colleagues[26]: type I, type II, and type III.

Type I Measures

Type I measures include rating scales and checklists administered to parents, teach-ers, and the child in the form of self-report measures. Some of the commonly used type I measures used in clinical and research settings have recently been updated to reflect information needed in effective intervention planning, such as the recent up-date to the Social Skills Rating System (SSRS).[70] Type I measures among the most common measures currently used to assess social functioning and include behavior rating scales and interviews that measure social competence or perception of social performance from key stakeholders such as teachers and parents. There are many advantages to type I measures. Type I measures are efficient and make it easy to obtain information regarding social behaviors in multiple settings and from a variety of sources. However, a disadvantage of type I measures is that they often provide general information about the development of social behaviors over time, but are not as helpful in tracking improvement during intervention when data must be collected frequently.[71]

There are several standardized social skills assessments that rely heavily on type I measures, such as rating scales completed by parents and teachers, that are used most commonly to assess social functioning of individuals with ASD. One of the most commonly used, and most researched, social skills assessments is the SSRS.[70] However, in 2008, an updated version of the assessment was released, called the Social Skills Improvement System (SSIS).[72] The SSIS is a rating scale for youth ages 3 to 18 that produces subscale scores on 3 dimensions:

1. Social skills
2. Problem behaviors
3. Academic competence.

The scales are used to screen for social difficulties and to assist in intervention planning, but are not specifically designed for individuals with ASD.[71]

Another social skills assessment that has been recently updated is the Social Responsiveness Scale. The Social Responsiveness Scale-2 (SRS-2)[73] includes self, parent, and teacher report scales that have been normed for use with youth between the ages of three and 18 years of age. Although the SSIS is not designed specifically for ASD, the SRS-2 is designed to measure social deficits in individuals with ASD from that age of 2 and one-half into adulthood. The SRS-2 produces an overall score to reflect the level of social functioning as well as scores on 5 treatment subscales: social awareness, social cognition, social communication, social motivation, and restricted interests and repetitive behavior. These new subscales were designed to align closely with the new DSM-5 criteria for ASD.

Type II Measures

Although type I measures assess the judgments and perspective of parents and teachers, type II measures include direct assessments of the individual's social functioning and behaviors. Type II measures are ideally suited for progress monitoring. Teachers and clinicians may wish to use type II measures when they would like to measure change in behavior after the implementation of an intervention. For example, observing a child in the classroom and collecting data on their behavior may be an example of a type II measure. Type II measures are effective in assessing current levels of functioning in a child's natural environment. These measures continue to be used extensively in applied research studies using a single-subject methodology to investigate the effectiveness of social skills interventions.

Type III Measures

The last of Gresham's 3 categories of social skills assessment are type III measures. Type III measures are assessments that use role-play scenarios and address questions regarding social cognition. Type III measures are highly useful in the measurement of social cognitive skills. For example, clinicians working in social skills groups can teach perspective-taking skills by creating scenarios in which the child is asked to infer the feelings and thoughts of others. A common example of a type III measure is the Sally-Anne false belief task[74] in which a child must predict the search behavior of a child that does not know his or her toy has been moved. Type II measures address social cognition and are not intended to be used to predict behavior in a natural setting. Type III measures are considered the least psychometrically sound of the 3 types of social skills assessment. In addition, research has not established a clear relationship between performance on type III measures and type I (ie, rating scales) or type II (ie, direct observation) measures.

Looking to the future, some researchers suggest that the number of social skills measures may, in fact, be overwhelming. Therefore, similar measures that have been shown to be reliable and valid should be combined.[75] Social skills measurement would benefit from comprehensive scales that are evidence-based that can be supplemented by more specific assessments that target precise social behaviors that are of interest to a particular case. In addition, future research should seek to develop more psychometrically sound social cognitive assessment measures.

SUMMARY

Social communication remains one of the core deficits associated with ASD. Given the increase in prevalence in recent years as well as the negative outcomes associated with limited social skills, it is important for practitioners to be knowledgeable of the EBPs that can be used to address these deficits. Fortunately, since 2008, the identification and dissemination of resources regarding the use of EBPs have been on the forefront of research efforts, allowing researchers and practitioners to make confident decisions regarding practices that may be efficacious. Not only are there several interventions for practitioners to choose from that have strong empirical support, information on them is readily available. In addition, assessment measures have been updated to identify social deficits and to align more closely with DSM-5 diagnostic criteria. Further research may focus on establishing best practices for SST interventions as well as developing comprehensive assessment tools.

REFERENCES

1. Kanner L. Autistic disturbances of affective contact. Nervous Child 1943;2: 217–50.
2. Autism and Developmental Disabilities Monitoring Network Surveillance Year 2010 Principal Investigators. Prevalence of autism spectrum disorder among children aged 8 years- Autism and Developmental Disabilities Monitoring Network, 11 sites, United States, 2010. Centers for Disease Control and Prevention. 2014. Available at http://www.cdc.gov/mmwr/preview/mmwrhtml/ss6302a1.htm?s_cid=ss6302a1_w. Accessed September 20, 2014.
3. American Psychiatric Association. Diagnostic and statistical manual of mental disorders. 5th edition. Arlington (VA): American Psychiatric Publishing; 2013.
4. Attwood T. Strategies for improving the social integration of children with Asperger Syndrome. Autism 2000;4(1):85–100.
5. Carrington S, Templeton E, Papinczak T. Adolescents with Asperger syndrome and perceptions of friendship. Focus Autism Other Dev Disabl 2003;18(4): 211–8.
6. Ochs E, Kremer-Sadlik T, Sirota K, et al. Autism and the social world: an anthropological perspective. Discourse Stud 2004;6(2):147–83.
7. Kroeger KA, Schultz JR, Newsom C. A comparison of two group-delivered social skills programs for young children with autism. J Autism Dev Disord 2006;37:808–17.

8. Lopata C, Thomeer ML, Volker MA, et al. Effectiveness of a manualized summer social treatment program for high-functioning children with autism spectrum disorders. J Autism Dev Disord 2007;38:890–904.
9. Bellini S, Peters J, Benner L, et al. A meta-analysis of school based social skills interventions for children with autism spectrum disorders. Remedial Spec Educ 2007;28:153–62.
10. Cappadocia MC, Weiss JA, Pepler D. Bullying experiences among children and youth with autism spectrum disorders. J Autism Dev Disord 2012;42(2):266–77. http://dx.doi.org/10.1007/s10803-01101241-x.
11. Tantam D. Adolescence and adulthood of individuals with Asperger syndrome. In: Klin A, Volkmar FR, Sparrow SS, editors. Asperger syndrome. New York: Guilford Press; 2000. p. 367–99.
12. Welsh M, Park RD, Widaman K, et al. Linkages between children's social and academic competence: a longitudinal analysis. J Sch Psychol 2001;39:463–81.
13. Bellini S. The development of social anxiety in high functioning adolescents with autism spectrum disorders. Focus Autism Other Dev Disabl 2006;21:138–45.
14. Bellini S, Peters J. Social skills training for youth with autism spectrum disorders. Child Adolesc Psychiatr Clin N Am 2008;17:857–73.
15. McConnell SR. Interventions to facilitate social interaction for young children with autism: review of available research and recommendations for educational intervention and future research. J Autism Dev Disord 2002;32:351–72.
16. Duncan AW, Klinger LG. Autism spectrum disorders: building social skills in group, school and community settings. Soc Work Groups 2010;33(2):175–93.
17. Rao PA, Beidel DC, Murray MJ. Social skills interventions for children with Asperger's syndrome or high-functioning autism: a review and recommendations. J Autism Dev Disord 2008;38:353–61.
18. Reichow B, Volkmar FR. Social skills interventions for individuals with autism: evaluation for evidence-based practices within a best evidence synthesis framework. J Autism Dev Disord 2010;40(2):149–66. http://dx.doi.org/10.1007/s10803-009-0842-0.
19. Wong C, Odom SL, Hume K, et al. Evidence-based practices for children, youth and young adults with autism spectrum disorder. Chapel Hill (NC): The University of North Carolina; Frank Porter Graham Child Development Institute; Autism Evidence-Based Practice Review Group; 2014.
20. National Autism Center. Findings and conclusions. National standards project. Randolph (MA): National Autism Center; 2009.
21. Rogers SJ, Vismara LA. Evidence-based comprehensive treatments for early autism. J Clin Child Adolesc Psychol 2008;37(1):8–38. http://dx.doi.org/10.1080/15374410701817808.
22. Collet-Klingenberg L. Overview of social skills groups. Madison (WI): The National Professional Development Center on Autism Spectrum Disorders; Waisman Center, University of Wisconsin; 2009.
23. Wang P, Spillane A. Evidence-based social sills interventions for children with autism: a meta-analysis. Educ Train Dev Disabil 2009;44(3):318–42.
24. de Bruin C, Deppeler J, Moore D, et al. Public school-based interventions for adolescents and young adults with an autism spectrum disorder: a meta-analysis. Rev Educ Res 2013;83(4):521–50.
25. Wang S, Parilla R, Cui Y. Meta-analysis of social skills interventions of single-case research for individuals with autism spectrum disorder: results from three-level HLM. J Autism Dev Disord 2013;43:1701–16. http://dx.doi.org/10.1007/s10803-012-1726-2.

26. Gresham FM, Sugai G, Horner RH. Interpreting outcomes of social skills training for students with high-incidence disabilities. Except Child 2001; 67(3):331–44.
27. Brock ME. Cognitive behavioral intervention (CBI) fact sheet. Chapel Hill (NC): The University of North Carolina; Frank Porter Graham Child Development Institute; The National Professional Development Center on Autism Spectrum Disorders; 2013.
28. Cappadocia MC, Weiss JA. Review of social skills training groups for youth with Asperger Syndrome and high-functioning autism. Res Autism Spectr Disord 2011;5(1):70–8.
29. Cotugno AJ. Social competence and social skills training and intervention for children with autism spectrum disorders. J Autism Dev Disord 2009;39(9):1268–77.
30. White SW, Albano AM, Johnson CR, et al. Development of a cognitive-behavioral intervention program to treat anxiety and social deficits in teens with high-functioning autism. Clin Child Fam Psychol Rev 2010;13(1):77–90. http://dx.doi.org/10.1007/s10567-009-0062-3.
31. Stitcher JP, Herzog MJ, Visovsky K, et al. Social competence intervention for youth with Asperger syndrome and high-functioning autism: an initial investigation. J Autism Dev Disord 2010;40(9):1067–79. http://dx.doi.org/10.1007/s10803-010-0959-1.
32. Koning C, Magill-Evans J, Volden J, et al. Efficacy of cognitive behavior therapy-based social skills intervention for school aged boys with autism spectrum disorders. Res Autism Spectr Disord 2011;7(10):1183–290.
33. Landa RJ, Holman KC, O'Neill AH, et al. Intervention targeting development of socially synchronous engagement in toddlers with autism spectrum disorder: a randomized controlled trial. J Child Psychol Psychiatry 2011;52(1):13–21. http://dx.doi.org/10.1111/j.1469-7610.2010.02288.x.
34. Schrandt JA, Townsend DB, Poulson CL. Teaching empathy skills to children with autism. J Appl Behav Anal 2009;42(1):17–32. http://dx.doi.org/10.1901/jaba.2009.42-17.
35. Wilson KP. Teaching social-communication skills to preschoolers with autism: efficacy of video versus in vivo modeling in the classroom. J Autism Dev Disord 2013;43(8):1819–31.
36. Dawson G, Jones EJH, Merkle K, et al. Early behavioral intervention is associated with normalized brain activity in young children with autism. J Am Acad Child Adolesc Psychiatry 2012;51(11):1150–9.
37. Ingersoll B, Meyer K, Bonter N, et al. A comparison of developmental social-pragmatic and naturalistic behavioral interventions on language use and social engagement in children with autism. J Speech Lang Hear Res 2010;55(5):1301–13.
38. Wong C. Pivotal response training (PRT) fact sheet. Chapel Hill (NC): The University of North Carolina; Frank Porter Graham Child Development Institute; The National Professional Development Center on Autism Spectrum Disorders; 2013.
39. Lydon H, Healy O, Leader G. A comparison of video modeling and pivotal response training to teach pretend play skills to children with autism spectrum disorder. Res Autism Spectr Disord 2011;5(2):872–84.
40. Koegel LK, Koegel RL, Harrower JK, et al. Pivotal response intervention I: overview of approach. J Assoc Pers Sev Handicaps 1999;24:174–85.
41. Genc GB, Vuran S. Examination of studies targeting social skills with pivotal response treatment. Educ Sci Theory Pract 2013;13(3):1730–42.

42. Coolican J, Smith IM, Bryson SE. Brief parent training in pivotal response treatment for preschoolers with autism. J Child Psychol Psychiatry 2010;51(12): 1321–30. http://dx.doi.org/10.1111/j.1469-7610.2010.02326.x.
43. Minjarez MB, Williams SE, Mercier EM, et al. Pivotal response group treatment program for parents of children with autism. J Autism Dev Disord 2011;41(1): 92–101.
44. Nefdt N, Koegel R, Singer G, et al. The use of a self-directed learning program to provide introductory training in pivotal response treatment to parents of children with autism. J Posit Behav Interv 2010;12(1):23–32.
45. Robinson SE. Teaching paraprofessionals of students with autism to implement pivotal response treatment in inclusive school settings using a brief video feedback training package. Focus Autism Other Dev Disabl 2011;26:105–18. http://dx.doi.org/10.1177/1088357611407063.
46. Rafferty L. Step-by-step: teaching students to self-monitor. Teaching Exceptional Children 2010;43(2):50–8.
47. Ganz JB. Self-monitoring across age and ability levels: teaching students to implement their own positive behavioral interventions. Prev Sch Fail 2008; 53(1):39–48.
48. Mooney P, Ryan JB, Uhing BB, et al. A review of self-management interventions targeting academic outcomes for students with emotional and behavioral disorders. J Behav Educ 2005;14(3):203–21.
49. Briesch AM, Chafouleas SM. A review and analysis of the literature on self-management interventions to promote appropriate classroom behaviors (1988-2008). Sch Psychol Q 2009;24:106–18.
50. Southall CM, Gast DL. Self-management procedures: a comparison across the autism spectrum. Educ Train Dev Disabil 2011;46(2):155–71.
51. Deitchman C, Reeve SA, Reeve KF, et al. Incorporating video feedback into self-management training to promote generalization of social initiations by children with autism. Educ Treat Children 2010;33:475–88.
52. Kokina A, Kern L. Social story™ interventions for students with autism spectrum disorders: a meta-analysis. J Autism Dev Disord 2010;40:812–26. http://dx.doi.org/10.1007/s10803-009-0931-0.
53. What are social stories™? The Gray Center website. Available at: http://www.thegraycenter.org/social-stories/what-are-social-stories. Accessed January 5, 2014.
54. Gray C. Social stories 10.0: the new defining criteria and guidelines. Jenison Autism Journal 2004;15:2–21.
55. Gagnon E. Power cards: using special interests to motivate children and youth with Asperger syndrome and autism. Shawnee Mission (KS): Autism Asperger Publishing; 2001.
56. Spencer V, Simpson CG, Day M, et al. Using the power cards strategy to teach social skills to a child with autism. Teaching Exceptional Children Plus 2008;5(1): 2–10.
57. Davis KM, Boon RT, Cihak DF, et al. Power cards to improve conversational skills of adolescents with Asperger syndrome. Focus Autism Other Dev Disabl 2010; 25:12–22.
58. Odom SL. Technology-aided instruction and intervention (TAII) fact sheet. Chapel Hill (NC): The University of North Carolina; Frank Porter Graham Child Development Institute; The National Professional Development Center on Autism Spectrum Disorders; 2013.
59. DiGennaro Reed FD, Hyman SR, Hirst JM. Applications of technology to teach social skills to children with autism. Res Autism Spectr Disord 2011;5:1003–10.

60. Ramdoss S, Machalicek W, Rispoli M, et al. Computer-based interventions to improve social and emotional skills in individuals with autism spectrum disorders: a systematic review. Dev Neurorehabil 2012;15(2):119–35.
61. Buggey T, Hoomes G, Sherberger ME, et al. Facilitating social initiations of preschoolers with autism spectrum disorders using video self-modeling. Focus Autism Other Dev Disabl 2011;26(1):25–36.
62. Shukla-Mehta S, Miller T, Callahan KJ. Evaluating the effectiveness of video instruction on social and communication skills training for children with autism spectrum disorders: a review of the literature. Focus Autism Other Dev Disabl 2010;25(1):23–36.
63. Plavnick JB, Sam AM, Hume K, et al. Effects of video-based group instruction for adolescents with autism spectrum disorder. Except Child 2013;80(1):67–83.
64. Van Laarhoven T, Kraus E, Karpman K, et al. A comparison of picture and video prompts to teach daily living skills to individuals with autism. Focus Autism Other Dev Disabl 2010;25(4):195–208. http://dx.doi.org/10.1177/1088357610380412.
65. Tereshko L, MacDonald R, Ahearn WH. Strategies for teaching children with autism to imitate response chains using video modeling. Res Autism Spectr Disord 2010;4(3):479–89. http://dx.doi.org/10.1016/j.rasd.2009.11.005.
66. Wang S, Cui Y, Parrila R. Examining the effectiveness of peer-mediated and video-modeling social skills interventions for children with autism spectrum disorders: a meta-analysis in single-case research using HLM. Res Autism Spectr Disord 2011;5(1):562–9. http://dx.doi.org/10.1016/j.rasd.2010.06.02.
67. Allen KD, Wallace DP, Renes D, et al. Use of video modeling to teach vocational skills to adolescents and young adults with autism spectrum disorders. Educ Treat Children 2010;33(3):339–49. http://dx.doi.org/10.1353/etc.0.0101.
68. Kleeberger V, Mirenda P. Teaching generalized imitation skills to a preschooler with autism using video modeling. J Posit Behav Interv 2010;12(2):116–27.
69. Buggey T. Effectiveness of video self-modeling to promote social initiations by 3-year-olds with autism spectrum disorders. Focus Autism Other Dev Disabl 2012;27(2):102–10.
70. Gresham FM, Elliot SN. Social skills rating system manual. Circle Pines (MN): American Guidance Service; 1990.
71. Gillis JM, Callahan EH, Romanczyk RG. Assessment of social behavior in children with autism: the development of the behavioral assessment of social interactions in young children. Res Autism Spectr Disord 2011;5(1):351–60.
72. Gresham F, Elliott S. Social skills improvement system (SSIS). Minneapolis (MN): Pearson Assessments; 2008.
73. Constantino JN, Gruber CP. Social responsiveness scale, 2nd edition (SRS-2). Torrance (CA): Western Psychological Services; 2012.
74. Baron-Cohen S, Leslie AM, Frith U. Does the autistic child have a "theory of mind?". Cognition 1985;21(1):37–46.
75. Matson JL, Wilkins J. Psychometric testing methods for children's social skills. Res Dev Disabil 2009;30(2):249–74.

Complementary and Alternative Medicine Treatments for Children with Autism Spectrum Disorders

Susan E. Levy, MD, MPH[a],*, Susan L. Hyman, MD[b]

KEYWORDS

- Autism • Autism spectrum • Complementary and alternative treatments
- Evidence based

KEY POINTS

- Families of children with autism spectrum disorders (ASD) commonly use complementary and alternative medical (CAM) treatments.
- CAM treatments are selected to promote wellness, treat specific symptoms, avoid side effects of conventional medicine, or promote resolution of core symptoms of ASD.
- Commonly used categories of CAM are natural products, mind and body therapies and other biomedical treatments.
- Conventional studies document that some CAM treatments are ineffective, whereas others require further study.

OVERVIEW

Autism spectrum disorders (ASD) are common neurodevelopmental disorders (affecting 1 in 68 children)[1] with a significant impact on the quality of life of child and family, owing to the constellation of core and associated symptoms. ASDs

Disclosures: Dr S.E. Levy was supported in part by National Institutes of Health R01 ES016443, Centers for Disease Control and Prevention U01-DD-000752, National Institute of Child Health and Human Development R01HD073258, and Autism Speaks – Autism Treatment Network; Dr S.L. Hyman was supported in part by Health Resources and Services Administration 2T73 MC00029-16-00 and UA3MC1105, National Institutes of Health R01 DC009439-02, and 1R34 MH100254 and Autism Speaks – Autism Treatment Network.
a Division of Developmental & Behavioral Pediatrics, The Children's Hospital of Philadelphia, Perelman School of Medicine, University of Pennsylvania, 3550 Market Street, 3rd Floor, Philadelphia, PA 19104, USA; b Neurodevelopmental and Behavioral Pediatrics, Golisano Children's Hospital, School of Medicine and Dentistry, University of Rochester School of Medicine and Dentistry, Rochester, NY 14642, USA
* Corresponding author.
E-mail address: levys@email.chop.edu

Child Adolesc Psychiatric Clin N Am 24 (2015) 117–143
http://dx.doi.org/10.1016/j.chc.2014.09.004
1056-4993/15/$ – see front matter © 2015 Elsevier Inc. All rights reserved.
childpsych.theclinics.com

Abbreviations	
ASD	Autism spectrum disorders
CAM	Complementary and alternative medical (treatments)
NCCAM	National Center for Complementary and Alternative Medicine
NHIS	National Health Interview Survey

have characteristic core deficits in communication-socialization and behavior, with a wide range of severity of symptoms.[2] Many treatments are recommended through collaborative medical, behavioral, and educational practice, but selection of treatment strategies is complicated by the impact of core deficits and frequently associated comorbid psychopathology.[3] Current scientific evidence strongly supports multifactorial genetic etiology,[4,5] with environmental factors also having an etiologic impact.[6] Thus for many children the specific causes are often not known. Furthermore, symptoms are behaviorally defined and heterogeneous, and will change over time with acquisition of developmental skills. As a result, families of children with autism and related disorders may find that the clinicians who diagnose their child's autism may sound vague about both cause and prognosis. This vagueness may turn families to therapies not based on conventional medical or psychological practice, proponents of which may present the treatment options as more concrete, definitive in etiology, and optimistic in outcome.[7]

This article provides an overview of commonly used complementary, alternative, or integrative health treatments that families of children with ASD may pursue. Many of these health care approaches are conceptualized outside of mainstream Western or conventional medicine[8] either to replace standard medical care or to supplement it. The combination of conventional practice and complementary techniques is often called integrative medicine. For ease of discussion, this article uses the term complementary and alternative medicine (CAM) to encompass all treatments that would fall under this integrative medicine rubric (not just biologically based medical treatments). This review discusses the reasons why families seek CAM, review the commonly used CAM therapies for ASD, and describes how conventional practitioners might work with patients who use CAM treatments.

The National Center for Complementary and Alternative Medicine (NCCAM) was established in 1991 as part of the National Institutes of Health to promote scientific study of CAM treatments, which it has promoted through education and direct support of research (www.nccam.nih.gov). NCCAM groups CAM therapies into 2 domains: Natural Products and Mind and Body Practices. Not included in these categories is the use of biological or biomedical treatments, which would also refer to psychopharmacologic or other pharmacologic agents used off-label to address a nonstandard hypothesis.

The use of CAM treatments by adults in the United States remains high. Analysis of data from the 2002 and 2007 National Health Interview Survey (NHIS) revealed rates of 36% and 38%, respectively, of any type of CAM treatment (excluding prayer) by United States adults.[9,10] Population-based data on the use of CAM treatments in children were available for the first time from the 2007 NHIS, reporting that 11.8% of children used CAM therapy in the 12 months before the survey.[9] This figure is likely to be an underestimate. Other reviews have reported a wide range of CAM use (2%–50%) in children, but these data are derived from selected groups and are not population based (as in the NHIS survey)[11]

TYPES OF TREATMENTS IN USE

Table 1 lists the categories and types of CAM treatments classified according to NCCAM and how they are administered, empirical evidence for effectiveness, and advantages and disadvantages of each therapy. CAM in adults is big business. In 2007, adults in the United States spent $33.9 billion out of pocket on purchases of CAM products, practitioner visits, and other related activities,[12] an increase from $21.2 billion in 1997.[13] The most commonly used CAM treatments in adults are in the category of natural products (17.7%) and mind and body practices (6.1%–12.7%).[9] Most often, adults use CAM to treat musculoskeletal pain and other chronic conditions.

WHO USES COMPLEMENTARY AND ALTERNATIVE TREATMENTS AND WHY

Studies report that children with chronic illnesses, such as cancer, asthma, rheumatoid arthritis, attention-deficit/hyperactivity disorder, genetic disorders (eg, Down syndrome), cerebral palsy, and other neurodevelopmental disorders are treated with CAM therapies at higher rates (24%–75%).[7,14–17] Families of children with ASD have even higher rates of usage (28%–95%).[18–20] The occurrence of comorbid disorders and increased severity of symptoms of autism is associated with increased use of CAM.[18–20]

The most commonly used CAM treatments for ASD reflecting similar patterns of use in adults and children with other chronic disorders are[18,21]:

- With natural products: 13% to 54%
- Special diet: 17% to 33%
- Mind and body practices: 25% to 30%

As in adults, the most commonly used treatments in the 2007 NHIS survey of CAM use in children were mind and body practices and natural products. Children whose parents used CAM were 2 times more likely to use CAM than those whose parents did not.

CAM treatments include therapies used in combination with mainstream approaches (complementary) and, less commonly, in place of conventional treatments (alternative) (www.nccam.nih.org). Reasons for use of CAM treatments vary, but usually target treatment of hypothetical causes of specific disorders or illnesses or for general wellness purposes.[9,22] Studies of CAM in adults have started to differentiate these purposes, but studies in children have not advanced to this level. A recent study by Davis and colleagues[22] identified respondents to the NHIS 2007 survey as nonusers (75%) and CAM treatment users (25%). Users were categorized into treatment only, health promotion only, and mixed users, and the investigators identified different characteristics of health behaviors and utilization. It was estimated that:

- 17.4% of adults used CAM to treat illness
- 27.4% used CAM for health promotion
- 13% were mixed users

By self-report, health promotion users were healthier, treatment users had higher rates of conventional use of medical care, and treatment users consumed more services. As already described, it appears that few adults are using these treatments as alternative care.

There are more specific reasons for use of CAM treatments beyond treatment of disorders and general wellness. Goals of treatment may include[9]:

Table 1
Types of CAM treatments

Type of Products[a]	Provider Based or No Provider	Efficacy/Effectiveness	Advantage	Disadvantage	Cost
Natural Products Herbs Vitamins, minerals, supplements Probiotics	No provider	Little research validation of efficacy or documentation of side effects	Consumer driven	Not FDA regulated No oversight of potential side effects or management Consumer driven	Out-of-pocket expenses
Mind and Body Practices Auditory integration Acupuncture Equine therapy Healing touch Hypnotherapy Massage therapy, qigong Music therapy Physical manipulation Yoga	Provider based	Little research validation of efficacy or documentation of side effects	Consumer driven Low potential for negative side effects and complication	Guidance nonmedical Lack of knowledge by medical practitioners Lack of regulatory oversight in some treatment	Out-of-pocket expenses
Other Biomedical Treatments Off-label prescription medications Other medical treatments Specialized or elimination diets	Provider based	Little research validation of efficacy or documentation of side effects	Perception of "cure"	High potential for negative side effects and complications Most guidance for use in community, lay press, or Internet Guidance nonmedical Lack of knowledge by medical practitioners Lack of regulatory oversight for some treatments High cost may interfere with ability to obtain other treatments	Out of pocket, may be expensive

Abbreviation: FDA, US Food and Drug Administration.
[a] Classified according to the National Center for Complementary and Alternative Medicine (www.nccam.nih.gov).

- Relief of specific symptoms (eg, pain, musculoskeletal symptoms, gastrointestinal symptoms)
- Alleviation of side effects of conventional treatments
- Philosophic reasons (eg, holistic health philosophy)
- Wanting greater control over health management

Many CAM treatments are perceived as "natural," without the potential side effects of conventional medical treatments.[23,24]

Use of Complementary and Alternative Medical in Families of Children with Autism Spectrum Disorder

Families of children with ASD may have wellness promotion among their reasons for electing nonstandard therapies, but they use CAM to treat symptoms of autism in general, comorbid symptoms (such as attention, hyperactivity, irritability, moodiness, gastrointestinal symptoms, seizures, sleep, and tactile sensitivity).[25,26] In some instances they select CAM when conventional therapies do not seem to affect core symptoms in an attempt to provide more comprehensive treatment.[15] Other families report the use of CAM to address concerns about negative side effects of conventional treatments.[7] Most importantly, most families who use CAM use more than 1 CAM treatment. Clinicians must be aware of this and must monitor for interactions of therapies, and the impact the cost and energy to provide CAM therapies may have on prescribed treatments.[19,27]

Despite the increasing trend for children with chronic illnesses such as ASD to be served in a primary care practice that can be a "medical home" where families can develop relationships with a clinician, most families continue to obtain their information about CAM from other sources. A survey of parents by Wong and Smith[28] reported the frequency of sources of information about CAM treatment:

- Family and the community members: 35%
- Physicians: 23%
- Other nonmedical professionals: 4% to 27%
- Internet: 23%
- Books: 15%

It is most notable that families reported that they rarely asked physicians for information about CAM. The proliferation of Internet-based lay communities and Web sites that are promoting untested treatments have increased the exposure of families to large volumes of information about treatments with potential harm. Sites often promote the use of bioactive substances without medical monitoring, and this has added stress to the relationship between families and medical providers. Conventional clinicians may not feel comfortable advising patients about treatments with little scientific basis in the conventional literature,[15] and this has a direct negative impact on the likelihood of shared decision making between medical providers and families about treatment choices. Many families do not tell their physician that they are using CAM. Reasons for lack of disclosure include a perception of physician's lack of knowledge about CAM therapies, lack of time for discussion, not seeing the necessity of reporting the use of other therapies, and concern regarding disapproval by the physician.[15,28]

EVIDENCE FOR COMPLEMENTARY AND ALTERNATIVE THERAPIES

Given the frequency of use of CAM treatments and that many families may not inform their provider of such use, practitioners must be aware of factors associated with the use, methods to evaluate evidence for efficacy and/or effectiveness, and how to negotiate with families for safe care. **Table 1** lists categories of CAM treatments and examples of each, providing an overview of available research, and advantages and disadvantages of the treatments.

For the purposes of this article, the authors have reviewed the available literature regarding CAM treatments (with emphasis on advances since the previous article)[7] and have assigned a grade for the strength of the research. In many instances a comprehensive systematic review was not possible because the evidence or studies did not exist and could not be compared. The authors have followed the recommendations of the GRADE (Grading of Recommendations Assessment, Development and Evaluation) Working Group, focused on rating the quality of evidence through systematic review to enable providers to develop and present recommendations for treatment.[29] The working group has graded evidence as[30]:

- High: several high-quality studies or randomized trials
- Moderate: one high-quality study or several with some limitations
- Low: study or studies with severe limitations
- Very low: no direct research evidence or expert opinion

For consistency, after reviewing the evidence for different treatments (consistent with the rubric of GRADE ratings) the authors have assigned scores for studies involving CAM treatments (**Box 1**). **Table 2** provides an overview of evidence-based support for selected treatments.

Natural Products

Natural products include a variety of products available to consumers over the counter, for which no prescription or recommendation by a licensed clinician is needed. These products may be administered as an oral or topical preparation, and are often sold as dietary supplements or neutraceuticals. Such products are consumer driven; that is, there is easy access by families. However, in many cases guidance or encouragement for their use may come from non–peer-reviewed sources (such as the community, lay press, or Internet), and this may play a role in lack of guidance or monitoring for potential side effects. Medical practitioners often lack the knowledge to guide consumers if they are informed by families of these products.

Mind and Body Practices

Mind and body practices are a diverse group of procedures or techniques administered or taught by a trained practitioner or teacher, on an individual or group basis. Most require ongoing treatment or support by trained practitioner. Acupuncture is administered individually, by a licensed acupuncturist. Hypnotherapy may be administered by a licensed provider (therapist or medical provider). Equine therapy may be provided in the context of a physical or occupational therapy treatment program or by an independent provider. Massage therapy is singular, administered by a variety of

Box 1 Scores for studies involving CAM treatments	
Score	**Qualifications**
A	>1 high-quality study with consistent results *or* 1 large multicenter trial
B	1 high-quality study *or* several studies with mild limitations
C	1 study with severe limitations
D	No evidence/theories/multiple studies with very severe limitations

Table 2
Evidence-based support for treatments

Treatments	Evidence	Comments	Rating of Evidence
Natural Products			
Herbal products[34]	No specific studies of herbs and autism	No studies; no recommendations	D
Vitamins/minerals/supplements[35,36]	Randomized DB/PC trials with vitamin mineral supplement. Outcome measures included PGI-R and symptoms of hyperactivity, tantruming, and changes in biotin and vitamin K	Significant methodological problems	C
Vitamin A[37]	No evidence; theories	No evidence of effectiveness; significant potential for harm	D
Vitamin C[38-40]	2 DB PC trials showing improved sensorimotor, sleep, and GI symptoms and differences in vitamin C levels Other reference theoretic, ascribing cause(s) of ASD associated with oxidative stress	Some preliminary evidence; toxicity not significant	B
Vitamin D[35,41-47]	Treatment based on circumstantial evidence: symptoms of ASD during 2nd and 3rd year of life when vitamin D may be low; correlation of UV-B doses in USA with prevalence; relationship of vitamin D hormone (calcitriol) and serotonin and correlations of 25(OH)-vitamin concentration and scores on the Autism-Spectrum Quotient	Primarily hypothetical theories. Methodological problems: observational, epidemiologic assumptions	D
Vitamin B$_6$ and magnesium[38,48-54]	Cochrane review 2005 of existing studies: 3 studies; Owing to small number of studies, methodological quality of studies, and small sample sizes, no recommendation can be advanced regarding the use of B$_6$-Mg as a treatment for autism. Update in 2010 came to same conclusion.[52] Study in 2006 with 33 children, poorly defined diagnosis, changes seen in blood studies; control by typical children; unblinded	Poor quality of studies precludes recommendations for treatment Potential neurotoxicity of B$_6$ and/or magnesium; report of death from combination of multiple supplements with magnesium	D

(continued on next page)

Table 2
(continued)

Treatments	Evidence	Comments	Rating of Evidence
DMG[55–57]	2 studies published: 1999 DB/PC crossover pilot of low-dose DMG, N = 8; no differences between groups. 2001 DB/PC trial, N = 37 no difference	Small studies, without benefit; no further evidence Parents report side effects of hyperactivity	C+
Amino acids[7,58,59]	No peer-reviewed studies of taurine, lysine, GABA administration Carnosine: most literature based on bench research. One study in humans, of L-carnosine (2002) DB/PC trial N = 31 children, improvement in GARS and other measures. No further trials reported	Inadequate study to make recommendations for treatment	C
Omega-3 FA[60–67]	Several systematic reviews examining nutritional and environmental factors. Studies of supplements have reported benefits, but many methodological problems. Cochrane review reported 3 studies (N = 37 children) with randomized, DB/PC; other studies excluded owing to nonrandomization or no controls. No evidence impact on social interaction, communication, stereotypy of hyperactivity	Not yet high-quality evidence that omega-3 FA supplementation is effective for improving core and associated symptoms of ASD. More study needed based on promising effects in other populations	C
Vitamin B$_{12}$[39,68–77]	Except for a small pilot study, with open-label extension. No additional studies since 2008 review Bertoglio study: 12 wk DB/PC, crossover clinical trial of injectable methyl B$_{12}$. N = 30; no differences in behavioral measures or laboratory tests; in a subgroup 30% improvement. No correlations of response to number of infections, GI symptoms, or food allergies	Need further study to delineate a responder group; may be related to measures used to examine outcome in a group of children with intellectual challenges	C+

Treatment	Studies	Evidence/Recommendations	Grade
Melatonin[78-89]	Multiple studies including (1) cohort study (Anderson, 2008); (2) open-label dose escalation (Malow, 2012); (3) biochemical analyses and susceptibility genes in ASD vs controls, showing differences in the 2 groups	Good physiologic evidence and some medium-quality observational and open-label studies. Few side effects	B
Probiotics[90-95]	No specific studies of treatment of children with ASD. Literature explores link between gastrointestinal dysfunction and associated symptoms. Theory that probiotic bacteria would restore normal gut microbiota or that probiotics would provide "detoxification"	No evidence to support need for detoxification. No recommendations for treatment	D+
Mind and Body Practices			
Auditory integration[96-100]	7 clinical trials with varied outcome measures; 5 do not demonstrate benefit	Randomized, blinded trial with adequate sample size, manualized approach, and valid outcome measures would be needed to demonstrate support. Risk low, unlikely benefit	B
Acupuncture[101,102]	RCTs suggest benefit when combined with language and other therapies; varying results when compared with wait-list controls	Randomized trials of adequate size with characterized patients and valid outcome data are needed. Risk for infection, injury in uncooperative patients. Potential for benefit for comorbid conditions possible. No evidence to support use for ASD	B
Equine therapy[103]	Case series identified improvement in teacher-reported behavioral scales while riding program in effect	Randomized trial with appropriate control activity with valid outcome measures needed. With appropriate attention to safety (helmet, trained assistants) risk is relatively low; potential benefit for symptoms or as leisure activity	C

(continued on next page)

Table 2
(continued)

Treatments	Evidence	Comments	Rating of Evidence
Hypnotherapy	Case reports only	Randomized trials of adequate size with characterized patients, manualized treatment, and valid outcome data needed Low risk, potential benefit	D+
Massage[104–106] Qigong[104,105,107–110]	Small studies without characterization of participants, standardization of treatments, or valid outcome measures. Benefits reported in parental perception and sensory and behavioral skills	Randomized trials of adequate size with characterized patients, manualized treatment, and valid outcome data needed Low risk, potential benefit	C
Music therapy[111,112]	Small trials and case series with suggestion of increased verbalizations in melodic-based interventions. Data do not demonstrate improvement in language or behavior	Randomized trials of adequate size with characterized patients, manualized approaches, and valid outcome measures needed Low risk, limited evidence for potential therapeutic benefit. (Note: outcome measures on use of music as cue for behavior may be warranted, eg, effect of Barney "Clean Up" song)	B
Chiropractic[113,114]	No trials in the literature to inform a recommendation for chiropractic for symptoms of ASD	Randomized trials of adequate size with characterized patients, manualized treatment, and valid outcome data needed Low risk (if no spinal abnormalities, eg, atlanto-occipital instability of Down syndrome), potential benefit for comorbid medical conditions possible	D
Craniosacral manipulation	No adequate clinical trials support this intervention in ASD. No evidence that external manipulation alters flow of spinal fluid	No clinical trials support this intervention or the underlying construct Risk low, no evidence of benefit	D

Yoga[115,116]	Small study or manualized approach with measured benefit in behavior using standard outcome measures	Randomized trials of adequate size with characterized patients needed to extend beyond pilot data Low risk, potential benefit	C
Biologically Based Practices			
Anti-infectives (antibiotics, antifungal, antivirals),[117–130] minocycline[131]	Antibiotics for intestinal overgrowth unproven Antiviral therapies untested Trial of minocycline may affect neurotrophic growth factors but did not affect clinical symptoms	No evidence for antibiotic or antifungal use for intestinal overgrowth, no studies on antiviral therapies Larger DB PC trial of minocycline indicated it as a psychopharmacologic agent No FDA-approved product on market with this clinical indication at present	C
Immunoglobulins[78,87,92,122,132–142]	IVIG did not alter behavioral symptoms in small open trials using valid outcome measures; a DB PC clinical trial of oral IgG did not affect behavior or GI symptoms	Data do not support using immunoglobulins for treatment of symptoms of ASD. Current research suggests that prenatal immune events may affect fetal brain development placing infants at risk for ASD No FDA-approved product on market with the clinical indication of altering immune function at present	C
Chelation agents: DMSA[92,143–150]	One case report of death with intravenous NaEDTA. Trial of DMSA chelation terminated because of concern about toxicity. Case series with methodological compromise suggested improvement after 6 mo of chelation	No evidence supporting the use of chelation Risk high. Use is not recommended outside of approved DB PC trials No FDA-approved product on market with this clinical indication at present	D
Digestive enzymes[151,152]	One RCT (N = 43) did not demonstrate clinical improvement, slight improvement in food variety	No FDA-approved product on market with this clinical indication at present	D

(continued on next page)

Table 2
(continued)

Treatments	Evidence	Comments	Rating of Evidence
Oxytocin[153,154]	7 RCTs, small samples; benefits in emotional recognition, eye gaze. One trial with benefit at 6 wk	Longer-lasting products needed that can be tested in appropriate clinical trials No FDA-approved product on market with this clinical indication at present	C+
Secretin[92,155–171]	>900 children have been evaluated in DB PC trials. No behavioral benefit	No FDA-approved product on market with this clinical indication at present Risk from intravenous route, stress. No benefit documented	A
Gluten-free/casein-free diet[93,172–190]	Single-blind trials suggested potential benefit in children 5–7 y of age with GI symptoms DB trial without demonstrable benefit	Provided by parents with/without professional guidance DB randomized trial with characterization of patients and standard outcome data would be needed to clarify utility of this intervention Risk for nutritional compromise with restriction of calcium, vitamin D in milk products, and other nutrients with additional restrictions. Can be delivered in a nutritionally sound fashion. Suggest consultation with registered dietitian	B
Hyperbaric oxygen therapy[76,191–196]	Two randomized trials, conflicting results. Statistics might be interpreted differently, impact of other therapies possible	Randomized trial, DB of well-characterized patients using manualized approach and valid outcome measures would be needed to determine efficacy No FDA-approved product on market with this clinical indication at present	B

Stem cell transplantation[197–200]	Open-label treatment claims improvement in 21 of 36 patients in one report and 23 of 37 in another. Seizures as side effect reported to be managed with medications	No FDA-approved product on market with this clinical indication at present	D
Transcranial magnetic stimulation[106,201–207]	Dorsomedial prefrontal cortex activation improved social relatedness and anxiety in adults with ASD over 2-wk trial with short-term follow-up, compared with sham treatment. Data supported by other small series. Safe in context of clinical trials	DB randomized trial with characterization of patients and standard outcome data would be needed to clarify utility of this intervention. Long-term efficacy and safety data needed to support pediatric use. No FDA-approved product on market with this clinical indication at present for general clinical use in children. Potential for risk, potential for benefit	B
Vagus nerve stimulation[208–210]	Anecdotal case reports for improved behavior. Prospective data suggest that patients with ASD may have improved mood	Use of questionnaires and direct observation may be helpful in documenting behavioral change with implantation of vagal nerve stimulators in patients with ASD and epilepsy. If demonstrable benefit, may justify trials for behavior alone. Risk with procedure, benefit unknown relative to ASD, benefit for seizure control	D

Abbreviations: ASD, autism spectrum disorders; DB, double-blind; DMG, dimethylglycine; DMSA, dimercaptosuccinic acid; FA, fatty acid; FDA, US Food and Drug Administration; GABA, γ-aminobutyric acid; GARS, Gilliam Autism Rating Scale; GI, gastrointestinal; IgG, immunoglobulin G; IVIG, intravenous immunoglobulin; NaEDTA, sodium ethylenediaminetetraacetic acid; PC, placebo-controlled; PGI-R, Parental Global Impressions—Revised; RCT, randomized controlled trial; UV-B, ultraviolet B.

individuals ranging from trained massage therapists to parents, and there may be inconsistencies in the administration, making study challenging. Music therapy may be provided on an individual or group basis by a music therapist, who may not be trained in working with children with ASD. Chiropractic manipulation is administered individually by a licensed chiropractor. Craniofacial manipulation is administered by a variety of licensed professionals including chiropractors, occupational therapists, and physical therapists.

These treatments are also consumer driven, with direct access by families (but not necessarily covered by insurance). Guidance for or promotion of their use for the treatment of symptoms of autism may come from non–peer-reviewed sources (community, lay press, or Internet). Again, medical practitioners may not be sufficiently knowledgable about these therapies to guide consumers in terms of their application in the treatment of autism symptoms. Owing to their lack of knowledge or experience, clinicians may not be open to reciprocal discussion (shared decision making). Some treatments (especially those involving physical manipulation) may not be adequately regulated by an oversight body or certification of providers.

Other Biomedical Treatments

Readers are referred to a recent review of biomedical complementary treatment approaches for autism by Robert Hendren[31] for further details about biomedical treatments and the purported mechanisms that they would target. Biomedical treatments represent diverse types of medical or biologically based therapy, which likely present the most potential for negative side effects. These agents may be divided into 2 broad categories: off-label prescribed medications (eg, anti-infectives, immunoglobulins, chelation agents, digestive enzymes, oxytocin, secretin) and other medical treatments (eg, specialized diets without known medical indications, hyperbaric oxygen therapy, stem cell transplantation, transcranial magnetic therapy, vagus nerve stimulation). These treatments require a licensed clinician (physician, nurse practitioner) to prescribe the medication or administer the treatment.

Off-label medications may be over the counter (such as digestive enzymes and certain chelation agents) but are most often prescribed by a licensed medical provider, but used for an unapproved indication, age, or dosage as indicated by the Food and Drug Administration. Depending on the medication, they may be provided orally (antibiotics, antifungals, antivirals, chelation agents, immunoglobulins, among others), intranasal (oxytocin), rectal (chelation), intravenous (immunoglobulins, secretin) or transdermal (secretin). A frequently used intervention without medical guidance is elimination diet(s), most commonly the gluten-free/casein-free diet. This therapy may be totally consumer driven, and may be implemented without medical support for monitoring side effects such as nutritional deficiency. Other procedures such as hyperbaric oxygen therapy are implemented using a hyperbaric chamber, administered by a technician. The patient may be alone or with a caregiver. This treatment is often prescribed by a medical provider, but units can be purchased online or consumers can find directions to build one. Stem cell transplantation is intravenous or intrathecal, prescribed by complementary medical professionals. Families may travel to other countries to obtain stem cell transplantation that does not have the oversight that professional practice does in the United States. Transcranial magnetic therapy is provided individually, directed by a licensed medical professional as part of a registered clinical trial. It is not commercially available for ASD at present. Vagus nerve stimulation is derived from a specialized treatment for intractable seizures, using a medically implanted device for seizure control, with demonstrated efficacy for seizure control.

These treatments all have high potential for negative side effects and complications. Complementary providers and families may lack a mechanism to monitor for side effects. Most promotion for use comes from the community, lay press, or Internet, and precludes adequate peer review for evidence of efficacy. Medical practitioners are often not knowledgable enough to guide consumers and may not be open to reciprocal discussion (shared decision making). These treatments are expensive (usually out of pocket), although in some instances insurance companies might cover some of the costs. Another cost to the patient is that the expenses to obtain these treatments may interfere with the ability to obtain other treatments (costs = time and money).

Some novel interventions, such as transcranial magnetic therapy, are investigational so may demonstrate a therapeutic effect after appropriate clinical trials. Many CAM approaches are rapid responses to new scientific observations that have not been critically examined or appropriately tested using appropriate clinical trial methodology.

WORKING WITH FAMILIES WHO CHOOSE COMPLEMENTARY AND ALTERNATIVE MEDICAL

The literature indicates that families of children with ASD often do not tell their health care provider that they are using nonstandard therapies unless directly asked. Many families do not think that their allopathic providers are knowledgable about CAM while others do not want to tell their providers they are using products or approaches the provider might not approve of. It is important for the health care provider to routinely and nonjudgmentally ask about all interventions that a family is using to ensure that potential side effects are considered and families helped to navigate the choices related to expense and time commitment. It is common for users of CAM to assume that there are no or few side effects. Loose stool, for example, may be a side effect of supplements containing magnesium. This sign may be perceived as a medical comorbidity of the ASD if a full evaluation of supplements used does not take place. The American Academy of Pediatrics published recommendations for clinicians working with families who elect to use CAM for their children with special health care needs. The tenets of this document are: respect for family beliefs, listening to concerns, maintaining a dialogue with the family, ensuring the safety of the child, and being knowledgable about how to evaluate the literature used to support CAM interventions.[13,32]

Health care providers need to understand how to interpret the literature regarding novel therapies. Clinical trials evaluating new therapies are increasingly published in peer-reviewed sources. Physicians use print literature (68%) and colleagues (60%) as their most common sources for updating their medical information, and report that medical conferences and physician-directed Web sites (both 42%) are also common sources of new information. This percentage is the same as that for the use of general Web-based searches.[33] By contrast, the Internet is the first source of medical information in almost two-thirds of families. The lay literature often used to promote CAM therapies may be based on anecdotal evidence and scant data, thus the health care provider may need to counsel the family regarding the components of an acceptable clinical trial. Peer-reviewed scientific reports should include information on the recruitment and characterization of the participants. The methods of study need to be described, and it should be noted if group assignment was random and the assessment and treatment was double-blinded. Treatments should use consistent dosing. If a nonbiological intervention was used, it should be described and noted if delivered in a standard fashion. Outcome measures need to be valid (ie, measure what they say they measure).[15] If no high-quality clinical trials inform the safety or efficacy of an intervention, the clinician can help the family understand the available data to enable them

Table 3
Working with families who select CAM use

Principles	What to Do

Discussion with families
    Family disclosure of CAM use to provider[15]
    Choice of treatments
	Ask about all treatments
	Partnering to promote discussion
	Shared decision making

Selection of non–evidence-based treatment	Educating about evidence and informed consumer practices[15]

Sources of information[26]	Provider awareness of potential sources of
	    information (family, friends, nonmedical
	    community, Internet)[15]

Provider comfort and knowledge about CAM treatments	Seek out sources of education Reviews of CAM treatment Educational opportunities

to make an informed choice on whether to use a novel therapy. **Table 3** lists some suggestions about working with families.

MONITORING INTERVENTIONS

Regardless of whether the literature supports an intervention, it may or may not be successful for an individual patient. It is important to establish the symptoms a novel therapy is used to address, and to define the expected benefits and potential side effects. Families should be counseled on the expected length of time until a therapeutic effect can be expected. With this knowledge they, and the program staff, can determine the impact of a specific intervention. It is important for interventions to be introduced one by one so that the effects can be correctly attributed.

SUMMARY

There are many treatments in current use for core and associated symptoms of ASD. This review discusses categories of CAM treatments commonly used for children with ASD, including natural products, mind and body practices, and other biomedical treatments. The focus is on factors associated with the use of CAM, the empirical evidence for the most frequently used treatments, and how to work with families who choose CAM treatments. Families choose CAM to promote wellness, to treat specific symptoms or co-occurring disorders of ASD, to avoid untoward symptoms of conventional medicine, and, in some cases, under the hope or assumption of resolution of core symptoms of ASD. Some treatments have been proved to be ineffective, some have unacceptable potential side effects, and others require more study in depth.

REFERENCES

1. Autism and Developmental Disabilities Monitoring Network Surveillance Year 2010 Principal Investigators, Centers for Disease Control and Prevention. Prevalence of autism spectrum disorder among children 8 years—Autism and Developmental Disabilities Monitoring Network, 11 sites, United States, 2010. MMWR Surveill Summ 2014;63(2):1–21.
2. American Psychiatric Association. Diagnostic and statistical manual of mental disorders, fifth edition (DSM-5). Arlington (VA): American Psychiatric Publishing; 2013.

3. Matson JL, Cervantes PE. Commonly studied comorbid psychopathologies among persons with autism spectrum disorder. Res Dev Disabil 2014;35(5): 952–62.
4. Persico AM, Napolioni V. Autism genetics. Behav Brain Res 2013;251:95–112.
5. Murdoch JD, State MW. Recent developments in the genetics of autism spectrum disorders. Curr Opin Genet Dev 2013;23(3):310–5.
6. Konopka G. Preface: the neurobiology of autism: integrating genetics, brain development, behavior, and the environment. Int Rev Neurobiol 2013;113:xi–xii.
7. Levy SE, Hyman SL. Complementary and alternative medicine treatments for children with autism spectrum disorders. Child Adolesc Psychiatr Clin N Am 2008;17(4):803–20, ix.
8. National Center for Complementary and Alternative Medicine. CAM basics: complementary, alternative, or integrative health: what's in a name? 2014. Available at: http://nccam.nih.gov/sites/nccam.nih.gov/files/CAM_Basics_What_Are_ CAIHA.pdf. Accessed September 17, 2014.
9. Barnes PM, Bloom B, Nahin RL. Complementary and alternative medicine use among adults and children: United States, 2007. Natl Health Stat Report 2008;(12):1–23.
10. Barnes PM, Powell-Griner E, McFann K, et al. Complementary and alternative medicine use among adults: United States, 2002. Adv Data 2004;(343):1–19.
11. Davis MP, Darden PM. Use of complementary and alternative medicine by children in the United States. Arch Pediatr Adolesc Med 2003;157(4):393–6.
12. Nahin RL, Barnes PM, Stussman BJ, et al. Costs of complementary and alternative medicine (CAM) and frequency of visits to CAM practitioners: United States, 2007. Natl Health Stat Report 2009;(18):1–14.
13. Huang A, Seshadri K, Matthews TA, et al. Parental perspectives on use, benefits, and physician knowledge of complementary and alternative medicine in children with autistic disorder and attention-deficit/hyperactivity disorder. J Altern Complement Med 2013;19(9):746–50.
14. Treat L, Liesinger J, Ziegenfuss JY, et al. Patterns of complementary and alternative medicine use in children with common neurological conditions. Glob Adv Health Med 2014;3(1):18–24.
15. Akins RS, Angkustsiri K, Hansen RL. Complementary and alternative medicine in autism: an evidence-based approach to negotiating safe and efficacious interventions with families. Neurotherapeutics 2010;7(3):307–19.
16. Liptak GS. Complementary and alternative therapies for cerebral palsy. Ment Retard Dev Disabil Res Rev 2005;11(2):156–63.
17. Roizen NJ. Complementary and alternative therapies for Down syndrome. Ment Retard Dev Disabil Res Rev 2005;11(2):149–55.
18. Akins RS, Krakowiak P, Angkustsiri K, et al. Utilization patterns of conventional and complementary/alternative treatments in children with autism spectrum disorders and developmental disabilities in a population-based study. J Dev Behav Pediatr 2014;35(1):1–10.
19. Perrin JM, Coury DL, Hyman SL, et al. Complementary and alternative medicine use in a large pediatric autism sample. Pediatrics 2012;130(Suppl 2):S77–82.
20. Christon LM, Mackintosh VH, Myers BA. Use of complementary and alternative medicine (CAM) treatments by parents of children with autism spectrum disorders. Res Autism Spectr Disord 2010;4:249–59.
21. Lofthouse N, Hendren R, Hurt E, et al. A review of complementary and alternative treatments for autism spectrum disorders. Autism Res Treat 2012;2012: 870391.

22. Davis MA, West AN, Weeks WB, et al. Health behaviors and utilization among users of complementary and alternative medicine for treatment versus health promotion. Health Serv Res 2011;46(5):1402–16.

23. McCaffrey AM, Pugh GF, O'Connor BB. Understanding patient preference for integrative medical care: results from patient focus groups. J Gen Intern Med 2007;22(11):1500–5.

24. Mathew E, Muttappallymyalil J, Sreedharan J, et al. Self-reported use of complementary and alternative medicine among the health care consumers at a Tertiary Care Center in Ajman, United Arab Emirates. Ann Med Health Sci Res 2013; 3(2):215–9.

25. Hanson E, Kalish LA, Bunce E, et al. Use of complementary and alternative medicine among children diagnosed with autism spectrum disorder. J Autism Dev Disord 2007;37(4):628–36.

26. Senel HG. Parents' views and experiences about complementary and alternative medicine treatments for their children with autistic spectrum disorder. J Autism Dev Disord 2010;40(4):494–503.

27. Green VA, Pituch KA, Itchon J, et al. Internet survey of treatments used by parents of children with autism. Res Dev Disabil 2006;27(1):70–84.

28. Wong HH, Smith RG. Patterns of complementary and alternative medical therapy use in children diagnosed with autism spectrum disorders. J Autism Dev Disord 2006;36(7):901–9.

29. Guyatt GH, Oxman AD, Kunz R, et al. What is "quality of evidence" and why is it important to clinicians? BMJ 2008;336(7651):995–8.

30. GRADE Working Group. Grading quality of evidence and strength of recommendations. BMJ 2004;328(7454):1490.

31. Hendren RL. Autism: biomedical complementary treatment approaches. Child Adolesc Psychiatr Clin N Am 2013;22(3):443–56, vi.

32. Golnik A, Maccabee-Ryaboy N, Scal P, et al. Shared decision making: improving care for children with autism. Intellect Dev Disabil 2012;50(4):322–31.

33. Wolters Kluwer Health. Wolters Kluwer Health 2011 point-of-care survey. 2011. Available at: http://www.wolterskluwerhealth.com/News/Documents/White% 20Papers/Wolters%20Kluwer%20Health%20Survey%20Executive%20Summary-Media.pdf. Accessed November 2, 2013.

34. Kemper KJ, O'Connor KG. Pediatricians' recommendations for complementary and alternative medical (CAM) therapies. Ambul Pediatr 2004;4(6): 482–7.

35. Adams JB, Audhya T, McDonough-Means S, et al. Effect of a vitamin/mineral supplement on children and adults with autism. BMC Pediatr 2011;11:111.

36. Adams JB, Audhya T, McDonough-Means S, et al. Nutritional and metabolic status of children with autism vs. neurotypical children, and the association with autism severity. Nutr Metab (Lond) 2011;8(1):34.

37. Megson MN. Is autism a G-alpha protein defect reversible with natural vitamin A? Med Hypotheses 2000;54(6):979–83.

38. Adams JB, Holloway C. Pilot study of a moderate dose multivitamin/mineral supplement for children with autistic spectrum disorder. J Altern Complement Med 2004;10(6):1033–9.

39. McGinnis WR. Oxidative stress in autism. Altern Ther Health Med 2004;10(6): 22–36 [quiz: 37, 92].

40. Dolske MC, Spollen J, McKay S, et al. A preliminary trial of ascorbic acid as supplemental therapy for autism. Prog Neuropsychopharmacol Biol Psychiatry 1993;17(5):765–74.

41. Patrick RP, Ames BN. Vitamin D hormone regulates serotonin synthesis. Part 1: relevance for autism. FASEB J 2014;28:2398–413.
42. Cannell JJ, Grant WB. What is the role of vitamin D in autism? Dermatoendocrinol 2013;5(1):199–204.
43. Cannell JJ. Autism, will vitamin D treat core symptoms? Med Hypotheses 2013; 81(2):195–8.
44. Whitehouse AJ, Holt BJ, Serralha M, et al. Maternal vitamin D levels and the autism phenotype among offspring. J Autism Dev Disord 2013;43(7):1495–504.
45. Kocovska E, Fernell E, Billstedt E, et al. Vitamin D and autism: clinical review. Res Dev Disabil 2012;33(5):1541–50.
46. Becker KG. Autism, immune dysfunction and vitamin D. Acta Psychiatr Scand 2011;124(1):74 [author reply: 74–5].
47. Grant WB, Soles CM. Epidemiologic evidence supporting the role of maternal vitamin D deficiency as a risk factor for the development of infantile autism. Dermatoendocrinol 2009;1(4):223–8.
48. Nye C, Brice A. Combined vitamin B6-magnesium treatment in autism spectrum disorder. Cochrane Database Syst Rev 2005;(4):CD003497.
49. Kleijnen J, Knipschild P. Niacin and vitamin B6 in mental functioning: a review of controlled trials in humans. Biol Psychiatry 1991;29(9):931–41.
50. Martineau J, Barthelemy C, Garreau B, et al. Vitamin B6, magnesium, and combined B6-Mg: therapeutic effects in childhood autism. Biol Psychiatry 1985; 20(5):467–78.
51. Martineau J, Garreau B, Barthelemy C, et al. Effects of vitamin B6 on averaged evoked potentials in infantile autism. Biol Psychiatry 1981;16(7):627–41.
52. Murza KA, Pavelko SL, Malani MD, et al. Vitamin B6-magnesium treatment for autism: the current status of the research. Magnes Res 2010;23(2):115–7.
53. Mousain-Bosc M, Roche M, Polge A, et al. Improvement of neurobehavioral disorders in children supplemented with magnesium-vitamin B6. II. Pervasive developmental disorder-autism. Magnes Res 2006;19(1):53–62.
54. Adams JB, George F, Audhya T. Abnormally high plasma levels of vitamin B6 in children with autism not taking supplements compared to controls not taking supplements. J Altern Complement Med 2006;12(1):59–63.
55. Kidd PM. Autism, an extreme challenge to integrative medicine. Part 2: medical management. Altern Med Rev 2002;7(6):472–99.
56. Kern JK, Miller VS, Cauller PL, et al. Effectiveness of N,N-dimethylglycine in autism and pervasive developmental disorder. J Child Neurol 2001;16(3):169–73.
57. Bolman WM, Richmond JA. A double-blind, placebo-controlled, crossover pilot trial of low dose dimethylglycine in patients with autistic disorder. J Autism Dev Disord 1999;29(3):191–4.
58. Frye RE, Rossignol D, Casanova MF, et al. A review of traditional and novel treatments for seizures in autism spectrum disorder: findings from a systematic review and expert panel. Front Public Health 2013;1:31.
59. Chez MG, Buchanan CP, Aimonovitch MC, et al. Double-blind, placebo-controlled study of L-carnosine supplementation in children with autistic spectrum disorders. J Child Neurol 2002;17(11):833–7.
60. Curtis LT, Patel K. Nutritional and environmental approaches to preventing and treating autism and attention deficit hyperactivity disorder (ADHD): a review. J Altern Complement Med 2008;14:79–85.
61. Kidd PM. Omega-3 DHA and EPA for cognition, behavior, and mood: clinical findings and structural-functional synergies with cell membrane phospholipids. Altern Med Rev 2007;12(3):207–27.

62. Gilbert DL. Regarding "omega-3 fatty acids supplementation in children with autism: a double-blind randomized, placebo-controlled pilot study". Biol Psychiatry 2008;63:e13.

63. Amminger GP, Berger GE, Schafer MR, et al. Omega-3 fatty acids supplementation in children with autism: a double-blind randomized, placebo-controlled pilot study. Biol Psychiatry 2007;61(4):551–3.

64. Young G, Conquer J. Omega-3 fatty acids and neuropsychiatric disorders. Reprod Nutr Dev 2005;45(1):1–28.

65. Vancassel S, Durand G, Barthelemy C, et al. Plasma fatty acid levels in autistic children. Prostaglandins Leukot Essent Fatty Acids 2001;65(1):1–7.

66. James S, Montgomery P, Williams K. Omega-3 fatty acids supplementation for autism spectrum disorders (ASD). Cochrane Database Syst Rev 2011;(11):CD007992.

67. Tan ML, Ho JJ, Teh KH. Polyunsaturated fatty acids (PUFAs) for children with specific learning disorders. Cochrane Database Syst Rev 2012;(12):CD009398.

68. Moretti P, Sahoo T, Hyland K, et al. Cerebral folate deficiency with developmental delay, autism, and response to folinic acid. Neurology 2005;64(6):1088–90.

69. Williams TA, Mars AE, Buyske SG, et al. Risk of autistic disorder in affected offspring of mothers with a glutathione S-transferase P1 haplotype. Arch Pediatr Adolesc Med 2007;161(4):356–61.

70. McGinnis WR. Could oxidative stress from psychosocial stress affect neurodevelopment in autism? J Autism Dev Disord 2007;37(5):993–4.

71. Deth R, Muratore C, Benzecry J, et al. How environmental and genetic factors combine to cause autism: a redox/methylation hypothesis. Neurotoxicology 2008;29:190–201.

72. James SJ, Melnyk S, Jernigan S, et al. Metabolic endophenotype and related genotypes are associated with oxidative stress in children with autism. Am J Med Genet B Neuropsychiatr Genet 2006;141(8):947–56.

73. Chauhan A, Chauhan V. Oxidative stress in autism. Pathophysiology 2006;13(3):171–81.

74. McGinnis WR. Oxidative stress in autism. Altern Ther Health Med 2005;11(1):19.

75. Chauhan A, Chauhan V, Brown WT, et al. Oxidative stress in autism: increased lipid peroxidation and reduced serum levels of ceruloplasmin and transferrin-the antioxidant proteins. Life Sci 2004;75(21):2539–49.

76. Rossignol DA, Rossignol LW, James SJ, et al. The effects of hyperbaric oxygen therapy on oxidative stress, inflammation, and symptoms in children with autism: an open-label pilot study. BMC Pediatr 2007;7(1):36.

77. Bertoglio K, James JS, Deprey L, et al. Pilot study of the effect of methyl B12 treatment on behavioral and biomarker measures in children with autism. J Altern Complement Med 2010;16(5):555–60.

78. Melke J, Goubran Botros H, Chaste P, et al. Abnormal melatonin synthesis in autism spectrum disorders. Mol Psychiatry 2008;13(1):90–8.

79. Pandi-Perumal SR, Srinivasan V, Spence DW, et al. Role of the melatonin system in the control of sleep: therapeutic implications. CNS Drugs 2007;21(12):995–1018.

80. Tordjman S, Anderson GM, Pichard N, et al. Nocturnal excretion of 6-sulphatoxymelatonin in children and adolescents with autistic disorder. Biol Psychiatry 2005;57(2):134–8.

81. Gupta R, Hutchins J. Melatonin: a panacea for desperate parents? (Hype or truth). Arch Dis Child 2005;90(9):986–7.

82. Owens JA, Rosen CL, Mindell JA. Medication use in the treatment of pediatric insomnia: results of a survey of community-based pediatricians. Pediatrics 2003;111(5 Pt 1):e628–635.
83. Hayashi E. Effect of melatonin on sleep-wake rhythm: the sleep diary of an autistic male. Psychiatry Clin Neurosci 2000;54(3):383–4.
84. Lord C. What is melatonin? Is it a useful treatment for sleep problems in autism? J Autism Dev Disord 1998;28(4):345–6.
85. Jan JE, O'Donnell ME. Use of melatonin in the treatment of paediatric sleep disorders. J Pineal Res 1996;21(4):193–9.
86. Chamberlain RS, Herman BH. A novel biochemical model linking dysfunctions in brain melatonin, proopiomelanocortin peptides, and serotonin in autism. Biol Psychiatry 1990;28(9):773–93.
87. Malow B, Adkins KW, McGrew SG, et al. Melatonin for sleep in children with autism: a controlled trial examining dose, tolerability, and outcomes. J Autism Dev Disord 2012;42(8):1729–37 [author reply: 1738].
88. Wright B, Sims D, Smart S, et al. Melatonin versus placebo in children with autism spectrum conditions and severe sleep problems not amenable to behaviour management strategies: a randomised controlled crossover trial. J Autism Dev Disord 2011;41(2):175–84.
89. Andersen IM, Kaczmarska J, McGrew SG, et al. Melatonin for insomnia in children with autism spectrum disorders. J Child Neurol 2008;23(5):482–5.
90. Gilbert Jack A, Krajmalnik-Brown R, Porazinska Dorota L, et al. Toward effective probiotics for autism and other neurodevelopmental disorders. Cell 2013; 155(7):1446–8.
91. Critchfield JW, van Hemert S, Ash M, et al. The potential role of probiotics in the management of childhood autism spectrum disorders. Gastroenterol Res Pract 2011;2011:161358.
92. Levy SE, Hyman SL. Novel treatments for autistic spectrum disorders. Ment Retard Dev Disabil Res Rev 2005;11(2):131–42.
93. Garvey J. Diet in autism and associated disorders. J Fam Health Care 2002; 12(2):34–8.
94. Linday LA. *Saccharomyces boulardii*: potential adjunctive treatment for children with autism and diarrhea. J Child Neurol 2001;16(5):387.
95. Brudnak MA. Probiotics as an adjuvant to detoxification protocols. Med Hypotheses 2002;58(5):382–5.
96. van der Smagt MJ, van Engeland H, Kemner C. Brief report: can you see what is not there? low-level auditory-visual integration in autism spectrum disorder. J Autism Dev Disord 2007;37(10):2014–9.
97. Smith EG, Bennetto L. Audiovisual speech integration and lipreading in autism. J Child Psychol Psychiatry 2007;48(8):813–21.
98. Dawson G, Watling R. Interventions to facilitate auditory, visual, and motor integration in autism: a review of the evidence. J Autism Dev Disord 2000;30(5): 415–21.
99. Auditory integration training and facilitated communication for autism. American Academy of Pediatrics. Committee on Children with Disabilities. Pediatrics 1998;102(2 Pt 1):431–3.
100. Sinha Y, Silove N, Hayen A, et al. Auditory integration training and other sound therapies for autism spectrum disorders (ASD). Cochrane Database Syst Rev 2011;(12):CD003681.
101. Lo SY. Diagnosis, treatment and prevention of autism via meridian theory. Am J Chin Med 2012;40(1):39–56.

102. Lee M, Choi TY, Shin BC, et al. Acupuncture for children with autism spectrum disorders: a systematic review of randomized clinical trials. J Autism Dev Disord 2012;42(8):1671–83.

103. Ward S, Whalon K, Rusnak K, et al. The association between therapeutic horse-back riding and the social communication and sensory reactions of children with autism. J Autism Dev Disord 2013;43(9):2190–8.

104. Silva LM, Cignolini A, Warren R, et al. Improvement in sensory impairment and social interaction in young children with autism following treatment with an original Qigong massage methodology. Am J Chin Med 2007;35(3):393–406.

105. Silva LM, Cignolini A. A medical qigong methodology for early intervention in autism spectrum disorder: a case series. Am J Chin Med 2005;33(2):315–27.

106. Cullen LA, Barlow JH, Cushway D. Positive touch, the implications for parents and their children with autism: an exploratory study. Complement Ther Clin Pract 2005;11(3):182–9.

107. Silva L, Schalock M. Treatment of tactile impairment in young children with autism: results with qigong massage. Int J Ther Massage Bodywork 2013; 6(4):12–20.

108. Silva LM, Schalock M, Gabrielsen K. Early intervention for autism with a parent-delivered Qigong massage program: a randomized controlled trial. Am J Occup Ther 2011;65(5):550–9.

109. Silva LM, Schalock M, Ayres R, et al. Qigong massage treatment for sensory and self-regulation problems in young children with autism: a randomized controlled trial. Am J Occup Ther 2009;63(4):423–32.

110. Silva LM, Ayres R, Schalock M. Outcomes of a pilot training program in a qigong massage intervention for young children with autism. Am J Occup Ther 2008; 62(5):538–46.

111. Sandiford GA, Mainess KJ, Daher NS. A pilot study on the efficacy of melodic based communication therapy for eliciting speech in nonverbal children with autism. J Autism Dev Disord 2013;43(6):1298–307.

112. Simpson K, Keen D. Music interventions for children with autism: narrative review of the literature. J Autism Dev Disord 2011;41(11):1507–14.

113. Sherman KJ, Cherkin DC, Connelly MT, et al. Complementary and alternative medical therapies for chronic low back pain: what treatments are patients willing to try? BMC Complement Altern Med 2004;4:9.

114. Simon GE, Cherkin DC, Sherman KJ, et al. Mental health visits to complementary and alternative medicine providers. Gen Hosp Psychiatry 2004;26(3):171–7.

115. Koenig KP, Buckley-Reen A, Garg S. Efficacy of the get ready to learn yoga program among children with autism spectrum disorders: a pretest-posttest control group design. Am J Occup Ther 2012;66(5):538–46.

116. Rosenblatt LE, Gorantla S, Torres JA, et al. Relaxation response-based yoga improves functioning in young children with autism: a pilot study. J Altern Complement Med 2011;17(11):1029–35.

117. Niehus R, Lord C. Early medical history of children with autism spectrum disorders. J Dev Behav Pediatr 2006;27(2 Suppl):S120–127.

118. Fallon J. Could one of the most widely prescribed antibiotics amoxicillin/clavulanate "augmentin" be a risk factor for autism? Med Hypotheses 2005;64(2): 312–5.

119. Manev R, Manev H. Aminoglycoside antibiotics and autism: a speculative hypothesis. BMC Psychiatry 2001;1:5.

120. Sandler RH, Finegold SM, Bolte ER, et al. Short-term benefit from oral vancomycin treatment of regressive-onset autism. J Child Neurol 2000;15(7):429–35.

121. Nicolson GL, Gan R, Nicolson NL, et al. Evidence for *Mycoplasma* ssp., *Chlamydia pneunomiae*, and human herpes virus-6 coinfections in the blood of patients with autistic spectrum disorders. J Neurosci Res 2007;85(5):1143–8.
122. Libbey JE, Coon HH, Kirkman NJ, et al. Are there altered antibody responses to measles, mumps, or rubella viruses in autism? J Neurovirol 2007;13(3):252–9.
123. Bonthius DJ, Perlman S. Congenital viral infections of the brain: lessons learned from lymphocytic choriomeningitis virus in the neonatal rat. PLoS Pathog 2007;3(11):e149.
124. Cohly HH, Panja A. Immunological findings in autism. Int Rev Neurobiol 2005;71:317–41.
125. Wakefield AJ. Enterocolitis, autism and measles virus. Mol Psychiatry 2002;7(Suppl 2):S44–46.
126. Uhlmann V, Martin CM, Sheils O, et al. Potential viral pathogenic mechanism for new variant inflammatory bowel disease. Mol Pathol 2002;55(2):84–90.
127. O'Leary JJ, Uhlmann V, Wakefield AJ. Measles virus and autism. Lancet 2000;356(9231):772.
128. Finegold SM. State of the art; microbiology in health and disease. Intestinal bacterial flora in autism. Anaerobe 2011;17(6):367–8.
129. Finegold SM. Therapy and epidemiology of autism–clostridial spores as key elements. Med Hypotheses 2008;70(3):508–11.
130. Finegold SM, Molitoris D, Song Y, et al. Gastrointestinal microflora studies in late-onset autism. Clin Infect Dis 2002;35(Suppl 1):S6–16.
131. Pardo CA, Buckley A, Thurm A, et al. A pilot open-label trial of minocycline in patients with autism and regressive features. J Neurodev Disord 2013;5(1):9.
132. Thompson WW, Price C, Goodson B, et al. Early thimerosal exposure and neuropsychological outcomes at 7 to 10 years. N Engl J Med 2007;357(13):1281–92.
133. Feasby T, Banwell B, Benstead T, et al. Guidelines on the use of intravenous immune globulin for neurologic conditions. Transfus Med Rev 2007;21(2 Suppl 1):S57–107.
134. Dochniak MJ. Autism spectrum disorders—exogenous protein insult. Med Hypotheses 2007;69(3):545–9.
135. Stern L, Francoeur MJ, Primeau MN, et al. Immune function in autistic children. Ann Allergy Asthma Immunol 2005;95(6):558–65.
136. Sperner-Unterweger B. Immunological aetiology of major psychiatric disorders: evidence and therapeutic implications. Drugs 2005;65(11):1493–520.
137. Murch S. Diet, immunity, and autistic spectrum disorders. J Pediatr 2005;146(5):582–4.
138. Krause I, He XS, Gershwin ME, et al. Brief report: immune factors in autism: a critical review. J Autism Dev Disord 2002;32(4):337–45.
139. Warren RP, Odell JD, Warren WL, et al. Brief report: immunoglobulin A deficiency in a subset of autistic subjects. J Autism Dev Disord 1997;27(2):187–92.
140. Singh VK, Warren R, Averett R, et al. Circulating autoantibodies to neuronal and glial filament proteins in autism. Pediatr Neurol 1997;17(1):88–90.
141. Persico AM, Van de Water J, Pardo CA. Autism: where genetics meets the immune system. Autism Res Treat 2012;2012:486359.
142. Handen BL, Melmed RD, Hansen RL, et al. A double-blind, placebo-controlled trial of oral human immunoglobulin for gastrointestinal dysfunction in children with autistic disorder. J Autism Dev Disord 2009;39(5):796–805.
143. Ng DK, Chan CH, Soo MT, et al. Low-level chronic mercury exposure in children and adolescents: meta-analysis. Pediatr Int 2007;49(1):80–7.

144. Geier DA, Geier MR. A prospective study of mercury toxicity biomarkers in autistic spectrum disorders. J Toxicol Environ Health A 2007;70(20):1723–30.

145. Geier DA, Geier MR. A case series of children with apparent mercury toxic encephalopathies manifesting with clinical symptoms of regressive autistic disorders. J Toxicol Environ Health A 2007;70(10):837–51.

146. Hussain J, Woolf AD, Sandel M, et al. Environmental evaluation of a child with developmental disability. Pediatr Clin North Am 2007;54(1):47–62, viii.

147. Sinha Y, Silove N, Williams K. Chelation therapy and autism. BMJ 2006;333(7571):756.

148. Doja A, Roberts W. Immunizations and autism: a review of the literature. Can J Neurol Sci 2006;33(4):341–6.

149. Mitka M. Chelation therapy trials halted. JAMA 2008;300(19):2236.

150. Brent J. Commentary on the abuse of metal chelation therapy in patients with autism spectrum disorders. J Med Toxicol 2013;9(4):370–2.

151. Munasinghe SA, Oliff C, Finn J, et al. Digestive enzyme supplementation for autism spectrum disorders: a double-blind randomized controlled trial. J Autism Dev Disord 2010;40(9):1131–8.

152. Brudnak MA, Rimland B, Kerry RE, et al. Enzyme-based therapy for autism spectrum disorders—is it worth another look? Med Hypotheses 2002;58(5):422–8.

153. Green JJ, Hollander E. Autism and oxytocin: new developments in translational approaches to therapeutics. Neurotherapeutics 2010;7(3):250–7.

154. Preti A, Melis M, Siddi S, et al. Oxytocin and autism: a systematic review of randomized controlled trials. J Child Adolesc Psychopharmacol 2014;24(2):54–68.

155. Levy SE, Souders MC, Ittenbach RF, et al. Relationship of dietary intake to gastrointestinal symptoms in children with autistic spectrum disorders. Biol Psychiatry 2007;61(4):492–7.

156. Williams KW, Wray JJ, Wheeler DM. Intravenous secretin for autism spectrum disorder. Cochrane Database Syst Rev 2005;(3):CD003495.

157. Sturmey P. Secretin is an ineffective treatment for pervasive developmental disabilities: a review of 15 double-blind randomized controlled trials. Res Dev Disabil 2005;26(1):87–97.

158. Sandler A. Placebo effects in developmental disabilities: implications for research and practice. Ment Retard Dev Disabil Res Rev 2005;11(2):164–70.

159. Ratliff-Schaub K, Carey T, Reeves GD, et al. Randomized controlled trial of transdermal secretin on behavior of children with autism. Autism 2005;9(3):256–65.

160. Jayachandra S. Is secretin effective in treatment for autism spectrum disorders (ASD)? Int J Psychiatry Med 2005;35(1):99–101.

161. Koves K, Kausz M, Reser D, et al. Secretin and autism: a basic morphological study about the distribution of secretin in the nervous system. Regul Pept 2004;123(1–3):209–16.

162. Kern JK, Espinoza E, Trivedi MH. The effectiveness of secretin in the management of autism. Expert Opin Pharmacother 2004;5(2):379–87.

163. Dogrukol-Ak D, Tore F, Tuncel N. Passage of VIP/PACAP/secretin family across the blood-brain barrier: therapeutic effects. Curr Pharm Des 2004;10(12):1325–40.

164. Levy SE, Souders MC, Wray J, et al. Children with autistic spectrum disorders. I: comparison of placebo and single dose of human synthetic secretin. Arch Dis Child 2003;88(8):731–6.

165. Unis AS, Munson JA, Rogers SJ, et al. A randomized, double-blind, placebo-controlled trial of porcine versus synthetic secretin for reducing symptoms of autism. J Am Acad Child Adolesc Psychiatry 2002;41(11):1315–21.

166. Sponheim E, Oftedal G, Helverschou SB. Multiple doses of secretin in the treatment of autism: a controlled study. Acta Paediatr 2002;91(5):540–5.
167. Patel NC, Yeh JY, Shepherd MD, et al. Secretin treatment for autistic disorder: a critical analysis. Pharmacotherapy 2002;22(7):905–14.
168. Molloy CA, Manning-Courtney P, Swayne S, et al. Lack of benefit of intravenous synthetic human secretin in the treatment of autism. J Autism Dev Disord 2002; 32(6):545–51.
169. Kern JK, Van Miller S, Evans PA, et al. Efficacy of porcine secretin in children with autism and pervasive developmental disorder. J Autism Dev Disord 2002; 32(3):153–60.
170. Kaminska B, Czaja M, Kozielska E, et al. Use of secretin in the treatment of childhood autism. Med Sci Monit 2002;8(1):RA22–6.
171. Williams K, Wray JA, Wheeler DM. Intravenous secretin for autism spectrum disorders (ASD). Cochrane Database Syst Rev 2012;(4):CD003495.
172. Elder JH, Shankar M, Shuster J, et al. The gluten-free, casein-free diet in autism: results of a preliminary double blind clinical trial. J Autism Dev Disord 2006; 36(3):413–20.
173. Pynnonen PA, Isometsa ET, Verkasalo MA, et al. Gluten-free diet may alleviate depressive and behavioural symptoms in adolescents with coeliac disease: a prospective follow-up case-series study. BMC Psychiatry 2005;5(1):14.
174. Millward C, Ferriter M, Calver S, et al. Gluten- and casein-free diets for autistic spectrum disorder. Cochrane Database Syst Rev 2004;(2):CD003498.
175. Ashwood P, Anthony A, Torrente F, et al. Spontaneous mucosal lymphocyte cytokine profiles in children with autism and gastrointestinal symptoms: mucosal immune activation and reduced counter regulatory interleukin-10. J Clin Immunol 2004;24(6):664–73.
176. Ashwood P, Anthony A, Pellicer AA, et al. Intestinal lymphocyte populations in children with regressive autism: evidence for extensive mucosal immunopathology. J Clin Immunol 2003;23(6):504–17.
177. Knivsberg AM, Reichelt KL, Hoien T, et al. A randomised, controlled study of dietary intervention in autistic syndromes. Nutr Neurosci 2002;5(4):251–61.
178. Cornish E. Gluten and casein free diets in autism: a study of the effects on food choice and nutrition. J Hum Nutr Diet 2002;15(4):261–9.
179. Knivsber AM, Reichelt KL, Nodland M. Reports on dietary intervention in autistic disorders. Nutr Neurosci 2001;4(1):25–37.
180. Whitely P, Rodgers J, Shattock P. A gluten-free diet as an intervention for autism and associated spectrum disorders: preliminary findings. Autism 1999;3(1):45–65.
181. Ek J, Stensrud M, Reichelt KL. Gluten-free diet decreases urinary peptide levels in children with celiac disease. J Pediatr Gastroenterol Nutr 1999;29(3):282–5.
182. Mari-Bauset S, Zazpe I, Mari-Sanchis A, et al. Evidence of the gluten-free and casein-free diet in autism spectrum disorders: a systematic review. J Child Neurol 2014. [Epub ahead of print].
183. Dosman C, Adams D, Wudel B, et al. Complementary, holistic, and integrative medicine: autism spectrum disorder and gluten- and casein-free diet. Pediatr Rev 2013;34(10):e36–41.
184. Pedersen L, Parlar S, Kvist K, et al. Data mining the ScanBrit study of a gluten- and casein-free dietary intervention for children with autism spectrum disorders: behavioural and psychometric measures of dietary response. Nutr Neurosci 2014;17:207–13.
185. Whiteley P, Shattock P, Knivsberg AM, et al. Gluten- and casein-free dietary intervention for autism spectrum conditions. Front Hum Neurosci 2012;6:344.

186. Pennesi CM, Klein LC. Effectiveness of the gluten-free, casein-free diet for children diagnosed with autism spectrum disorder: based on parental report. Nutr Neurosci 2012;15(2):85–91.
187. Whiteley P, Haracopos D, Knivsberg AM, et al. The ScanBrit randomised, controlled, single-blind study of a gluten- and casein-free dietary intervention for children with autism spectrum disorders. Nutr Neurosci 2010;13(2):87–100.
188. Hsu CL, Lin CY, Chen CL, et al. The effects of a gluten and casein-free diet in children with autism: a case report. Chang Gung Med J 2009;32(4):459–65.
189. Marcason W. What is the current status of research concerning use of a gluten-free, casein-free diet for children diagnosed with autism? J Am Diet Assoc 2009; 109(3):572.
190. Elder JH. The gluten-free, casein-free diet in autism: an overview with clinical implications. Nutr Clin Pract 2008–2009;23(6):583–8.
191. Rossignol DA. Hyperbaric oxygen therapy might improve certain pathophysiological findings in autism. Med Hypotheses 2007;68(6):1208–27.
192. Rossignol DA, Rossignol LW. Hyperbaric oxygen therapy may improve symptoms in autistic children. Med Hypotheses 2006;67(2):216–28.
193. Sampanthavivat M, Singkhwa W, Chaiyakul T, et al. Hyperbaric oxygen in the treatment of childhood autism: a randomised controlled trial. Diving Hyperb Med 2012;42(3):128–33.
194. Rossignol DA, Bradstreet JJ, Van Dyke K, et al. Hyperbaric oxygen treatment in autism spectrum disorders. Med Gas Res 2012;2(1):16.
195. Ghanizadeh A. Hyperbaric oxygen therapy for treatment of children with autism: a systematic review of randomized trials. Med Gas Res 2012;2:13.
196. Bent S, Bertoglio K, Ashwood P, et al. Brief report: hyperbaric oxygen therapy (HBOT) in children with autism spectrum disorder: a clinical trial. J Autism Dev Disord 2012;42(6):1127–32.
197. Ichim TE, Solano F, Glenn E, et al. Stem cell therapy for autism. J Transl Med 2007;5:30.
198. Liu EY, Scott CT. Great expectations: autism spectrum disorder and induced pluripotent stem cell technologies. Stem Cell Rev 2014;10(2):145–50.
199. Aigner S, Heckel T, Zhang JD, et al. Human pluripotent stem cell models of autism spectrum disorder: emerging frontiers, opportunities, and challenges towards neuronal networks in a dish. Psychopharmacology 2014;231(6):1089–104.
200. Siniscalco D, Sapone A, Cirillo A, et al. Autism spectrum disorders: is mesenchymal stem cell personalized therapy the future? J Biomed Biotechnol 2012; 2012:480289.
201. Helm D. Psychodynamic and behavior modification approaches to the treatment of infantile autism empirical similarities. J Autism Child Schizophr 1976;6(1):27–41.
202. Enticott PG, Fitzgibbon BM, Kennedy HA, et al. A double-blind, randomized trial of deep repetitive transcranial magnetic stimulation (rTMS) for autism spectrum disorder. Brain Stimul 2014;7(2):206–11.
203. Oberman LM, Rotenberg A, Pascual-Leone A. Use of transcranial magnetic stimulation in autism spectrum disorders. J Autism Dev Disord 2013. [Epub ahead of print].
204. Panerai S, Tasca D, Lanuzza B, et al. Effects of repetitive transcranial magnetic stimulation in performing eye-hand integration tasks: four preliminary studies with children showing low-functioning autism. Autism 2013;18:638–50.
205. Casanova MF, Baruth JM, El-Baz A, et al. Repetitive transcranial magnetic stimulation (rTMS) modulates event-related potential (ERP) indices of attention in autism. Transl Neurosci 2012;3(2):170–80.

206. Enticott PG, Kennedy HA, Zangen A, et al. Deep repetitive transcranial magnetic stimulation associated with improved social functioning in a young woman with an autism spectrum disorder. J ECT 2011;27(1):41–3.

207. Tsai SJ. Could repetitive transcranial magnetic stimulation be effective in autism? Med Hypotheses 2005;64(5):1070–1.

208. Warwick TC, Griffith J, Reyes B, et al. Effects of vagus nerve stimulation in a patient with temporal lobe epilepsy and Asperger syndrome: case report and review of the literature. Epilepsy Behav 2007;10(2):344–7.

209. Danielsson S, Viggedal G, Gillberg C, et al. Lack of effects of vagus nerve stimulation on drug-resistant epilepsy in eight pediatric patients with autism spectrum disorders: a prospective 2-year follow-up study. Epilepsy Behav 2008; 12:298–304.

210. Levy ML, Levy KM, Hoff D, et al. Vagus nerve stimulation therapy in patients with autism spectrum disorder and intractable epilepsy: results from the vagus nerve stimulation therapy patient outcome registry. J Neurosurg Pediatr 2010;5(6): 595–602.

Primary Sleep Disorders in People with Epilepsy

Clinical Questions and Answers

Madeleine M. Grigg-Damberger, MD[a],*,
Nancy Foldvary-Schaefer, DO[b]

KEYWORDS

- Sleep disorders and epilepsy • Sleep apnea and epilepsy
- Sleepwalking and frontal lobe epilepsy • Insomnia and epilepsy

KEY POINTS

- Identifying and treating sleep disorders in people with epilepsy often improves seizure control and quality of life.
- Comorbid neurodevelopmental disorders increased the likelihood for sleep complaints in adults with epilepsy.
- Sleep disruption in children with epilepsy compared with adults is more likely multifactorial, including varying combinations of epilepsy per se, frequent nocturnal seizures disrupting nocturnal sleep organization, effects of antiepileptic medications on daytime alertness and nighttime sleep, and treatable primary sleep disorders.
- Cosleeping reduces risk for sudden unexpected death in epilepsy.
- Fifty percent to 80% of patients with temporal lobe epilepsy have nocturnal seizures, but nearly all have seizures when awake.

Sleep is the golden chain that ties health and our bodies together.
—*Thomas Dekker*

Sleep and epilepsy are common but often poor bedfellows. Many primary sleep disorders such as obstructive sleep apnea (OSA), excessive daytime sleepiness (EDS), and sleep-maintenance insomnia are 2 to 3 times more common in people with

Financial disclosure and conflict of interest obligations: the authors have no conflicts of interest to declare regarding this article. The use of melatonin to treat insomnia in children with epilepsy is discussed.

This article is reproduced for psychiatric professionals; it originally appeared in *Sleep Medicine Clinics*, volume 7, issue 1.

[a] Department of Neurology, University of New Mexico School of Medicine, MSC10 5620, One University of New Mexico, Albuquerque, NM 87131-0001, USA; [b] Section of Sleep Medicine, Department of Neurology, Cleveland Clinic, S51, 9500 Euclid Avenue, Cleveland, OH 44195, USA
* Corresponding author.
E-mail address: mgriggd@salud.unm.edu

1056-4993/15/$ – see front matter © 2015 Elsevier Inc. All rights reserved.

Abbreviations/Acronyms: Sleep disorders and epilepsy	
AASM	American Academy of Sleep Medicine
AED	Antiepileptic drug
AHI	Apnea-hypopnea index
AWE	Adults with epilepsy
BMI	Body mass index
CAP	Cyclic alternating pattern
CPAP	Continuous positive airway pressure
DoA	Disorders of arousal
EDS	Excessive daytime sleepiness
EEG	Electroencephalography
ESS	Epworth Sleepiness Scale
FLE	Frontal lobe epilepsy
IED	Interictal epileptiform discharges
JME	Juvenile myoclonic epilepsy
NFLE	Nocturnal frontal lobe
NREM	Non–rapid eye movement
OSA	Obstructive sleep apnea
OSDB	Obstructive sleep disordered breathing
PGE	Primary generalized epilepsy
PLMS	Periodic limb movements in sleep
PNE	Paroxysmal nocturnal behaviors
PSG	Polysomnography
RBD	Rapid eye movement sleep behavior disorder
REM	Rapid eye movement
RLS	Restless legs syndrome
RS	Rett syndrome
SA-SDQ	Sleep Apnea-Sleep Disorders Questionnaire
SD	Sleep deprivation
TLE	Temporal lobe epilepsy
TSC	Tuberous sclerosis complex
VNS	Vagal nerve stimulation
V-PSG	Video-PSG
WASO	Wake time after sleep onset

epilepsy than the general population.[1–14] AWE and sleep complaints have significantly lower quality of life than those without sleep problems.[11–13,15,16]

Sleep problems in children and adolescents with epilepsy are associated with negative effects on daytime behavior and academic performance.[17–19] Recognition of this situation has led to more patients referred to sleep centers to evaluate whether untreated sleep disorders may be contributing to their seizures. Late onset or worsening seizure control in older adults often heralds OSA.[20,21] Identifying and treating sleep disorders in people with epilepsy often improves seizure control and quality of life. The recent evidence for this theory is review in this article.

QUESTIONNAIRE-BASED STUDIES OF THE PREVALENCE OF PRIMARY SLEEP DISORDERS IN ADULTS WITH EPILEPSY

Sleep disorders are 2 to 3 times more common in adults[11–14] and children[1–10] with epilepsy compared with the general age-matched population, especially when their seizures are poorly controlled or complicated by comorbid neurologic conditions.

Most recent studies examining the prevalence of sleep complaints in AWE are based on sleep questionnaires, sometimes coupled with structured clinical interviews, neuropsychological testing, or psychiatric evaluation.[11–13,21–24] **Table 1** summarizes these studies.

Table 1 Questionnaire-based studies evaluating sleep problems in adults with epilepsy			
Authors, Year	**Study Design**	**Study Population**	**Findings**
Manni et al,[22] 2000	Large case-control	244 focal or generalized epilepsy vs 205 controls	Higher scores on ESS in those with snoring, apneas, or recurrent seizures past year
Malow et al,[23] 1997	Large case-control	158 with focal or generalized epilepsy vs 68 patients with other neurologic disorders	ESS $\geq$10 in 28% with epilepsy vs 18% controls Symptoms of sleep apnea or RLS independent predictors of ESS >10
Vignatelli et al,[24] 2006	Small case-control	33 with nocturnal FLE (36% seizures nightly) vs 27 controls	36% NFLE tired most mornings vs 11% controls; 50% awoke most nights vs 22% controls
De Weerd et al,[11] 2004	Large case-control	492 with epilepsy vs controls	39% of people with epilepsy complained of sleep disturbances last 6 mo vs 18% controls Quality of life most impaired in epilepsy patients with sleep complaints
Khatami et al,[12] 2006	Prospective large case-control (questionnaire and structured clinical interview)	100 consecutive patients with either generalized or focal epilepsy compared with controls	30% of people with epilepsy had sleep complaints vs 10 controls. Loud snoring and restless legs independent predictors of EDS in patients with epilepsy
Xu et al,[15] 2006	Large case series	201 people with refractory partial epilepsy on $\geq$2 AEDS	34% reported diagnosed with sleep disturbances last 6 mo 10% prescribed hypnotics Those reporting sleep disturbances were more likely to endorse symptoms of depression or anxiety, have poorer quality of life, and have had a seizure in the past week
Piperdou et al,[13] 2008	Large case series	124 consecutive patients with focal or generalized epilepsy: 42% nocturnal seizures	28% had scores suggest OSA; 25% insomnia and 17% EDS; Insomnia independent predictor of reduced quality of life Insomnia correlated with seizure frequency
Haut et al,[21] 2009	Small case-control retrospective study included extensive neuropsychological testing	31 elders with epilepsy compared with 31 age-matched healthy controls	18% with epilepsy depressed vs 0% controls Poor sleeper complained more of EDS, awakening short of breath or with headache

(continued on next page)

Table 1
(continued)

Authors, Year	Study Design	Study Population	Findings
Zanzerma et al,[142] 2012	Prospective case-control study with actigraphy	40 patients (median age 18 y) with epilepsy, 20 well-controlled; 20 medically refractory epilepsy	Patients with medically refractory epilepsy had longer sleep duration at home, more daytime napping, more 24-hour sleep time, EDS. ESS scores did not distinguish medically refractory from well controlled
Foldvary-Schaefer et al,[164] 2012	Prospective cross-sectional study with polysomnographic confirmation of OSA	130 consecutive adults with epilepsy seen in a tertiary epilepsy center	Prevalence of OSA (AHI ≥10 per h of sleep) was 30%, moderate to severe (AHI ≥15/h) in 16%, rates that markedly exceed general population estimates. Male gender, older age, higher BMI, hypertension, and dental problems were associated with higher AHI. Risk for OSA increased with age and antiepileptic drug load
Wigg et al,[131] 2014	Prospective study	98 unselected adults with epilepsy	Prevalence of suicidal ideation was 13%. Reports of poor sleep quality and depression were good predictors of suicidal risk

Abbreviations: AEDs, antiepileptic drugs; AHI, apnea-hypopnea index; BMI, body mass index; ESS, Epworth Sleepiness Scale; FLE, frontal lobe epilepsy; NFLE, nocturnal frontal lobe epilepsy; RLS, restless legs syndrome.

Difficulty staying asleep (sleep-maintenance insomnia) is perhaps the most common sleep complaint in AWE. A prospective study[12] found that 52% of 100 consecutive Greek AWE endorsed symptoms of sleep-maintenance insomnia versus 38% of 90 age-matched controls; however, another study[13] found insomnia in only 25% of Greek AWE. Another study[15] found that 10% of 201 adults with medically refractory partial epilepsies were prescribed hypnotics for complains of insomnia. Recent prospective case-control studies find that poor sleep quality, difficulty sleeping, or EDS are 2 to 3 times more common in AWE than healthy controls.[11–14] The most common sleep/wake complaint among AWE is sleep-maintenance insomnia (difficulty staying asleep). One prospective study found that 30% of 100 AWE reported sleep complaints compared with 10% of 90 controls[12]:

- Sleep-maintenance insomnia: 52% versus 38%
- Sleep-onset insomnia: 34% versus 28%
- EDS: 19% versus 14%
- Restless legs: 18% versus 12%
- Sleep apnea: 9% versus 3%

Another study of 486 adults with focal epilepsy found that 39% reported sleep complaints versus 18% of controls.[11]

Two questionnaire-based studies have reported that EDS was statistically more common in people with epilepsy versus controls.[13,23] Eighteen percent to 28% of AWE complained of EDS (Epworth Sleepiness Scale [ESS] score >10) compared with 12% to 17% of controls.[13,23] An international cross-sectional survey of 35,327 adults found that 24% reported that they did not sleep well and 12% complained of severe or dangerous EDS.[25] Although sleepiness in AWE is more likely multifactorial, symptoms suggestive of OSA or restless legs syndrome (RLS) were independent predictors of an increased ESS greater than 10.[22,23,26]

Several studies have found that EDS in people with epilepsy is more likely to be associated with depression or anxiety. Depression and anxiety are more common among AWE than healthy controls.[27] Scores on the Beck Depression Inventory suggestive of moderate to severe depression best predicted a complaint of EDS in patients with epilepsy, whereas sleep apnea scores contributed only minor independent effects.[14] Thirty-two percent of 201 patients with refractory partial epilepsy were also taking medications to treat depression, 21% for anxiety; those taking psychotropics were more likely to complain of sleep problems than those who did not take these.[15] A retrospective study found that 31 elders with partial epilepsies endorsed more symptoms of EDS depression, anxiety, daytime sleepiness, and awakening short of breath or with a headache than age-matched and gender-matched controls.[21] Complaints of EDS reported by 48% of 99 unselected adult patients with epilepsy correlated best with anxiety (and neck circumference).[28]

Comorbid neurodevelopmental disorders increased the likelihood for sleep complaints in AWE. Thirty-one percent of 35 adults with tuberous sclerosis complex (TSC) complained of insomnia, 71% of whom also had a history of epilepsy.[26] Complaints of insomnia were associated with OSA and RLS scores. Daytime sleepiness was associated with depression, antisocial behavior, and psychotropic medications. Patients treated with antiepileptic drugs AED were more likely to report daytime sleepiness, attention deficits, and anxiety.

Sleep hygiene may contribute to sleep/wake complaints in people with epilepsy. A study examining sleep hygiene in 270 AWE compared with controls found among the patients with epilepsy:

1. 23% smoked at bedtimes;
2. 29% had irregular sleep/wake schedules or varying degrees of sleep deprivation (SD);
3. 17% engaged in high concentration/upsetting activities at bedtime.[22]

Controls had many (if not more) poor sleep habits. However, the AWE were more likely to drink coffee before bedtime (50% of patients with epilepsy vs 30% controls) and nap after dinner (16% epilepsy vs 6% controls).

Another study of 108 AWE[29] found that many did not practice healthy lifestyle behaviors (including sleep hygiene), even if they were compliant with their AED medication.

Factors that do not contribute to more sleep complaints in AWE:

1. Most studies do not find gender a risk factor for sleep problems in people with epilepsy,[12,13,22] except 1 study that found that women with refractory partial epilepsy reported more severe sleep problems than men[15];
2. Neither EDS nor insomnia was particularly more common in adults with partial-onset or primary generalized epilepsies[12,13,22,23]; and
3. Nocturnal seizures were not more likely to be associated with sleep problems,[15,23] except in people with nocturnal frontal lobe epilepsy (NFLE), who only reported more midsleep awakenings than controls.[24]

IS SLEEP ARCHITECTURE ALTERED IN ADULTS WITH EPILEPSY?

Several older studies[30,31] reported abnormalities in sleep architecture in AWE, but few of these controlled either for seizures or medication. These studies found:

1. Reduced time spent in rapid eye movement (REM) sleep;
2. Prolonged REM latency;
3. Increased wake time after sleep onset (WASO), resulting in reduced total sleep time and sleep efficiency;
4. Increased number of arousals, awakenings, and stage shifts[30,31] and in even the absence of seizures the night of the polysomnography (PSG).[31]

Abnormalities in Rapid Eye Movement Sleep Often Seen in Adults with Epilepsy

REM sleep may be particularly susceptible to the occurrence of seizures in people with partial epilepsy. One study found that percentage of REM sleep decreased from a mean of 18% to 12% if the patient had a seizure that day, and 16% to 7% if the seizure occurred during nighttime sleep.[32] Night seizures (but not day seizures) significantly reduced sleep efficiency, increased REM latency, increased stage 1, reduced stage 2 and 4 sleep, and increased drowsiness on the maintenance of wakefulness test.[32] With daytime seizures, the percent of total sleep time spent in REM sleep the following night decreased from 18% at baseline to 12%.[32] If the seizure occurred at night, the decrease in REM sleep time was greater (7% vs 16%). The reduced sleep efficiency and prolonged REM latency were even greater if the temporal lobe seizure occurred before the first REM period. Both diurnal and nocturnal seizures prolonged REM sleep latency. Nocturnal, but not diurnal, seizures increased stage non–rapid eye movement 1 (NREM 1) and decreased deeper NREM 3 sleep.

If a motor convulsion occurs during a night of PSG in a person with epilepsy (regardless of whether it is primary generalized or focal in onset), changes in sleep architecture observed may include a prolonged REM latency, decreased total sleep time and REM sleep time and increased WASO, arousals, NREM 1 and 2 sleep.[31,33]

Sleep Architecture May Be More Disrupted in People with Temporal Lobe Epilepsy

Some studies suggest that sleep architecture is more disturbed in adults with temporal lobe epilepsy (TLE) compared with those whose seizures emanate from the frontal lobes (frontal lobe epilepsy [FLE]) or are primary generalized convulsions (primary generalized epilepsy [PGE]).[31,33,34] Crespel and colleagues[34] found that sleep architecture was more disturbed in 15 patients with mesial TLE compared with 15 with FLE. The patients with TLE had reduced sleep efficiency, increased WASO, and more arousals. These investigators also found that patients with TLE often had dysmorphic sleep spindles in the epileptic hemisphere. Even although FLE seizures most occurred in sleep, the macroarchitecture and microarchitecture of their sleep was normal. Although seizures in people with TLE most often occurred awake, their sleep architecture was disrupted, especially by reduced sleep efficiency. These differences persisted even after SD or AEDs were discontinued. **Fig. 1** shows 2 illustrative sleep histograms, one from a patient with FLE, the other from a patient with TLE.

Abnormalities in Non–Rapid Eye Movement Sleep Microarchitecture Identified Using Cyclic Alternating Pattern Analysis in People with Epilepsy

For more than 2 decades, primarily Italian sleep researchers[35–45] have used cyclic alternating pattern (CAP) analysis of NREM sleep microarchitecture to confirm that

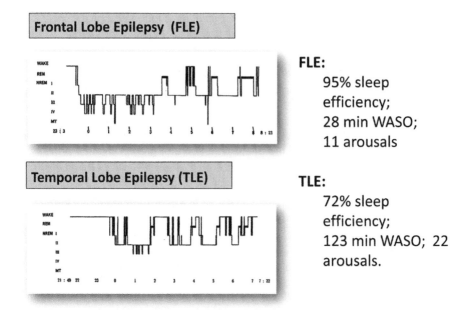

Frontal Lobe Epilepsy (FLE)

FLE:
95% sleep efficiency;
28 min WASO;
11 arousals

Temporal Lobe Epilepsy (TLE)

TLE:
72% sleep efficiency;
123 min WASO; 22 arousals.

Fig. 1. Two illustrative histograms, one from a patient with FLE, the other with TLE. (*Modified from* Crespel A, Baldy-Moulinier M, Coubes P. The relationship between sleep and epilepsy in frontal and temporal lobe epilepsies: practical and physiopathologic considerations. Epilepsia 1998;39(2):150–7.)

instability of NREM sleep is present in a variety of sleep disorders, including different epilepsies. NREM sleep using CAP analysis can be divided into 2 phases (A and B). In patients with epilepsy, interictal epileptiform discharges (IEDs) more often occur in the transition from NREM1 and 2 to NREM 3 sleep, less in NREM 3, and least in REM sleep. CAP studies show:

1. Most IEDs occur during phase A1 of CAP, when NREM sleep was dominated by either K-complexes or δ bursts
2. Studies in primary generalized and frontotemporal partial epilepsies show that IEDs are most inhibited during phase B of CAP
3. Nocturnal convulsions or motor seizures most often arise concomitant with phase A of CAP
4. Partial seizures occurring in clusters during sleep more often occurred during CAP, and
5. An increase in CAP rate has been observed during the 30-minute period after a partial sleep-related seizure

These findings are nonspecific; similar abnormalities in CAP are seen in patients with OSA, periodic limb movements in sleep (PLMS), RLS, and NREM parasomnias.

SLEEP DISORDERS CONFIRMED BY POLYSOMNOGRAPHY IN ADULTS WITH EPILEPSY

Sleep studies in AWE are most often for suspected OSA, occasionally to characterize nocturnal spells, rarely for suspected REM sleep behavior, or unexplained hypersomnia. A few studies[19,20,46–48] have suggested that OSA is found in 10% of unselected adult patients with epilepsy and 30% of patients with medically refractory epilepsy.

If an apnea-hypopnea index (AHI) score of 5 or greater is found in approximately 24% of men and 9% of women in the general adult population (ages 30–60 years),[49,50] then, OSA is more prevalent in AWE.

Obstructive Sleep Apnea in Adults with Epilepsy Often Mild

Manni and colleagues[46] found OSA (AHI ≥5) in 10% of 283 unselected AWE; however, OSA was mild (AHI 5–14/h) in 67%, moderate (15–29/h) in 22%, and severe (>30) in only 11%. Using the Sleep Apnea-Sleep Disorders Questionnaire (SA-SDQ), Weatherwax and colleagues[51] found OSA (AHI >5) in 45% of 125 unselected AWE. These investigators validated the use of the SA-SDQ: a score of greater than 29 provided a sensitivity of 75% and a specificity of 65% in men, 80% and 67%, respectively, in women with epilepsy.

Obstructive Sleep Apnea More Likely to Be Found in Adults with Medically Refractory, Late Onset, or Worsening Epilepsy

Three recent studies[20,46,47] have suggested that OSA is more likely to be found in AWE who are older, heavier, male, or have late onset, medically refractory, or worsening epilepsy. A study by Manni and colleagues[46] reported that OSA was more likely to be found on PSG in AWE who were male (15.4% men, 5.4% women), older (46 ± 15 vs 33 ± 12 years), sleepier (23% vs 9%), heavier (28.5 ± 3.6 vs 23.3 ± 3.7 kg/m^2), and had experienced their first seizure at an older age (32 vs 19 years).

Chihorek and colleagues[20] prospectively recorded PSG in 21 older adults, comparing results of 11 with late onset or worsening seizures with 10 who were seizure free or had improving seizure control. The group of patients who had late onset or worsening seizures had higher AHI and higher scores on the SA-SDQ and ESS than the group with better-controlled epilepsy. The 2 groups were similar in age, body mass index (BMI, calculated as weight in kilograms divided by the square of height in meters), neck circumference, number of prescribed AEDs, and frequency of nocturnal seizures. The investigators concluded that OSA in older adults is associated with seizure exacerbation. A retrospective chart review by Hollinger and colleagues[47] found that the appearance of OSA symptoms in 21 of 29 older adults (median age 56 years, 86% men) coincided with a clear increase in seizure frequency or the first episode of status epilepticus. A prospective pilot study found OSA (AHI >10) in 46% of 13 adults with refractory epilepsy.[48] Larger prospective studies are needed to confirm these findings.

Periodic Limb Movements and Restless Legs in Adults with Epilepsy

PLMS are common and often nonspecific in adults who do not endorse symptoms of RLS, REM sleep behavior disorder (RBD), narcolepsy with cataplexy, or take psychotropic medications. A few studies have been published reporting PLMS in PSG in adults or children with epilepsy. Sleep studies were most often performed for sleep complaints suggestive of OSA, less often for limb jerking or RLS. Khatami and colleagues[12] found that complaints of RLS were not more prevalent in AWE than healthy controls (18% vs 12%), but they screened for RLS using only a single question. Malow and colleagues[23] found that 35% of 158 AWE endorsed symptoms of RLS, but so did 29% of controls with other neurologic disorders. These investigators recorded PSG in 27 of the 42 AWE who complained of RLS; periodic limb movement arousal index (PLMI) scores higher than 10 were found in only 15%. Another retrospective study by the same group recorded PSG in 63 AWE with sleep complaints: PLMI 20 or greater in 17% (45% of whom had PLMI >30)[52]; however, most of the PLMS did not cause arousal or need treatment.

Rapid Eye Movement Sleep Behavior Disorder Occasionally Found in Older Adults with Epilepsy

Two case series have been published reporting RBD coexisting with epilepsy in older adults. The first[53] described 2 men (ages 60 and 75 years) who developed late onset sleep-related motor convulsions and who also had symptoms and PSG findings of RBD. RBD preceded the onset of their epilepsy by 5 to 10 years. A prospective study[54] found RBD in 10 (12.5%) of 80 older adults (mean age 71 ± 7 years, 47 men) with epilepsy. RBD episodes preceded seizure onset by 4.5 years in 6 patients, and followed it by 9.7 years in 4.

Given the prevalence of OSA in late onset or worsening epilepsy, RBD needs to be distinguished from pseudo-RBD caused by severe OSA. Iranzo and Santamaria[55] reported on 16 adults with severe OSA (mean AHI of 68 ± 19/h) who were believed likely to have RBD because they complained of dream-enacting behaviors and unpleasant dreams. However, skeletal atonia was preserved during REM sleep in these patients with pseudo-RBD and continuous positive airway pressure (CPAP) therapy eliminated the abnormal behaviors, unpleasant dreams, daytime sleepiness, and snoring.

QUESTIONNAIRE-BASED STUDIES ON THE PREVALENCE OF SLEEP DISORDERS IN CHILDREN WITH EPILEPSY

Like AWE, children with it are more likely to have sleep problems than the general pediatric population.[1–10] Sleep disruption in children with epilepsy is more likely multifactorial, including varying combinations of epilepsy per se, frequent nocturnal seizures disrupting nocturnal sleep organization, effects of antiepileptic medications on daytime alertness and nighttime sleep, and treatable primary sleep disorders. Comorbidities such as physical disability,[8] intellectual disability,[2,56,57] neurodevelopmental syndromes,[58,59] autism spectrum disorder,[60] and behavioral disorders[1,7–9,61] may add to the likelihood of sleep disorders in a child with epilepsy. Sleep complaints in children with epilepsy are rarely brought up at a pediatric visit and often misdiagnosed.[62] A case-control parental report study of 43 children with idiopathic benign rolandic epilepsy (ages 6–16 years) found that those with epilepsy had significantly shorter sleep duration, more frequent parasomnias, and daytime sleepiness than the controls.[5]

Cortesi and colleagues[1] prospectively evaluated whether sleep or daytime behavior problems were more common in children with epilepsy than their siblings or healthy age-matched controls. Using post hoc comparisons, these investigators found that the 89 children with idiopathic partial or generalized epilepsy had significantly more sleep problems than their 49 siblings or 321 healthy controls for parasomnias, bedtime difficulties, sleep fragmentation, and daytime drowsiness. Using multiple regression analysis, the investigators further found that sleep complaints, longer sleep latencies, and shorter sleep times were more likely to be found in the children whose seizures were not controlled. Daytime seizures and high nighttime IED discharge rates predicted daytime drowsiness, explaining 15% of its variance.

Cortesi and colleagues further found that behavior problems (inattention, hyperactivity, impulsivity, oppositional defiant disorder) greatly increased the likelihood that sleep problems would be reported in children with epilepsy. Three variables significantly associated with greater sleep problems in these otherwise normal children with epilepsy were:

1. Length of freedom from seizures
2. Age
3. Higher rates of IEDs during sleep (accounting for 24% of the variance)

The investigators concluded that the presence of epilepsy in a highly selected sample of children (without other comorbidities and whose epilepsy was more often well controlled) was associated with sleep, behavior, and adjustment problems beyond those seen in their siblings or healthy controls.

A case-control study found that children with epilepsy (n = 79, mean age 10.1 ± 3.1 years) had a mean of 4 ± 3 sleep problems compared with 2 ± 2 among 73 controls matched for age and gender (P<.001).[7] Reports of frequent unsound sleep, snoring, daytime hyperactivity, sudden daytime sleep attacks, limb movements during sleep, bedtime refusal, were all more commonly reported in the children with epilepsy. Mean scores for sleep-disordered breathing (SDB) symptoms were 2 times higher among the children with epilepsy compared with controls (10.5 vs 5.0). Other questionnaire-based studies have found:

1. Symptoms of OSA were 15 times more likely to be reported by the parents of 26 children with epilepsy (mean age 14.6 years) than 26 healthy controls (65% vs 4%)[6];
2. Children with epilepsy compared with control individuals had more daytime sleepiness, less on-task behavior, and less attention.[57];
3. Children with rolandic epilepsy had significantly shorter sleep duration, more frequent parasomnias, and daytime sleepiness than a reference sample of children.[5]

Poor sleep hygiene may also contribute to sleep problems in children with epilepsy. Batista and colleagues[2] prospectively evaluated sleep habits in 121 children compared with a similar number of healthy Brazilian schoolchildren. Compared with controls, the children with epilepsy were more likely to need to be put to bed by their parents, have an afternoon nap, wake during the night, take more than 30 minutes to fall asleep, express fear of the dark, awake with a distressing dream or worry, call out for the parent during the night, or visit the parental bed. The children whose seizures were poorly controlled were more likely to have poor sleep habits when compared with those children whose epilepsy was controlled. Compared with the children whose seizures usually occurred when awake, children whose seizures were primarily nocturnal (47%) had significantly more difficulty falling asleep, afternoon napping, nocturnal awakenings, awakening with fear or a dream, calling out for their parents at night, or visiting the parental bed.

Parental fear and anxiety about seizure recurrence often results in a return to cosleeping in families of children with epilepsy. One study found that 22% of 179 children with epilepsy changed to less independent sleep arrangements after onset of their epilepsy compared with 8% of 155 children with juvenile diabetes.[10] Cosleeping reduces risk for sudden unexpected death in epilepsy.

IS SLEEP ARCHITECTURE ABNORMAL IN CHILDREN WITH EPILEPSY?

Five case-control studies[35,40,63–65] and 6 case series[61,66–69] have been published evaluating sleep architecture in children with various epilepsies. A study comparing sleep complaints in 40 children with epilepsy referred for various sleep complaints with 11 children who had moderate obstructive sleep disordered breathing (OSDB) (AHI 5–10/h) found that the children whose seizures were poorly controlled had significantly lower sleep efficiency, a higher arousal index, and a higher percent of time spent in REM sleep compared with the children with OSA or those whose epilepsy was controlled. Sleep studies were normal in 7.5% of the children with epilepsy.

A case-control PSG study[64] recording 2 nights of video-PSG (V-PSG) study with 24-channel electroencephalography (EEG) in 17 children with partial epilepsy and

11 controls found that the group of children who had seizure(s) during their PSG had significantly less time in bed and sleep time. Children with epilepsy also had significantly fewer stage shifts per hour of sleep than controls (mean 4/h vs 6/h, respectively). Another recent 2-night V-PSG study[65] found significantly more NREM 1 and long REM sleep latency in 11 children with PGE who were seizure free and 8 age-matched and gender-matched controls. A case-control V-PSG study found reduced total sleep time, sleep efficiency, and percent REM sleep in 10 children with benign rolandic epilepsy compared with age-matched normal controls.[35]

Another small case-control PSG study[70] found that 10 patients with idiopathic generalized epilepsy (most had absence) had reduced sleep efficiency, total sleep time, and stage 4 sleep compared with 10 patients with idiopathic focal epilepsy and 12 age-matched normal controls when overnight PSG was recorded. However, 2 other studies[43,71] found no abnormalities in sleep architecture in children with absence seizures (which typically occur awake). Abnormalities in sleep spindles were reported in 1 case-control PSG study[72] recording sleep in 15 children with primary generalized epilepsies (9 untreated, 6 treated) and 47 healthy controls. These investigators found some abnormalities in sleep spindle density and frequency in children whose epilepsy was untreated (none in the treated). Another small PSG study[37] in 10 patients with Lennox-Gastaut syndrome (medically refractory epilepsy that begins in early childhood with multiple seizure types and intellectual disability) found reduced REM and stage 2 and decreased stage 3 compared with age-matched controls.

Girls with Rett syndrome (RS) often have epilepsy and severe sleep problems. A large study of 202 girls with RS[73] found that more than 80% had sleep problems, and these problems are more often severe and persistent. Sleep problems in girls with RS include:

- Nocturnal laughter: 59%
- Bruxism: 55%
- Long spells of screaming: 36%
- Nocturnal seizures: 26%
- Sleep terrors: 18%
- Sleep talking: 18%

Nocturnal seizures peaked between ages 13 and 17 years, and nocturnal screaming decreased to 30% in those older than 18 years. Frequent nighttime awakenings occurred in 54% up to age 7 years, decreasing to 40% by age 18 years. Compared with age-matched controls, girls with RS did not show the age-related decrease in total sleep time. They also continued to nap during the day: 75% of those 8 years and older took daytime naps, and 85% of the over-18-year-olds. Because of their often severe and persistent sleep/wake complaints, girls with RS are referred to pediatric sleep specialists to evaluate which of their nighttime behaviors are seizures or not.

PREVALENCE OF SLEEP APNEA AND OTHER PRIMARY SLEEP DISORDERS ON SLEEP STUDIES IN CHILDREN WITH EPILEPSY

A retrospective analysis by Kaleyias and colleagues[63] compared PSG findings in 40 children with epilepsy referred for symptoms suggestive of OSA with 11 children with moderate uncomplicated OSA (AHI 5–10/h). PSG abnormalities in the children with epilepsy were: OSA (AHI >1) in 20%, obstructive hypoventilation in 33%, upper airway resistance syndrome in 8%, primary snoring in 18%, and PLMS in 10%. These findings are not particularly revelatory, given that the children were symptomatic.

However, the children with epilepsy and OSA compared with the children with uncomplicated moderate OSA had significantly higher BMI (29 vs 2), were more often obese (BMI >95th percentile 62% vs 18%), had longer sleep latency (51 vs 16 minutes), higher arousal index (49 vs 21/h of sleep), and lower nadir Spo_2 (86% vs 90%) despite having a lower mean AHI (3/h) compared with those with uncomplicated moderate OSA (7/h). The children with poor seizure control had significantly lower sleep efficiency, a higher arousal index, and a higher percentage of REM sleep compared with children who were seizure free or showed good seizure control.

Another study of 30 children with epilepsy recruited for symptoms of OSA found varying degrees of OSA in 80% (AHI ≥1.5, mean AHI 8 ± 9/h).[61] The mean duration of respiratory events was significantly longer in the children who had more frequent epileptic seizures (mean apnea duration as a group was 22 ± 20 seconds).

Several PSG studies have been published screening for OSA and other sleep disorders in children with epilepsy and comorbid neurologic or neurodevelopmental disorders. Miano and colleagues[40] compared PSG findings in 11 Italian children with mental retardation and epilepsy (mean age 13 ± 4 years) and 11 healthy controls without sleep/wake complaints. PSG findings among the children with intellectual disability and epilepsy were: a mean AHI of 5 ± 3/h, but only 3 had an AHI greater than 5 (AHI 9–11/h), and 27% had PLMI greater than 5. Compared with controls, the children with epilepsy were longer sleep latency, higher percentage of WASO and NREM 3 sleep, lower sleep efficiency, more awakenings and stage shifts, a higher CAP rate, increased A1 index, and long and less numerous CAP sequences.

Bruni and colleagues[74] compared PSG findings in 10 children (mean age 11 years) with TSC and 10 healthy controls. These investigators found reduced sleep efficiency (60%–88%) in 9 and WASO greater than 10% in 7 of the children TSC. Frequent nocturnal awakenings occurred in 6 and poorly organized sleep cycles in 3. Compared with controls, the TSC group showed shorter sleep time, lower sleep efficiency, higher number of awakenings and stage shifts, increased NREM 1 and WASO, and decreased REM sleep. Sleep architecture was significantly more disrupted in the 3 children who had at least 1 seizure recorded during their PSG (sleep efficiency 69%, WASO 24%, mean awakenings 16/h) compared with the children with TSC who did not (sleep efficiency 88%, WASO 5%, and mean awakenings 3/h).

Although girls with RS have peculiar patterns of hyperventilation and apnea awake, they usually do not have OSA. Marcus and colleagues[75] found that sleep architecture, sleep efficiency, and breathing were normal in 30 girls with RS (median age 7 years) and age-matched controls. The investigators emphasized that unless there are clinical symptoms suggestive of SDB (such as scoliosis, present in 65% of patients), the diagnostic yield of PSG is low in patients with RS.[75] A particular EEG pattern of rhythmic theta (4–6 Hz) activity over the central regions, particularly during NREM sleep, often accompanied by central spikes is characteristic of RS.[76] Patients with RS have a higher incidence of sudden unexplained death (often during sleep) compared with age-matched controls; this factor may reflect their loss of heart rate variability and impaired cardiac autonomic regulation.[77]

ARE PARASOMNIAS MORE COMMON IN PEOPLE WITH EPILEPSY?

A prospective case-control study[1] found a higher incidence of parasomnias among 89 children with idiopathic epilepsy compared with 49 siblings and 321 healthy control children using parental sleep questionnaires. Parasomnias were not more common in a prospective study[12] of adults with a wide variety of different epilepsies and seizure types compared with healthy controls. Sixty percent with epilepsy and 58% of the controls complained of at least 1 parasomnia: most often nocturnal leg cramps (25% vs 17%), sleep starts (22% vs 17%), and sleep talking (21% vs 16%). Reports of sleep hallucinations, sleep paralysis, and violent acts during sleep occurred with equal frequency in patients and controls (16%, 4% and 2%, respectively), as were shouting out when sleeping (4% vs 3%). Nightmares and sleep-related bruxism were significantly more common, but among control individuals not the AWE (16% vs 6%, and 19% vs 10%, respectively). None of their study patients reported sleepwalking or bedwetting.

However, NREM disorders of arousal (DoA) (such as sleepwalking, sleep terrors, and confusional arousals) and sleep-related bruxism are significantly more common in patients and their relatives with NFLE.[78] An individual with NFLE has a 6-fold greater lifetime risk for DoA and 5-fold for sleep-related bruxism compared with controls. The lifetime prevalence of a DoA in relatives of patients with NFLE was 4.7 times greater and nightmares 2.6 times greater than compared with relatives of control individuals. NFLE predisposes patients and their relatives to the particular parasomnias (DoA and bruxism).

DIAGNOSTIC AND TECHNICAL CONSIDERATIONS WHEN PERFORMING SLEEP STUDIES IN PEOPLE WITH EPILEPSY

Comprehensive V-PSG is most often performed in people with epilepsy for suspected OSA or to identify primary sleep disorders contributing to complaints of EDS. Sometimes, we are asked to confirm whether paroxysmal nocturnal behaviors (PNE) are epileptic or not. The differential diagnosis of paroxysmal nocturnal events is shown in **Box 1**. The American Academy of Sleep Medicine (AASM) clinical practice parameters recommend in-laboratory V-PSG be used to evaluate parasomnias that are unusual or atypical because of patient's age at onset; the time, duration, or frequency of occurrence of the behavior; or the specifics of the particular motor patterns in question (eg, stereotypical, repetitive, or focal).[79]

A PSG is not needed if the nocturnal behavior events are typical, noninjurious, infrequent, and not disruptive to the child or family[79]; however, in children with sleep terrors or sleepwalking events occurring more than 2 to 3 times per week (and symptoms suggestive of OSA or PLMS), a PSG should be considered. Guilleminault and colleagues[80] found OSA in 58% of 84 children with frequent arousal parasomnias. Tonsillectomy eliminated OSA and arousals in those who had tonsillectomy.[80]

Box 1
Differential diagnosis of paroxysmal behavioral events in sleep

- NREM partial arousal disorder (confusional arousal; sleepwalking; sleep terror)
- Sleep-related epilepsy
- REM sleep behavior disorder
- Nightmare disorder
- Sleep-related dissociative disorder
- Sleep-related panic disorder
- Sleep-related choking, laryngospasm, or gastroesophageal reflux
- Sleep-related rhythmical movement disorder with vocalization
- Sleep-related expiratory groaning (catathrenia)

The diagnosis of epilepsy is usually known in most patients with epilepsy referred to sleep specialists. Symptoms that should prompt concern for sleep-related epileptic seizures include:

1. Events occur any time of the night, occur just after falling asleep, or shortly before awakening in the morning
2. Multiple events a night, or
3. Occasional occurrence of these events awake or during a brief nap

If we suspect that the nocturnal events are sleep-related epilepsy and the patient has no known diagnosis of epilepsy and has not had an EEG with sleep, we request one first. If a patient's spells occur only at night and are frequent, we may order V-PSG with expanded EEG before prolonged in-patient video-EEG monitoring, especially if concomitant OSA or RBD is suspected. If the first (or second with 24 hours of SD) routine EEG with sleep is normal and our clinical suspicion for a sleep-related epilepsy remains, we request continuous inpatient video-EEG monitoring (long-term monitoring) for 2 to 5 days. **Table 2** summarizes studies evaluating the diagnostic yield IEDs are found on various clinical neurophysiology tests in children with sleep-related seizures. Prolonged in-patient video-EEG monitoring is often a better choice in patients with undiagnosed paroxysmal nocturnal events when:

1. The nocturnal behaviors do not occur nightly or every other night
2. A primary sleep disorder (eg, OSA) is unlikely

Table 2
Likelihood of finding IEDs on a clinical neurophysiology test in children

Clinical Test	Diagnostic Yield
Routine EEG recording 20–30 min	IEDs found on initial EEG in 37% of children with definite epilepsy, and 13% suspected epilepsy (n = 534)[165] Initial EEG normal in 50% of children with clinically diagnosed epilepsy[166,167]
Routine EEG with video recording 25–30 min	Diagnosis determined in 45% referred for frequent paroxysmal events; 55% in the developmentally challenged[168] Confirmed staring spells, tics, stereotypias, tremor, paroxysmal eye movements, breath holding, or cyanotic spells[168]
Sleep-deprived EEG	Sleep deprivation increased likelihood NREM sleep observed NREM sleep observed in 57% of sleep-deprived, 44% partially sleep deprived, and 21% non–sleep deprived (n = 820 pediatric EEGs)[169] No increase in odds ratio of finding IEDs whether sleep occurred, partial, or total sleep deprivation[169] Need to test 11 children with sleep-deprived EEG to identify 1 additional child with IEDs[169]
Overnight diagnostic V-PSG	35% have full-blown event during 1 night of PSG, often need 2 nights to confirm diagnosis 41% of patients referred for minor events, 78% of 36 patients with known
Daytime video-EEG recording for 4–8 h	80% diagnostic yield if spells occur daily (n = 230)[170] Best reserved for children whose events occur daily[170,171]
Prolonged continuous in-patient video-EEG monitoring for 2–5 d	45%–80% of patients who have ≥1 event per week[170,172,173] Diagnostic in 53%, confirming epilepsy in 34%; nonepileptic behaviors in 96%[173] Likelihood of capturing an event was greater if a patient had an event frequency of at least 1 per week

3. A history exists of postictal agitation or wandering, or
4. Cooperation of the patient is questionable

The AASM further recommends that V-PSGs be performed to diagnose parasomnias:

1. Additional EEG derivations in an expanded bilateral montage to diagnose paroxysmal arousals or other sleep disruptions believed to be seizure-related when the initial clinical evaluation and results of a standard EEG are inconclusive;
2. Recording surface electromyographic activity from the left and right anterior tibialis and extensor digitorum muscles;
3. Obtaining good audiovisual recording; and
4. Having a sleep technologist present throughout the study to observe and document events.[79]

The AASM encourages sleep specialists who are not experienced or trained in recognizing and interpreting both PSG and EEG abnormalities to seek appropriate consultation or refer patients to a center where this expertise is available.[79]

How Many Channels of Electroencephalography Are Needed to Identify Epileptiform and Ictal Activity in a Polysomnogram?

Regarding how many additional EEG derivations should be recorded in a PSG in a person with epilepsy, a study by Foldvary-Schaefer and colleagues[81] found that recording 18 channels of EEG during V-PSG did not improve the ability to recognize frontal lobe seizures. The ability to recognize frontal lobe seizures by EEG alone was not helped by more EEG channels, slower screen times, or midline electrodes. **Fig. 2** shows how difficult it is to recognize a frontal lobe seizure even recording 18 channels of EEG. However, Foldvary and colleagues found that 7 or 18 channels of EEG improved the accuracy of temporal lobe seizure detection (sensitivity 67% for 4 channels, 82% for 7, and 86% for 18). **Fig. 3** shows the electrographic appearance of a temporal seizure recording 4, 7, or 18 channels of EEG.

Challenges of Identifying and Scoring Interictal Epileptiform Activity in a Polysomnogram

It is important to increase the high-frequency filter to 70 Hz when reviewing EEG in V-PSG for IEDs and seizures. **Fig. 4** shows the effects of 15-Hz, 30-Hz, and 70-Hz high-frequency filter settings on IEDs in a PSG. We also review portions of the recording using vertical screen times (epochs) of 10 or 15 seconds, although we typically score sleep stages using 30-second epochs. Scoring sleep studies in patients with epilepsy can be difficult, especially when IEDs are frequent, and even more difficult when their sleep spindles are dysmorphic or low in amplitude or they have inappropriate α intrusions in their sleep EEG.[82] **Fig. 5** shows 30 seconds of NREM sleep in a child whose sleep is disrupted by almost continuous IEDs; staging this is a challenge.

More than One Night of Video-Polysomnography Often Needed to Capture the Habitual Paroxysmal Nocturnal Event

The habitual nocturnal event may not be captured by 1 night of in-laboratory V-PSG. One to 2 consecutive nights of V-PSG provided valuable diagnostic information in 69% of 41 patients whose paroxysmal motor behaviors were prominent, 41% of 11 patients referred for minor motor activity in sleep, and 78% of 36 patients with known epilepsy.[83] Another study found that V-PSG was diagnostic in 65% and helpful in another 26% of 100 consecutive adults referred for frequent sleep-related injuries;

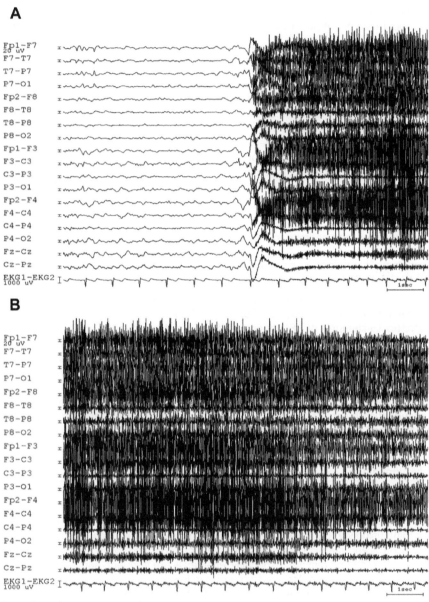

Fig. 2. (A–C) A sleep-related frontal seizure obscured by muscle artifact.

V-PSG identified DoA in 54, RBD in 36, sleep-related dissociative disorders in 7, nocturnal seizures in 2, and OSA in one.[84] Only one-third of patients with paroxysmal nocturnal events have a typical spell of a single night of V-PSG.[83,85]

Sleep researchers have found that they were able to increase the diagnostic yield of 1 night of V-PSG for recording NREM DoA by recording in-laboratory PSG after 25 hours of total SD, then ringing loud auditory stimuli. Patients arrived at their customary bedtime, remained awake the entire night, then were permitted to fall asleep 1 hour later than their usual wake time (ie, 25 hours of prior wakefulness). To

C

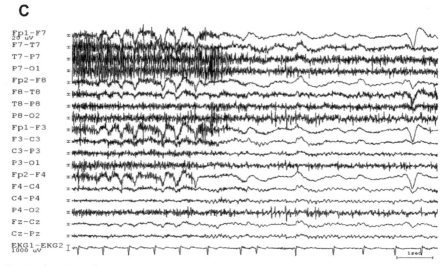

Fig. 2. (*continued*)

further provoke DoA events, patients are subjected to auditory stimuli delivered via earphones inserted in both ears. The auditory stimuli used was a pure sound lasting 3 seconds, and most often 40 to 90 dB was needed to arouse both sleepwalkers and healthy control individuals from NREM 3. Using this technique, the investigators found that they could trigger 1 to 3 sleepwalking events in 30% of 10 patients with DoA by sounding a 40-dB to 70-dB buzzer during NREM 3 sleep. After 25 hours of total SD, the auditory stimuli provoked DoA behaviors in 100% of their patients (and none of their controls). SD nearly tripled the percentage of auditory stimulus trials that induced a behavioral event (57% vs 20%).

Is One Night of In-Laboratory Polysomnography Sufficient to Confirm or Exclude Obstructive Sleep Apnea in People with Epilepsy?

Usually, 1 night of PSG is sufficient to confirm OSA in people with epilepsy. Two studies have evaluated first night effects recording 2 consecutive nights of comprehensive in-laboratory PSG in AWE. One study[86] found the only significant difference in sleep architecture was increased NREM 3 time and percent on the second night in 53 adults with medically refractory epilepsies. Another study compared median AHI recording 2 consecutive nights of PSG in 29 AWE and OSA (AHI >5).[87] These investigators found that:

1. Time spent in REM and NREM 3 and the percent time in REM sleep were greater on night 2
2. Median difference in AHI between nights 1 and 2 was 3.25/h for the group, and
3. First PSG confirmed (or excluded) OSA (AHI ≥5) in all but 1 patient

Recognizing the Effects of Vagal Nerve Stimulation on Respiration During Sleep

Vagal nerve stimulation (VNS, a treatment of medically refractory epilepsy) often alters the rate and amplitude of breathing when it activates during sleep. Numerous small case series have described this effect. Decreases in airflow and respiratory effort (and rarely, frank obstructive events) are observed during the 30-second period when the stimulator activates (typically every 5 minutes). These findings have been

A

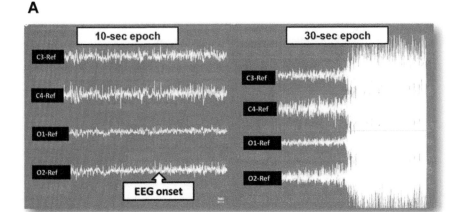

B

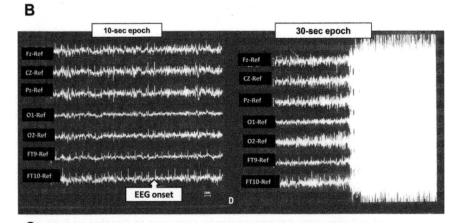

C

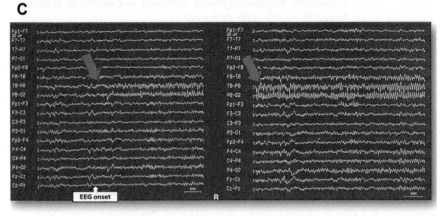

Fig. 3. (*A–C*) A temporal lobe seizure recorded using 4, 7, and 18 channels of EEG at screen times (paper speeds) of 10 mm/s and 30 mm/s. Arrows show EEG seizure onset. ([*B, C*] *Data from* Foldvary N, Caruso AC, Mascha E, et al. Identifying montages that best detect electrographic seizure activity during polysomnography. Sleep 2000;23(2):221–9.)

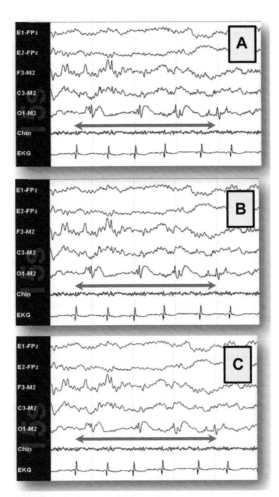

Fig. 4. The effects of and (*A*) 70-Hz, (*B*) 30-Hz, and (*C*) 15-Hz high-frequency filter settings on IEDs in a PSG.

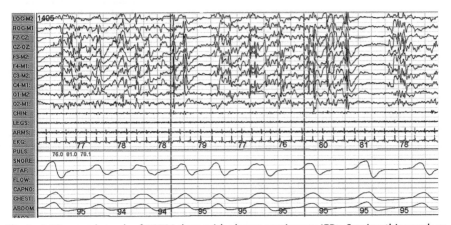

Fig. 5. A 30-second epoch of NREM sleep with almost continuous IEDs. Scoring this epoch as a particular stage of sleep is challenging.

observed in adults[88–90] and children[66,68,91–95] treated with the device. Most often, the respiratory change is an increase in the respiratory rate and decrease in respiratory amplitude when the device fires, which usually does not cause an arousal or desaturation.

Studies of the effects of VNS in children with epilepsy[91,92,94,95] describe:

1. The respiratory effort and tidal volume decrease when the VNS activates, which usually causes an increase in the respiratory rate, rarely a decrease, but no arousal or desaturation[91];
2. The reductions in the amplitude of the respiratory effort were most pronounced in the first 15 seconds (maximal decrease 47 ± 17%), although they persisted throughout in a few[94];
3. A rebound increase in respiratory amplitude is sometimes seen after the activation[94];
4. The effects are often more pronounced during NREM sleep compared with REM sleep[94]; and
5. Greater than 1% decreases in arterial oxygen saturation have been observed in a few children beginning 10 seconds after it fires, resolving quickly. Frank obstructive events with significant desaturation when the VNS activates are uncommon. When this situation is observed, consider reducing the VNS stimulation current from 1 to 2 mA. This strategy often suppresses the effect of VNS on respiration. The effects of VNS on breathing in sleep do not usually warrant its removal.

Less Common Clinical Presentations of Epileptic and Nonepileptic Parasomnias

The differential diagnosis of paroxysmal nocturnal events needs to include consideration that episodes of nocturnal choking can be caused by sleep-related panic attacks, NFLE, or other types of epilepsy.[96,97] However, NFLE can present with RLS-like symptoms.[98] Nonconvulsive status epilepticus can present as recurrent hypersomnia.[99] Partial seizures can mimic sleep terrors.[100] Psychogenic nonepileptic events (pseudoseizures) may arise during periods when the patients seem to be sleeping but the EEG showed them awake (a condition called pseudosleep).[101–103] Injuries and incontinence do not distinguish between epilepsy and pseudoseizures.[104]

Although longer-lasting, NFLE seizures can lead to episodic nocturnal wandering but more often are temporal lobe in origin.[105–109] Tai and colleagues[105] found that postictal wandering was predominantly associated with temporal rather than extratemporal seizures, particularly those arising from the nondominant temporal lobe. Patients prone to wandering did so in a few of their seizures (14%). Most temporal lobe seizures with postictal wandering began during wakefulness. The investigators speculated that relatively greater sparing of suprasylvian motor structures after temporal lobe seizures may favor complex automatic wandering behaviors in the postictal state. Fifty percent to 80% of patients with TLE have nocturnal seizures, but nearly all have seizures when awake. Nocturnal temporal lobe seizures tend to be less frequent, do not cluster, and usually do not have the hyperkinetic motor activity of NFLE. Most patients with NFLE and also those with RBD remain in the bed during episodes, whereas adults with sleepwalking, sleep terrors, or sleep dissociative events often leave the bed.

CLINICAL IMPACT OF TREATING SLEEP DISORDERS IN PEOPLE WITH EPILEPSY

A paucity of studies have been published examining the effects of treating primary sleep disorders on epilepsy. Large prospective trials of the impact of treating primary sleep disorders in people with epilepsy are greatly needed.

Treating Obstructive Sleep Apnea in People with Epilepsy

One prospective study examined the effects of treating OSA with CPAP in adults with medically refractory epilepsy.[110] Investigators found that seizures were reduced 50% or more compared with their baseline in 28% of patients treated with CPAP versus 15% treated with sham CPAP.[110] Seven other small retrospective case series have reported that CPAP improved epilepsy control in some (but not all) when used.[20,47,111–115]

CPAP in 12 AWE led to a significant reduction in EDS and seizure frequency in 4.[47] Three of 10 AWE became seizure free after their OSA was treated; 1 had a greater than 95% reduction in seizure frequency and 3 others greater than 50% when their OSA was treated (2 with positional therapy to avoid sleep supine and 8 with CPAP).[112] Four patients with medically refractory epilepsy had a greater than 50% reduction in their seizure frequency after CPAP use for 6 to 24 months, and antiepileptic medications were discontinued in 2 of these patients attributing their seizures to the OSA.[111] CPAP in 6 with OSA, and supplemental oxygen in 2 with snoring and chronic obstructive pulmonary disease, reduced interictal spiking rates during sleep in 8 AWE, especially those who had high spiking rates before treatment.[114] A 45% or greater reduction in seizure frequency was found in 3 of 6 AWE who used CPAP, and 60% or greater in 1 of 3 children who tolerated it.[48] Compliant use of CPAP 6 months or longer reduced seizure frequency by more than 150% in a retrospective study of 41 adults with OSA and epilepsy who had no change in their AED for 6 months.[115] Seizure frequency decreased from 1.8 to 1 per month in the group who used their CPAP (based on device compliance data), whereas seizure frequency was 2.1 per month at baseline and 1.8 per month at follow-up in the group who did not.

Melatonin to Treat Sleep Disorders in Children with Epilepsy

Alterations in the circadian rhythm secretion of melatonin and lower nocturnal melatonin levels have been reported in children with epilepsy, especially those with medically intractable epilepsy.[116,117] Melatonin may have anticonvulsant effects, shown in several different animal models of epilepsy.[4,118–128] Mechanisms by which melatonin may improve seizure control include its ability to reduce the electrical activity of neurons secreting glutamate (the primary central nervous system excitatory neurotransmitter) and enhance neuronal release of neurons that secrete γ-aminobutyric acid (the primary central nervous system inhibitory neurotransmitter). Moreover, melatonin is metabolized to kynurenic acid (an endogenous anticonvulsant). Melatonin and its metabolites may have neuroprotective effects, in that they can act as a free radical scavenger and antioxidant. However, relatively high doses of melatonin are needed to inhibit experimental seizures, and such doses are more likely to cause undesirable adverse effects of decreased body temperature and even cognitive and motor impairment.

Four randomized double-blind placebo-controlled studies of bedtime oral melatonin in children with epilepsy have shown positive effects on sleep.[4,120,129,130] These studies found:

1. Oral melatonin improved sleep latency and quality and reduced parasomnias by a mean of 60% in 31 children with epilepsy (ages 3–12 years)[129];
2. Nightly oral melatonin in 23 children with medically refractory epilepsy resulted in significant improvements in bedtime resistance, sleep duration, sleep latency, nocturnal arousals, sleepwalking, nocturnal enuresis, daytime sleepiness, and even seizure frequency[4];

3. Nightly use of oral melatonin (3 mg increased weekly to 9 mg as needed) in 25 children with epilepsy, mental retardation, and sleep/wake disorders (mean age 10.5 years) resulted in significant subjective improvements in sleep[130]; and
4. Significantly fewer nocturnal awakenings and better control of convulsions in 10 children with severe medically intractable epilepsy given 3 mg of oral melatonin before bed nightly for 3 months followed by placebo for 3 months.[120]

In humans, melatonin has relatively low toxicity, rare reports of nightmares, hypotension, and daytime sleepiness.

COMMENTARY: WHAT IS NEW IN SLEEP MEDICINE AND EPILEPSY
Complaint of Insomnia or Excessive Sleepiness in People with Epilepsy Warrants Consideration of Comorbid Depression, Anxiety, and Suicidal Ideation

A complaint of insomnia or EDS in AWE warrants consideration of comorbid depression, anxiety, and suicidal ideation.[96,131–133] Fifty-five percent of 152 consecutive AWE (mean age 46 years) complained of insomnia and correlated with the number of AEDs prescribed and depressive symptoms.[133] Reports of poor sleep quality and depression were good predictors of suicide in 98 unselected AWE.[131]

Pregabalin and Gabapentin May Improve Disturbed Sleep in People with Epilepsy and Insomnia

Pregabalin or gabapentin are 2 AEDs that have been shown to improve disturbed sleep in a variety of common conditions, including neuropathic pain,[134–136] postherpetic neuralgia,[137,138] fibromyalgia,[139,140] RLS,[141] general anxiety disorder,[142] sleep bruxism,[143] menopausal women with insomnia with or without hot flashes,[144–147] and autistic children with refractory insomnia.[148] The evidence suggests that the positive effects of pregabalin are distinct from its analgesic, anxiolytic, and anticonvulsant effects.[149] A double-blind, placebo-controlled crossover study showed pregabalin increased NREM 3, decreased NREM 1 sleep, and improved attention in 9 adults with well-controlled epilepsy and sleep-maintenance insomnia.[150]

Sleep Deprivation Most Likely to Trigger Seizures in People with Juvenile Myoclonic Epilepsy

Seventy-seven percent of 75 patients with juvenile myoclonic epilepsy (JME) reported that SD triggered their seizures,[151] and SD (often coupled with acute drug withdrawal or alcohol use) caused recurrence of seizures after a long period of remission in 105 patients with JME.[152] Seizures in JME are facilitated by SD and sudden arousal.[153] The mean number and duration of IEDs during sleep and on awakening has been shown to increase in JME after SD.[154]

Recommendations to have sufficient sleep and maintain regular bedtimes often go unheeded in patients with JME. Why unheeded given the dire consequences? Recent research provides clues. Compared with patients with TLE, patients with JME were more likely to prefer late bedtimes and wake times.[155] Night owl preferences predisposed them to SD and convulsions when not permitted to sleep late into the morning after a late night out. Abnormalities in frontal lobe executive function with difficulties making advantageous decisions in JME may explain their failure to follow adherence to treatment plans and regulate their sleep/wake habits.[153,156–160] Studies combining cognitive testing and functional magnetic imaging show that inadequate sleep, especially in adolescents or young adults, increases risk-taking and reward-seeking behaviors.[161,162]

Effective Control of Symptomatic Obstructive Sleep Apnea Can Improve Seizure Control

Effective control of symptomatic OSA in AWE can lead to improved seizure control. One recent study[115] found that seizure frequency decreased from a mean of 1.8 to 1 per month in 28 of 41 AWE with OSA who were CPAP compliant and 16 for at least 6 months. No decrease in seizure frequency was noted in the noncompliant group (2.1–1.8/mo). Sixteen of 28 CPAP-adherent patients became seizure free versus 3 of 13 nonadherent patients (relative risk 1.54). Another, albeit small, study[136] in 27 children (median age 5 years) with epilepsy found treating their OSA often improved symptom control. Three months after adenotonsillectomy, 37% were seizure free, and 11% had a greater than 50% reduction in seizure frequency.

Parental Fear and Anxiety of Seizure Recurrence Often Result in Return to Cosleeping

A recent large well-designed study[163] explored the effect of pediatric epilepsy on child sleep, parental sleep and fatigue, and parent-child sleeping arrangements, including room sharing and cosleeping. These investigators found increased rates of a return to cosleeping after a child developed epilepsy, especially if the seizures were nocturnal. Sixty-two percent of parents complained of decreased quantity or quality of sleep when cosleeping, and 44% reported rarely/never feeling rested because they were concerned about their child having seizures during sleep. Rates of both parent-child room sharing and cosleeping were significantly greater than controls. Nocturnal seizures were associated with parental sleep problems, whereas room sharing and cosleeping behavior were associated with child sleep problems. Pediatric epilepsy can significantly affect sleep patterns for both the affected child and their parents. Parents frequently room share or cosleep with their child, adaptations that may have detrimental effects for many households. Clinicians must be attentive not only to the sleep issues occurring in pediatric patients with epilepsy but also for the household as a whole. These data provide evidence of a profound clinical need for improved epilepsy therapeutics and the development of nocturnal seizure monitoring technologies.

SUMMARY

The relationship between sleep and epilepsy is a fruitful and rewarding area for research. More research and knowledge are needed to better understand:

1. Why sleep macroarchitecture and microarchitecture are altered in patients with epilepsy
2. Whether treating OSA in patients with epilepsy improves seizure control
3. The influence of circadian rhythms and chronotypes on different epilepsy syndromes, and
4. Whether frequent IEDs during sleep without few or no seizures should be treated

Better understanding of the link between particular epilepsies, nonepileptic parasomnias, sleep fragmentation, and arousal is needed to understand how to best improve overall function. A multidisciplinary model best serves patients with these disorders.

REFERENCES

1. Cortesi F, Giannotti F, Ottaviano S. Sleep problems and daytime behavior in childhood idiopathic epilepsy. Epilepsia 1999;40(11):1557–65.

2. Batista BH, Nunes ML. Evaluation of sleep habits in children with epilepsy. Epilepsy Behav 2007;11(1):60–4.

3. Ong LC, Yang WW, Wong SW, et al. Sleep habits and disturbances in Malaysian children with epilepsy. J Paediatr Child Health 2010;46(3):80–4.

4. Elkhayat HA, Hassanein SM, Tomoum HY, et al. Melatonin and sleep-related problems in children with intractable epilepsy. Pediatr Neurol 2010;42(4): 249–54.

5. Tang SS, Clarke T, Owens J, et al. Sleep behaviour disturbances in rolandic epilepsy. J Child Neurol 2011;26(2):239–43.

6. Maganti R, Hausman N, Koehn M, et al. Excessive daytime sleepiness and sleep complaints among children with epilepsy. Epilepsy Behav 2006;8(1): 272–7.

7. Stores G, Wiggs L, Campling G. Sleep disorders and their relationship to psychological disturbance in children with epilepsy. Child Care Health Dev 1998; 24(1):5–19.

8. Wirrell E, Blackman M, Barlow K, et al. Sleep disturbances in children with epilepsy compared with their nearest-aged siblings. Dev Med Child Neurol 2005; 47(11):754–9.

9. Byars AW, Byars KC, Johnson CS, et al. The relationship between sleep problems and neuropsychological functioning in children with first recognized seizures. Epilepsy Behav 2008;13(4):607–13.

10. Williams J, Lange B, Sharp G, et al. Altered sleeping arrangements in pediatric patients with epilepsy. Clin Pediatr (Phila) 2000;39(11):635–42.

11. de Weerd A, de Haas S, Otte A, et al. Subjective sleep disturbance in patients with partial epilepsy: a questionnaire-based study on prevalence and impact on quality of life. Epilepsia 2004;45(11):1397–404.

12. Khatami R, Zutter D, Siegel A, et al. Sleep-wake habits and disorders in a series of 100 adult epilepsy patients–a prospective study. Seizure 2006;15(5): 299–306.

13. Piperidou C, Karlovasitou A, Triantafyllou N, et al. Influence of sleep disturbance on quality of life of patients with epilepsy. Seizure 2008;17(7):588–94.

14. Jenssen S, Gracely E, Mahmood T, et al. Subjective somnolence relates mainly to depression among patients in a tertiary care epilepsy center. Epilepsy Behav 2006;9(4):632–5.

15. Xu X, Brandenburg NA, McDermott AM, et al. Sleep disturbances reported by refractory partial-onset epilepsy patients receiving polytherapy. Epilepsia 2006;47(7):1176–83.

16. Manni R, Tartara A. Evaluation of sleepiness in epilepsy. Clin Neurophysiol 2000; 111(Suppl 2):S111–4.

17. Chan S, Baldeweg T, Cross JH. A role for sleep disruption in cognitive impairment in children with epilepsy. Epilepsy Behav 2011;20(3):435–40.

18. Parisi P, Bruni O, Pia Villa M, et al. The relationship between sleep and epilepsy: the effect on cognitive functioning in children. Dev Med Child Neurol 2010;52(9): 805–10.

19. Manni R, Terzaghi M. Comorbidity between epilepsy and sleep disorders. Epilepsy Res 2010;90(3):171–7.

20. Chihorek AM, Abou-Khalil B, Malow BA. Obstructive sleep apnea is associated with seizure occurrence in older adults with epilepsy. Neurology 2007;69(19): 1823–7.

21. Haut SR, Katz M, Masur J, et al. Seizures in the elderly: impact on mental status, mood, and sleep. Epilepsy Behav 2009;14(3):540–4.

22. Manni R, Politini L, Sartori I, et al. Daytime sleepiness in epilepsy patients: evaluation by means of the Epworth sleepiness scale. J Neurol 2000;247(9):716–7.
23. Malow BA, Bowes RJ, Lin X. Predictors of sleepiness in epilepsy patients. Sleep 1997;20(12):1105–10.
24. Vignatelli L, Bisulli F, Naldi I, et al. Excessive daytime sleepiness and subjective sleep quality in patients with nocturnal frontal lobe epilepsy: a case-control study. Epilepsia 2006;47(Suppl 5):73–7.
25. Soldatos CR, Allaert FA, Ohta T, et al. How do individuals sleep around the world? Results from a single-day survey in ten countries. Sleep Med 2005;6(1):5–13.
26. van Eeghen AM, Numis AI, Staley BA, et al. Characterizing sleep disorders of adults with tuberous sclerosis complex: a questionnaire-based study and review. Epilepsy Behav 2011;20(1):68–74.
27. Stefanello S, Marin-Leon L, Fernandes PT, et al. Depression and anxiety in a community sample with epilepsy in Brazil. Arq Neuropsiquiatr 2011;69(2B):342–8.
28. Giorelli AS, Neves GS, Venturi M, et al. Excessive daytime sleepiness in patients with epilepsy: a subjective evaluation. Epilepsy Behav 2011;21(4):449–52.
29. Kobau R, DiIorio C. Epilepsy self-management: a comparison of self-efficacy and outcome expectancy for medication adherence and lifestyle behaviors among people with epilepsy. Epilepsy Behav 2003;4(3):217–25.
30. Manni R, Galimberti CA, Zucca C, et al. Sleep patterns in patients with late onset partial epilepsy receiving chronic carbamazepine (CBZ) therapy. Epilepsy Res 1990;7(1):72–6.
31. Touchon J, Baldy-Moulinier M, Billiard M, et al. Sleep organization and epilepsy. Epilepsy Res Suppl 1991;2:73–81.
32. Bazil CW, Castro LH, Walczak TS. Reduction of rapid eye movement sleep by diurnal and nocturnal seizures in temporal lobe epilepsy. Arch Neurol 2000; 57(3):363–8.
33. Montplaisir J, Laverdiere M, Saint-Hilaire JM, et al. Nocturnal sleep recording in partial epilepsy: a study with depth electrodes. J Clin Neurophysiol 1987;4(4): 383–8.
34. Crespel A, Baldy-Moulinier M, Coubes P. The relationship between sleep and epilepsy in frontal and temporal lobe epilepsies: practical and physiopathologic considerations. Epilepsia 1998;39(2):150–7.
35. Bruni O, Novelli L, Luchetti A, et al. Reduced NREM sleep instability in benign childhood epilepsy with centro-temporal spikes. Clin Neurophysiol 2010; 121(5):665–71.
36. De Gennaro L, Ferrara M, Spadini V, et al. The cyclic alternating pattern decreases as a consequence of total sleep deprivation and correlates with EEG arousals. Neuropsychobiology 2002;45(2):95–8.
37. Eisensehr I, Parrino L, Noachtar S, et al. Sleep in Lennox-Gastaut syndrome: the role of the cyclic alternating pattern (CAP) in the gate control of clinical seizures and generalized polyspikes. Epilepsy Res 2001;46(3):241–50.
38. Gigli GL, Calia E, Marciani MG, et al. Sleep microstructure and EEG epileptiform activity in patients with juvenile myoclonic epilepsy. Epilepsia 1992;33(5): 799–804.
39. Manni R, Zambrelli E, Bellazzi R, et al. The relationship between focal seizures and sleep: an analysis of the cyclic alternating pattern. Epilepsy Res 2005; 67(1–2):73–80.
40. Miano S, Bruni O, Arico D, et al. Polysomnographic assessment of sleep disturbances in children with developmental disabilities and seizures. Neurol Sci 2010;31(5):575–83.

41. Parrino L, Halasz P, Tassinari CA, et al. CAP, epilepsy and motor events during sleep: the unifying role of arousal. Sleep Med Rev 2006;10(4): 267–85.
42. Parrino L, Smerieri A, Spaggiari MC, et al. Cyclic alternating pattern (CAP) and epilepsy during sleep: how a physiological rhythm modulates a pathological event. Clin Neurophysiol 2000;111(Suppl 2):S39–46.
43. Terzano MG, Parrino L, Anelli S, et al. Effects of generalized interictal EEG discharges on sleep stability: assessment by means of cyclic alternating pattern. Epilepsia 1992;33(2):317–26.
44. Terzano MG, Parrino L, Garofalo PG, et al. Activation of partial seizures with motor signs during cyclic alternating pattern in human sleep. Epilepsy Res 1991; 10(2–3):166–73.
45. Zucconi M, Oldani A, Smirne S, et al. The macrostructure and microstructure of sleep in patients with autosomal dominant nocturnal frontal lobe epilepsy. J Clin Neurophysiol 2000;17(1):77–86.
46. Manni R, Terzaghi M, Arbasino C, et al. Obstructive sleep apnea in a clinical series of adult epilepsy patients: frequency and features of the comorbidity. Epilepsia 2003;44(6):836–40.
47. Hollinger P, Khatami R, Gugger M, et al. Epilepsy and obstructive sleep apnea. Eur Neurol 2006;55(2):74–9.
48. Malow BA, Weatherwax KJ, Chervin RD, et al. Identification and treatment of obstructive sleep apnea in adults and children with epilepsy: a prospective pilot study. Sleep Med 2003;4(6):509–15.
49. Young T, Palta M, Dempsey J, et al. The occurrence of sleep-disordered breathing among middle-aged adults. N Engl J Med 1993;328(17):1230–5.
50. Young T, Peppard P, Palta M, et al. Population-based study of sleep-disordered breathing as a risk factor for hypertension. Arch Intern Med 1997;157(15): 1746–52.
51. Weatherwax KJ, Lin X, Marzec ML, et al. Obstructive sleep apnea in epilepsy patients: the Sleep Apnea scale of the Sleep Disorders Questionnaire (SA-SDQ) is a useful screening instrument for obstructive sleep apnea in a disease-specific population. Sleep Med 2003;4(6):517–21.
52. Malow BA, Fromes GA, Aldrich MS. Usefulness of polysomnography in epilepsy patients. Neurology 1997;48(5):1389–94.
53. Manni R, Terzaghi M. REM behavior disorder associated with epileptic seizures. Neurology 2005;64(5):883–4.
54. Manni R, Terzaghi M, Zambrelli E. REM sleep behaviour disorder in elderly subjects with epilepsy: frequency and clinical aspects of the comorbidity. Epilepsy Res 2007;77(2–3):128–33.
55. Iranzo A, Santamaria J. Severe obstructive sleep apnea/hypopnea mimicking REM sleep behavior disorder. Sleep 2005;28(2):203–6.
56. Didden R, Korzilius H, van Aperlo B, et al. Sleep problems and daytime problem behaviours in children with intellectual disability. J Intellect Disabil Res 2002; 46(Pt 7):537–47.
57. Didden R, de Moor JM, Korzilius H. Sleepiness, on-task behavior and attention in children with epilepsy who visited a school for special education: a comparative study. Res Dev Disabil 2009;30(6):1428–34.
58. Conant KD, Thibert RL, Thiele EA. Epilepsy and the sleep-wake patterns found in Angelman syndrome. Epilepsia 2009;50(11):2497–500.
59. Segawa M, Nomura Y. Polysomnography in the Rett syndrome. Brain Dev 1992; 14(Suppl):S46–54.

60. Liu X, Hubbard JA, Fabes RA, et al. Sleep disturbances and correlates of children with autism spectrum disorders. Child Psychiatry Hum Dev 2006;37(2): 179–91.
61. Becker DA, Fennell EB, Carney PR. Daytime behavior and sleep disturbance in childhood epilepsy. Epilepsy Behav 2004;5(5):708–15.
62. Nunes ML. Sleep disorders. J Pediatr (Rio J) 2002;78(Suppl 1):S63–72 [in Portuguese].
63. Kaleyias J, Cruz M, Goraya JS, et al. Spectrum of polysomnographic abnormalities in children with epilepsy. Pediatr Neurol 2008;39(3):170–6.
64. Nunes ML, Ferri R, Arzimanoglou A, et al. Sleep organization in children with partial refractory epilepsy. J Child Neurol 2003;18(11):763–6.
65. Maganti R, Sheth RD, Hermann BP, et al. Sleep architecture in children with idiopathic generalized epilepsy. Epilepsia 2005;46(1):104–9.
66. Zaaimi B, Grebe R, Berquin P, et al. Vagus nerve stimulation induces changes in respiratory sinus arrhythmia of epileptic children during sleep. Epilepsia 2009; 50(11):2473–80.
67. Hallbook T, Lundgren J, Rosen I. Ketogenic diet improves sleep quality in children with therapy-resistant epilepsy. Epilepsia 2007;48(1):59–65.
68. Pruvost M, Zaaimi B, Grebe R, et al. Cardiorespiratory effects induced by vagus nerve stimulation in epileptic children. Med Biol Eng Comput 2006;44(4): 338–47.
69. Koh S, Ward SL, Lin M, et al. Sleep apnea treatment improves seizure control in children with neurodevelopmental disorders. Pediatr Neurol 2000;22(1):36–9.
70. Barreto JR, Fernandes RM, Sakamoto AC. Correlation of sleep macrostructure parameters and idiopathic epilepsies. Arq Neuropsiquiatr 2002;60(2-B):353–7.
71. Sato S, Dreifuss FE, Penry JK. The effect of sleep on spike-wave discharges in absence seizures. Neurology 1973;23(12):1335–45.
72. Myatchin I, Lagae L. Sleep spindle abnormalities in children with generalized spike-wave discharges. Pediatr Neurol 2007;36(2):106–11.
73. Young D, Nagarajan L, de Klerk N, et al. Sleep problems in Rett syndrome. Brain Dev 2007;29(10):609–16.
74. Bruni O, Cortesi F, Giannotti F, et al. Sleep disorders in tuberous sclerosis: a polysomnographic study. Brain Dev 1995;17(1):52–6.
75. Marcus CL, Carroll JL, McColley SA, et al. Polysomnographic characteristics of patients with Rett syndrome. J Pediatr 1994;125(2):218–24.
76. Niedermeyer E, Naidu SB, Plate C. Unusual EEG theta rhythms over central region in Rett syndrome: considerations of the underlying dysfunction. Clin Electroencephalogr 1997;28(1):36–43.
77. Sekul EA, Moak JP, Schultz RJ, et al. Electrocardiographic findings in Rett syndrome: an explanation for sudden death? J Pediatr 1994;125(1):80–2.
78. Bisulli F, Vignatelli L, Naldi I, et al. Increased frequency of arousal parasomnias in families with nocturnal frontal lobe epilepsy: a common mechanism? Epilepsia 2010;51(9):1852–60.
79. Kushida CA, Littner MR, Morgenthaler T, et al. Practice parameters for the indications for polysomnography and related procedures: an update for 2005. Sleep 2005;28(4):499–521.
80. Guilleminault C, Palombini L, Pelayo R, et al. Sleepwalking and sleep terrors in prepubertal children: what triggers them? Pediatrics 2003;111(1):e17–25.
81. Foldvary-Schaefer N, De Ocampo J, Mascha E, et al. Accuracy of seizure detection using abbreviated EEG during polysomnography. J Clin Neurophysiol 2006;23(1):68–71.

82. Marzec ML, Malow BA. Approaches to staging sleep in polysomnographic studies with epileptic activity. Sleep Med 2003;4(5):409–17.

83. Aldrich MS, Jahnke B. Diagnostic value of video-EEG polysomnography. Neurology 1991;41(7):1060–6.

84. Schenck CH, Milner DM, Hurwitz TD, et al. A polysomnographic and clinical report on sleep-related injury in 100 adult patients. Am J Psychiatry 1989; 146(9):1166–73.

85. Blatt I, Peled R, Gadoth N, et al. The value of sleep recording in evaluating somnambulism in young adults. Electroencephalogr Clin Neurophysiol 1991;78(6): 407–12.

86. Marzec ML, Selwa LM, Malow BA. Analysis of the first night effect and sleep parameters in medically refractory epilepsy patients. Sleep Med 2005;6(3):277–80.

87. Selwa LM, Marzec ML, Chervin RD, et al. Sleep staging and respiratory events in refractory epilepsy patients: is there a first night effect? Epilepsia 2008;49(12): 2063–8.

88. Malow BA, Edwards J, Marzec M, et al. Effects of vagus nerve stimulation on respiration during sleep: a pilot study. Neurology 2000;55(10):1450–4.

89. Marzec M, Edwards J, Sagher O, et al. Effects of vagus nerve stimulation on sleep-related breathing in epilepsy patients. Epilepsia 2003;44(7):930–5.

90. Holmes MD, Miller JW, Voipio J, et al. Vagal nerve stimulation induces intermittent hypocapnia. Epilepsia 2003;44(12):1588–91.

91. Nagarajan L, Walsh P, Gregory P, et al. Respiratory pattern changes in sleep in children on vagal nerve stimulation for refractory epilepsy. Can J Neurol Sci 2003;30(3):224–7.

92. Hsieh T, Chen M, McAfee A, et al. Sleep-related breathing disorder in children with vagal nerve stimulators. Pediatr Neurol 2008;38(2):99–103.

93. Zaaimi B, Grebe R, Berquin P, et al. Vagus nerve stimulation therapy induces changes in heart rate of children during sleep. Epilepsia 2007;48(5):923–30.

94. Zaaimi B, Heberle C, Berquin P, et al. Vagus nerve stimulation induces concomitant respiratory alterations and a decrease in SaO2 in children. Epilepsia 2005; 46(11):1802–9.

95. Khurana DS, Reumann M, Hobdell EF, et al. Vagus nerve stimulation in children with refractory epilepsy: unusual complications and relationship to sleep-disordered breathing. Childs Nerv Syst 2007;23(11):1309–12.

96. Hitomi T, Oga T, Tsuboi T, et al. Transient increase in epileptiform discharges after the introduction of nasal continuous positive airway pressure in a patient with obstructive sleep apnea and epilepsy. Intern Med 2012;51(17):2453–6.

97. Timofeev I, Bazhenov M, Seigneur J, et al. Neuronal Synchronization and Thalamocortical Rhythms in Sleep, Wake and Epilepsy. In: Noebels JL, Avoli M, Rogawski MA, et al, editors. Jasper's Basic Mechanisms of the Epilepsies [Internet]. 4th edition. Bethesda (MD): National Center for Biotechnology Information (US); 2012. Available from: http://www.ncbi.nlm.nih.gov/books/NBK98144/.

98. Seegmuller C, Deonna T, Dubois CM, et al. Long-term outcome after cognitive and behavioral regression in nonlesional epilepsy with continuous spike-waves during slow-wave sleep. Epilepsia 2012;53(6):1067–76.

99. Bazil CW, Dave J, Cole J, et al. Pregabalin increases slow-wave sleep and may improve attention in patients with partial epilepsy and insomnia. Epilepsy Behav 2012;23(4):422–5.

100. Andersen ML, Tufik S, Cavalheiro EA, et al. Lights out! It is time for bed. Warning: obstructive sleep apnea increases risk of sudden death in people with epilepsy. Epilepsy Behav 2012;23(4):510–1.

101. Koutroumanidis M, Tsiptsios D, Kokkinos V, et al. Focal and generalized EEG paroxysms in childhood absence epilepsy: topographic associations and distinctive behaviors during the first cycle of non-REM sleep. Epilepsia 2012; 53(5):840–9.
102. Ning ZS, Zhang J, Jiang Z, et al. Epileptiform discharges and sleep structure in children with nocturnal epilepsy. Zhongguo Dang Dai Er Ke Za Zhi 2012;14(2): 124–7 [in Chinese].
103. Serafini A, Kuate C, Gelisse P, et al. Sleep before and after temporal lobe epilepsy surgery. Seizure 2012;21(4):260–5.
104. Chen NC, Tsai MH, Chang CC, et al. Sleep quality and daytime sleepiness in patients with epilepsy. Acta Neurol Taiwan 2011;20(4):249–56.
105. Tai P, Poochikian-Sarkissian S, Andrade D, et al. Postictal wandering is common after temporal lobe seizures. Neurology 2010;74(11):932–3.
106. Plazzi G, Vetrugno R, Provini F, et al. Sleepwalking and other ambulatory behaviours during sleep. Neurol Sci 2005;26(Suppl 3):s193–8.
107. Mai R, Sartori I, Francione S, et al. Sleep-related hyperkinetic seizures: always a frontal onset? Neurol Sci 2005;26(Suppl 3):s220–4.
108. Nobili L, Cossu M, Mai R, et al. Sleep-related hyperkinetic seizures of temporal lobe origin. Neurology 2004;62(3):482–5.
109. Nobili L, Francione S, Cardinale F, et al. Epileptic nocturnal wanderings with a temporal lobe origin: a stereo-electroencephalographic study. Sleep 2002; 25(6):669–71.
110. Malow BA, Foldvary-Schaefer N, Vaughn BV, et al. Treating obstructive sleep apnea in adults with epilepsy: a randomized pilot trial. Neurology 2008;71(8): 572–7.
111. Beran RG, Holland GJ, Yan KY. The use of CPAP in patients with refractory epilepsy. Seizure 1997;6(4):323–5.
112. Vaughn BV, D'Cruz OF, Beach R, et al. Improvement of epileptic seizure control with treatment of obstructive sleep apnoea. Seizure 1996;5(1):73–8.
113. Devinsky O, Ehrenberg B, Barthlen GM, et al. Epilepsy and sleep apnea syndrome. Neurology 1994;44(11):2060–4.
114. Oliveira AJ, Zamagni M, Dolso P, et al. Respiratory disorders during sleep in patients with epilepsy: effect of ventilatory therapy on EEG interictal epileptiform discharges. Clin Neurophysiol 2000;111(Suppl 2):S141–5.
115. Vendrame M, Auerbach S, Loddenkemper T, et al. Effect of continuous positive airway pressure treatment on seizure control in patients with obstructive sleep apnea and epilepsy. Epilepsia 2011;52(11):e168–71.
116. Paprocka J, Dec R, Jamroz E, et al. Melatonin and childhood refractory epilepsy–a pilot study. Med Sci Monit 2010;16(9):CR389–96.
117. Ardura J, Andres J, Garmendia JR, et al. Melatonin in epilepsy and febrile seizures. J Child Neurol 2010;25(7):888–91.
118. Scorza FA, Colugnati DB, Arida RM, et al. Cardiovascular protective effect of melatonin in sudden unexpected death in epilepsy: a hypothesis. Med Hypotheses 2008;70(3):605–9.
119. Sanchez-Forte M, Moreno-Madrid F, Munoz-Hoyos A, et al. The effect of melatonin as anti-convulsant and neuron protector. Rev Neurol 1997;25(144): 1229–34 [in Spanish].
120. Uberos J, Augustin-Morales MC, Molina Carballo A, et al. Normalization of the sleep-wake pattern and melatonin and 6-sulphatoxy-melatonin levels after a therapeutic trial with melatonin in children with severe epilepsy. J Pineal Res 2011;50(2):192–6.

121. Fenoglio-Simeone K, Mazarati A, Sefidvash-Hockley S, et al. Anticonvulsant effects of the selective melatonin receptor agonist ramelteon. Epilepsy Behav 2009;16(1):52–7.
122. Molina-Carballo A, Munoz-Hoyos A, Sanchez-Forte M, et al. Melatonin increases following convulsive seizures may be related to its anticonvulsant properties at physiological concentrations. Neuropediatrics 2007;38(3):122–5.
123. Yahyavi-Firouz-Abadi N, Tahsili-Fahadan P, Riazi K, et al. Melatonin enhances the anticonvulsant and proconvulsant effects of morphine in mice: role for nitric oxide signaling pathway. Epilepsy Res 2007;75(2–3):138–44.
124. Yildirim M, Marangoz C. Anticonvulsant effects of melatonin on penicillin-induced epileptiform activity in rats. Brain Res 2006;1099(1):183–8.
125. Yahyavi-Firouz-Abadi N, Tahsili-Fahadan P, Riazi K, et al. Involvement of nitric oxide pathway in the acute anticonvulsant effect of melatonin in mice. Epilepsy Res 2006;68(2):103–13.
126. Ray M, Mediratta PK, Reeta K, et al. Receptor mechanisms involved in the anticonvulsant effect of melatonin in maximal electroshock seizures. Methods Find Exp Clin Pharmacol 2004;26(3):177–81.
127. Mevissen M, Ebert U. Anticonvulsant effects of melatonin in amygdala-kindled rats. Neurosci Lett 1998;257(1):13–6.
128. Lapin IP, Mirzaev SM, Ryzov IV, et al. Anticonvulsant activity of melatonin against seizures induced by quinolinate, kainate, glutamate, NMDA, and pentylenetetrazole in mice. J Pineal Res 1998;24(4):215–8.
129. Gupta M, Aneja S, Kohli K. Add-on melatonin improves sleep behavior in children with epilepsy: randomized, double-blind, placebo-controlled trial. J Child Neurol 2005;20(2):112–5.
130. Coppola G, Iervolino G, Mastrosimone M, et al. Melatonin in wake-sleep disorders in children, adolescents and young adults with mental retardation with or without epilepsy: a double-blind, cross-over, placebo-controlled trial. Brain Dev 2004;26(6):373–6.
131. Wigg CM, Filgueiras A, Gomes Mda M. The relationship between sleep quality, depression, and anxiety in patients with epilepsy and suicidal ideation. Arq Neuropsiquiatr 2014;72(5):344–8.
132. Kwan P, Yu E, Leung H, et al. Association of subjective anxiety, depression, and sleep disturbance with quality-of-life ratings in adults with epilepsy. Epilepsia 2009;50(5):1059–66.
133. Halasz P. Sleep and epilepsy. Handb Clin Neurol 2012;107:305–22.
134. Zhou JY, Tang XD, Huang LL, et al. The acute effects of levetiracetam on nocturnal sleep and daytime sleepiness in patients with partial epilepsy. J Clin Neurosci 2012;19(7):956–60.
135. Biyik Z, Solak Y, Atalay H, et al. Gabapentin versus pregabalin in improving sleep quality and depression in hemodialysis patients with peripheral neuropathy: a randomized prospective crossover trial. Int Urol Nephrol 2013;45(3):831–7.
136. Segal E, Vendrame M, Gregas M, et al. Effect of treatment of obstructive sleep apnea on seizure outcomes in children with epilepsy. Pediatr Neurol 2012;46(6):359–62.
137. Wang J, Chen YB, Liang D. Epilepsy with continuous spike and wave during slow wave sleep: a case report. Zhongguo Dang Dai Er Ke Za Zhi 2012;14(1):71–2 [in Chinese].
138. van Seventer R, Feister HA, Young JP Jr, et al. Efficacy and tolerability of twice-daily pregabalin for treating pain and related sleep interference in postherpetic neuralgia: a 13-week, randomized trial. Curr Med Res Opin 2006;22(2):375–84.

139. Jain SV, Horn PS, Simakajornboon N, et al. Obstructive sleep apnea and primary snoring in children with epilepsy. J Child Neurol 2013;28(1):77–82.

140. Russell IJ, Crofford LJ, Leon T, et al. The effects of pregabalin on sleep disturbance symptoms among individuals with fibromyalgia syndrome. Sleep Med 2009;10(6):604–10.

141. Misra UK, Kalita J, Kumar B, et al. Treatment of restless legs syndrome with pregabalin: a double-blind, placebo-controlled study. Neurology 2011;76(4):408 [author reply: 408–9].

142. Zanzmera P, Shukla G, Gupta A, et al. Markedly disturbed sleep in medically refractory compared to controlled epilepsy–a clinical and polysomnography study. Seizure 2012;21(7):487–90.

143. Sugiura C, Matsumura W, Togawa M, et al. Lamotrigine-induced sleep behavior disturbance in a case with intractable epilepsy. No To Hattatsu 2011;43(6):489–90 [in Japanese].

144. Agarwal N, Singh S, Kriplani A, et al. Evaluation of gabapentin in management of hot flushes in postmenopausal women. Post Reprod Health 2014;20(1):36–8.

145. Saadati N, Mohammadjafari R, Natanj S, et al. The effect of gabapentin on intensity and duration of hot flashes in postmenopausal women: a randomized controlled trial. Glob J Health Sci 2013;5(6):126–30.

146. Guttuso T Jr. Nighttime awakenings responding to gabapentin therapy in late premenopausal women: a case series. J Clin Sleep Med 2012;8(2):187–9.

147. Pinkerton JV, Kagan R, Portman D, et al. Phase 3 randomized controlled study of gastroretentive gabapentin for the treatment of moderate-to-severe hot flashes in menopause. Menopause 2014;21(6):567–73.

148. Robinson AA, Malow BA. Gabapentin shows promise in treating refractory insomnia in children. J Child Neurol 2013;28(12):1618–21.

149. Roth T, Arnold LM, Garcia-Borreguero D, et al. A review of the effects of pregabalin on sleep disturbance across multiple clinical conditions. Sleep Med Rev 2014;18(3):261–71.

150. Li P, Ghadersohi S, Jafari B, et al. Characteristics of refractory vs. medically controlled epilepsy patients with obstructive sleep apnea and their response to CPAP treatment. Seizure 2012;21(9):717–21.

151. da Silva Sousa P, Lin K, Garzon E, et al. Self-perception of factors that precipitate or inhibit seizures in juvenile myoclonic epilepsy. Seizure 2005;14(5):340–6.

152. Sokic D, Ristic AJ, Vojvodic N, et al. Frequency, causes and phenomenology of late seizure recurrence in patients with juvenile myoclonic epilepsy after a long period of remission. Seizure 2007;16(6):533–7.

153. Kossoff EH, Los JG, Boatman DF. A pilot study transitioning children onto levetiracetam monotherapy to improve language dysfunction associated with benign rolandic epilepsy. Epilepsy Behav 2007;11(4):514–7.

154. Sousa NA, Sousa Pda S, Garzon E, et al. EEG recording after sleep deprivation in a series of patients with juvenile myoclonic epilepsy. Arq Neuropsiquiatr 2005;63(2B):383–8.

155. Pung T, Schmitz B. Circadian rhythm and personality profile in juvenile myoclonic epilepsy. Epilepsia 2006;47(Suppl 2):111–4.

156. Northcott E, Connolly AM, McIntyre J, et al. Longitudinal assessment of neuropsychologic and language function in children with benign rolandic epilepsy. J Child Neurol 2006;21(6):518–22.

157. Clarke T, Strug LJ, Murphy PL, et al. High risk of reading disability and speech sound disorder in rolandic epilepsy families: case-control study. Epilepsia 2007;48(12):2258–65.

158. Canavese C, Rigardetto R, Viano V, et al. Are dyslexia and dyscalculia associated with Rolandic epilepsy? A short report on ten Italian patients. Epileptic Disord 2007;9(4):432–6.
159. Northcott E, Connolly AM, Berroya A, et al. The neuropsychological and language profile of children with benign rolandic epilepsy. Epilepsia 2005;46(6):924–30.
160. Polychronopoulos P, Argyriou AA, Papapetropoulos S, et al. Wilson's disease and benign epilepsy of childhood with centrotemporal (rolandic) spikes. Epilepsy Behav 2006;8(2):438–41.
161. Telzer EH, Fuligni AJ, Lieberman MD, et al. The effects of poor quality sleep on brain function and risk taking in adolescence. Neuroimage 2013;71:275–83.
162. Womack SD, Hook JN, Reyna SH, et al. Sleep loss and risk-taking behavior: a review of the literature. Behav Sleep Med 2013;11(5):343–59.
163. Larson AM, Ryther RC, Jennesson M, et al. Impact of pediatric epilepsy on sleep patterns and behaviors in children and parents. Epilepsia 2012;53(7):1162–9.
164. Foldvary-Schaefer N, Andrews ND, Pornsriniyom D, et al. Sleep apnea and epilepsy: who's at risk? Epilepsy Behav 2012;25(3):363–7.
165. Aydin K, Okuyaz C, Serdaroglu A, et al. Utility of electroencephalography in the evaluation of common neurologic conditions in children. J Child Neurol 2003;18(6):394–6.
166. Camfield P, Gordon K, Camfield C, et al. EEG results are rarely the same if repeated within six months in childhood epilepsy. Can J Neurol Sci 1995;22(4):297–300.
167. Gilbert DL, Gartside PS. Factors affecting the yield of pediatric EEGs in clinical practice. Clin Pediatr (Phila) 2002;41(1):25–32.
168. Watemberg N, Tziperman B, Dabby R, et al. Adding video recording increases the diagnostic yield of routine electroencephalograms in children with frequent paroxysmal events. Epilepsia 2005;46(5):716–9.
169. Gilbert DL. Interobserver reliability of visual interpretation of electroencephalograms in children with newly diagnosed seizures. Dev Med Child Neurol 2006;48(12):1009–10 [author reply: 1010–1].
170. Chen LS, Mitchell WG, Horton EJ, et al. Clinical utility of video-EEG monitoring. Pediatr Neurol 1995;12(3):220–4.
171. Valente KD, Freitas A, Fiore LA, et al. The diagnostic role of short duration outpatient V-EEG monitoring in children. Pediatr Neurol 2003;28(4):285–91.
172. Bye AM, Kok DJ, Ferenschild FT, et al. Paroxysmal non-epileptic events in children: a retrospective study over a period of 10 years. J Paediatr Child Health 2000;36(3):244–8.
173. Mohan KK, Markand ON, Salanova V. Diagnostic utility of video EEG monitoring in paroxysmal events. Acta Neurol Scand 1996;94(5):320–5.

Adolescent Eating Disorders
Update on Definitions, Symptomatology, Epidemiology, and Comorbidity

Beate Herpertz-Dahlmann, MD

KEYWORDS

- Anorexia nervosa • Bulimia nervosa • Binge-eating disorder • Adolescence
- Epidemiology • Comorbidity • Diagnostic classification

KEY POINTS

- Eating disorders are some of the most prevalent disorders in adolescence, often taking a chronic and disabling course.
- Most eating disorders imply a deep dissatisfaction with the subject's own body and shape; everyday live is often unduly preoccupied by eating and weight-control practices.
- There have been major changes from DSM-IV to DSM-5, leading to an increasing prevalence of anorexia and bulimia nervosa and a decreasing prevalence of eating disorders not otherwise classified. According to DSM-5, binge-eating disorder (BED) enters a distinct category of its own.
- In adolescence and childhood, the rates of eating disorders are on the increase. Every clinician working with this age group should be familiar with their symptomatology and medical/psychiatric assessment.
- Eating disorders are associated with high and sometimes life-threatening medical and psychiatric comorbidities.
- Severe and prolonged starvation, characteristic of chronic anorexia nervosa, can have profound consequences on brain and bone development.

INTRODUCTION

Eating disorders are the third most common chronic illness among adolescents, after obesity and asthma[1]; the peak age of onset occurs between 14 and 19 years. In this article, 5 categories of eating disorder are described according to the *Diagnostic and*

Disclosure: Dr B. Herpertz-Dahlmann has received industry research funding from Vifor and research funding from the German Ministry for Education and Research (Grants 01GV0602 and 01GV0623).
Department of Child and Adolescent Psychiatry, Psychosomatics, and Psychotherapy, RWTH Aachen University, Neuenhofer Weg 21, Aachen 52074, Germany
E-mail address: bherpertz-dahlmann@ukaachen.de

Child Adolesc Psychiatric Clin N Am 24 (2015) 177–196
http://dx.doi.org/10.1016/j.chc.2014.08.003
1056-4993/15/$ – see front matter © 2015 Elsevier Inc. All rights reserved.

Abbreviations	
ADHD	Attention-deficit/hyperactivity disorder
AN	Anorexia nervosa
BED	Binge-eating disorder
BMI	Body mass index
BN	Bulimia nervosa
DSM-5	*Diagnostic and Statistical Manual of Mental Disorders*, 5th edition
EDNOS	Eating disorders not otherwise specified
LOC	Loss of control of eating
OCD	Obsessive-compulsive disorder
OSFED	Other specified feeding or eating disorders

Statistical Manual of Mental Disorders, 5th edition (DSM-5)[2]: Anorexia Nervosa (AN), Bulimia Nervosa (BN), Binge-Eating Disorder (BED), Other Specified Feeding or Eating Disorders (OSFED), and Unspecified Feeding or Eating Disorders. All of these disorders are thought to exist within a broader spectrum, and patients frequently move among them.[3] Recent epidemiologic studies have suggested higher prevalence rates in youth than previously thought,[4,5] with a substantial increase in unspecified eating disorders over recent years. Although approximately 10% of the general population suffers from some type of eating disorder, only a minority of these individuals ever seek treatment.[6] Children and adolescents often become adults in whom these disorders persist: the chronic and disabling courses of these conditions generate high somatic and psychiatric comorbidity rates, along with substantial personal and societal costs.

This article provides an overview of the recent developments in definitions and diagnoses, including new classification issues, medical and psychiatric comorbidities, and current trends in the prevalence of the spectrum of eating disorders.

DEFINITION AND CLASSIFICATION

Definition of Eating Disorders

Most of the spectrum of eating disorders, especially AN, BN, and some OSFED, is characterized by a fear of fatness and a pathologic preoccupation with weight and shape. Self-evaluation is predominantly based on the perception of one's own body, and everyday life is unduly influenced by weight-control practices. In BED, negative feelings related to body weight and shape are also frequently prevalent.

Anorexia Nervosa

AN is a severe psychiatric disorder with substantial morbidity and the highest mortality of all mental disorders. The standardized mortality rate for AN is approximately 6,[7] which is higher than that for asthma and diabetes mellitus type 1.[8] About one-fifth of those who die commit suicide.[7]

Extreme dissatisfaction with the size or shape of one's body or some body parts leads to weight phobia and food aversion. Whereas some patients perceive their bodies as being fat despite of severe starvation, others are able to recognize their emaciated figures but find it attractive. Low body weight is the result of a strict diet and/or excessive hyperactivity. It is pursued beyond the bounds of reason and to the exclusion of age-appropriate activities. In very young patients, especially in those with prepubertal onset, low body weight may be achieved by increasing growth in height without corresponding weight gain. Most patients experience their symptoms as egosyntonic, and despite feeling weak and excluded from age-appropriate life, they feel distinguished by having AN.

Bulimia Nervosa

Similarly to AN, fear of fatness and attempts to lose weight are core symptoms of BN. In many patients, a body-image disturbance is present and can be characterized by a profound dissatisfaction with one's own body shape and weight. While permanently restricting calories, fasting is interrupted by binge-eating episodes accompanied by a feeling of losing control. Binges are followed by fear of weight gain and the desire to purge and, thus, compensate for the calories consumed. Patients with BN usually weigh within a normal range, although some fall in the upper or lower normal ranges. A lower body mass index (BMI; calculated as weight in kilograms divided by height in square meters [kg/m²]) is often associated with a history of AN. However, the percentage of overweight and adiposity in BN has increased during recent years,[9,10] rendering its treatment more demanding. Overweight patients with BN seek help for bingeing and purging in addition to weight loss,[10] which in turn might promote bingeing.

Binge-Eating Disorder and Loss of Control of Eating

BED is characterized by episodes of binge eating associated with feelings of loss of control, for example, eating a large amount of food in a discrete period of time but not followed by purging behavior. BED usually starts in adolescence but may already be prevalent in children.[11] In contrast to individuals with similar high BMI, individuals with BED often present with high psychiatric comorbidities, especially mood and anxiety disorders.[12] In children and adolescents, BED or any other type of disinhibited eating is often preceded by loss of control of eating (LOC).[13,14] LOC is defined as eating with the associated experience of being unable to control the amount of food, regardless of the size of the meal.

CLASSIFICATION OF ADOLESCENT EATING DISORDERS: CHANGES FROM *DIAGNOSTIC AND STATISTICAL MANUAL OF MENTAL DISORDERS*, 4TH EDITION TO *DIAGNOSTIC AND STATISTICAL MANUAL OF MENTAL DISORDERS*, 5TH EDITION

To reduce the frequency of eating disorders not otherwise specified (EDNOS in the *Diagnostic and Statistical Manual of Mental Disorders*, 4th edition, text revision [DSM-IV]),[15,16] the threshold for both AN and BN has been lowered, and BED has been introduced into DSM-5. Previous research has reported the stigmatization of individuals with eating disorders by both health professionals and the general public.[17] The stigmatization of AN was most likely supported by DSM-IV items implying a deliberate attitude of the patient and willful actions, such as "refusal to maintain body weight at or above a minimally normal weight for age and height" or a "denial of the seriousness of low body weight." In DSM-5 criteria for AN (**Box 1**), these items have been replaced by more neutral terms, such as "restriction of energy intake relative to requirements" and "persistent lack of recognition of the seriousness of the current low body weight." In item A of the new DSM-5 criteria, underweight must be judged in the context of "age, sex, developmental trajectory and physical health," which is especially important for diagnosing and treating children and adolescents. Moreover, it seems to be helpful for clinicians treating younger subjects to rely on the clinical symptom "persistent behavior that interferes with weight gain" because many underweight adolescent patients or children do not

> **Box 1**
> **Diagnostic criteria for anorexia nervosa according to DSM-5 (abbreviated form)**
>
> A. Restriction of energy intake relative to requirements, leading to a significantly low body weight in the context of age, sex, developmental trajectory, and physical health. For children and adolescents, significantly low weight is defined as a weight that is less than minimally expected
>
> B. Intense fear of gaining weight or becoming fat or persistent behavior that interferes with weight gain
>
> C. Body image disturbance, undue influence of weight and shape on self-confidence, or persistent lack of recognition of the seriousness of the illness
>
> Subtypes: Restricting and Binge Eating/Purging Type.

admit "an intense fear of gaining weight" or a distortion of body image.[18] However, especially in the younger patient groups, the lack of a standard or reference for the weight criterion is a problem. According to DSM-5, significantly low body weight in children and adolescents is defined as "weight that is less than minimally expected." For adults, a BMI of 18.5 is proposed as the lower limit of normal body weight,[2] which approximately corresponds to the 10th BMI percentile in United States and European adult populations. Accordingly, BMI below the 10th percentile is used in Germany[19,20] and by several United States[21] and international clinicians[22] as a weight threshold for minors.

In comparison with DSM-IV the amenorrhea criterion has been left out of DSM-5, which was the most important step in lowering the diagnostic threshold. DSM-IV amenorrhea was not applicable to prepubescent and premenarchal girls and to females on contraceptives, and is not relevant for male patients with AN. In addition, no important differences seem to exist between those with amenorrhea and those without. A significant minority of women (up to one-fourth in clinical samples) who fulfill all other criteria for AN and need clinical attention, menstruate.[23] It must be noted, however, that existence of amenorrhea might help to distinguish between constitutional thinness and AN.

DSM-5, similarly to DSM-IV, distinguishes between 2 subtypes of AN: the restricting type and the binge-eating/purging type. The restricting type is characterized by accomplishing weight loss primarily by fasting and/or excessive exercising, whereas patients with the binge-eating/purging type may engage in bingeing and purging, only bingeing (with intermittent periods of fasting or excessive exercising) or only purging (practicing self-induced vomiting, laxative abuse, diuretics, or other weight-loss–supporting medications, such as thyroid hormones, amphetamines, or enemas). However, in contrast to DSM-IV, the time frame is more specific; instead of referencing the "current episode" of the eating disorder, a duration of at least 3 months for either symptomatology is given, thus corresponding to the definitions for bingeing in BN and BED. The subtyping of AN is important, as both subgroups differ in somatic and psychiatric comorbidities and, most likely, in outcomes.

DSM-5 criteria for BN are very similar to those of DSM-IV. However, the symptom frequency of binge eating and subsequent compensatory behavior was relaxed to once a week for 3 months instead of twice a week (**Box 2**).

The major change from DSM-IV to DSM-5 is the official diagnostic classification of BED. The publication of preliminary criteria in DSM-IV was followed by extensive research in adult and youth populations. From many empirically derived results, it

---

Box 2
Diagnostic criteria for bulimia nervosa according to DSM-5 (abbreviated form)

A. Recurrent episodes of binge eating

B. Recurrent inappropriate compensatory behaviors, eg, self-induced vomiting, laxative or diuretics abuse, or fasting or excessive exercise

C. Frequency of binge eating at least once a week for 3 months

D. Self-confidence is contingent on weight and shape

E. Symptoms do not only occur during episodes of anorexia nervosa

---

was demonstrated that BED has sufficient clinical utility and validity.[24] In children and adolescents, a consistent relationship between binge eating and overweight/obesity and current and future comorbid psychopathologies was observed (**Box 3**).[25]

Other Specified Feeding or Eating Disorder

An eating disorder is classified under this diagnostic category if it does not fulfill all diagnostic criteria for one of the aforementioned categories but causes "clinically significant distress or impairment" in different types of functioning.[2] The following disorders are subsumed under this eating disorder class: atypical AN (weight criterion not fulfilled), atypical BN of low frequency and/or limited duration (time frame not fulfilled), atypical BED of low frequency and/or limited duration (time frame not fulfilled), purging disorder, and night eating syndrome.

In a recent study, no significant differences between AN and EDNOS-AN were found according to self-report or interview measures, with the exception that participants with AN reported higher rates of binge eating and purging compared with those with EDNOS-AN and more obvious somatic sequelae, such as lower white blood cell counts.[26]

Purging disorders are defined by recurrent self-induced vomiting and/or laxative abuse or other medications to lose weight, and an overvaluation of shape and weight in the absence of binge eating and low body weight.

Night eating is diagnosed in the presence of recurrent eating after awakening from sleep or excessive food consumption after evening dinner. The patient is aware of and remembers this food consumption.

Box 3
Diagnostic criteria for binge-eating disorders according to DSM-5 (abbreviated form)

A. Recurrent episodes of binge eating

B. Binge eating is associated with eating faster until feeling uncomfortably full, eating when not feeling hungry, eating alone due to being embarrassed, or feeling disgusted or depressed

C. Marked distress because of the symptoms

D. Frequency at least once a week for 3 months

E. Symptoms are not followed by compensatory behavior and do not occur in the context of bulimia nervosa or anorexia nervosa

---

Unspecified Feeding or Eating Disorder

This term applies to eating disorders that cause significant impairment but do not fulfill all diagnostic criteria enumerated under the other diagnostic classes already mentioned.

Eating Disorders: DSM-IV to DSM-5

The most important change from DSM-IV to DSM-5 is the reduction of the residual diagnosis of EDNOS by introducing the new specific diagnostic category for BED and by lowering the thresholds for AN, owing to the omission of the amenorrhea criterion, and for BN, because of the reduced symptom frequency in BN.

SYMPTOMS
Anorexia Nervosa

Dieting behaviors

AN almost always begins with dieting. Girls with AN will mostly eat so-called healthy food, such as fruit, vegetables, and salad; many of them become vegetarians. Persons with AN differentiate between "good" and "bad" foodstuffs, and are often influenced by magical or superstitious thinking. Several of them celebrate their eating by setting the table in a particular manner and practicing rituals while eating. Adolescents with AN often eat very slowly and show picky eating, taking very small bites, avoiding any fat and smearing food up to avoid eating it. Many of them excessively count calories. Some develop an extensive interest in recipes and cooking, or they may urge their family members to eat large meals so that those often complain of weight gain. Younger adolescents or children may even refuse to drink because of an intense fear of becoming fat.[27] Others do not dare to even touch fat because they fear it might be absorbed by the skin.

Anorexia Nervosa Pearl

The younger the girl and the quicker the weight loss, the higher the rate of medical complications.

Weight control and exercise

Patients with AN step on the scales several times a day and look in mirrors to assess their shape. Their moods will be heavily influenced by weight gain; often the pursuit of thinness escalates with increasing weight loss. Approximately 30% to 80% of individuals with AN can be characterized as hyperactive.[28] Many of them practice sports or commit themselves to fitness training or gymnastics. Exercise often becomes ritualized and may be used for regulating mood states, such as anxiety, anger, and depression. With increasing weight loss, active sports are often replaced or complemented by restlessness, which may express itself in a constantly active posture, fidgeting, or inability to sit still. Exercise is not only voluntarily driven; it is also induced by prolonged semistarvation. In the advanced stages of the illness, hyperactivity is largely triggered by hypoleptinemia[29,30] and other metabolic changes.[31] Hyperactive individuals with AN suffer from higher relapse rates[32] and often fall ill at a younger age.[30]

Physical Hyperactivity and Anorexia Nervosa
Hyperactivity is associated with
a. More severe psychopathology[33]
b. Lower BMI[29]
c. Higher dissatisfaction with one's own body[34]
d. Worse response to treatment[35]
e. A more chronic course[36]

Body image disturbance

Slade[37] defined body image as the "picture we have in our minds of the size, shape and form of our bodies; and our feelings concerning these characteristics and our constituent body parts." Today the conception of body image is based on a combination of perceptual, affective, and cognitive components with behavioral features. Although the results are somewhat contradictory in reports on adolescent patients, many individuals with AN (and BN) overestimate their body size in comparison with healthy controls. Certain body parts are more overestimated than others, especially the thighs and waist. Patients with the binge/purging type of AN seem to be more affected than those with the restrictive subtype. Some patients practice checking rituals, such as touching body parts repetitively or controlling their shape in the mirror (for a review see Legenbauer and colleagues[38]).

Bulimia Nervosa

Girls and young women with BN share the fear of obesity and exaggerated wish of thinness with individuals suffering from AN. Although body-image distortion is less pronounced than in emaciated AN, several patients with BN also tend to overestimate their body size. In most cases, BN starts with a longer episode of fasting, which is terminated by a loss of control resulting in binge attacks followed by an extreme fear of gaining weight and weight-loss practices, such as vomiting, laxative abuse, diuretics, the abuse of other medications, or, more rarely, the use of nonpurging strategies, such as exercising. Thus, a vicious circle is started. Binges and purges are mostly practiced in secret. Failure to adhere to a planned small amount of food is sometimes deliberately followed by a binge to facilitate vomiting. For the same purpose, patients drink fluid copiously during meals. A binge attack might comprise up to more than 10,000 calories and mostly consists of cold food that is easy to swallow, such as desserts, cake, and chocolate. In contrast to objective binges with high amounts of food, some patients may engage in so-called subjective binges with only small quantities of food, which nevertheless cause them to experience a loss of control. In short, a binge is the violation of one's personal conception of the amount and type of food he or she is allowed to eat. In the beginning, binge attacks and compensatory behaviors are often preceded by emotional stress and feelings of loneliness; during the course of the disorder, they become more and more habitual and are sometimes regularly scheduled in everyday life. Binges may occur from once a week to several times a day, with a higher medical risk associated with the latter. Some patients combine vomiting with taking laxatives. In contrast to AN patients, many individuals with BN can hide their disorder and avoid treatment for many years.[27]

Binge-Eating Disorder

BED in children and adolescents refers to eating an objectively large amount of food while experiencing a sense of loss of control. Similarly to BN, children and adolescents with BED seek food in the absence of hunger for example, after a full meal. Some of them use bingeing to regulate negative effects or as a reward; they may also hoard or hide food. However, several researchers have pointed out that BED is not easy to conceptualize in childhood, largely because of the difficult definition of "a large amount of food" in childhood or adolescence; for example, whether 3 pieces of cake would be too large for a 12-year old boy might be judged differently. In addition, the amount of food might be limited by caretakers so that the real quantity the child would have eaten cannot be assessed. Moreover, some children report a decreased awareness during the meal, resulting in a biased recall of the amount eaten. Tanofsky-Kraff and colleagues[39] have therefore proposed to better refer to "loss of control of eating" independently, rather than as measured by the quantity eaten, as they believe the former constitutes a more reliable criterion for an eating disorder in younger age groups. Indeed, recent studies have shown that LOC and not overeating was predictive of later overweight and obesity, and depression.[25] Children with LOC develop more general and eating disorder psychopathologies than those without LOC, and gain more weight over time.[40] Moreover, children with LOC make significantly higher use of dysfunctional emotion-regulation strategies.[41]

EPIDEMIOLOGY
Anorexia Nervosa

Very few community studies have assessed the incidence of eating disorders. Comparing these incidence rates with those of primary care, the former are significantly higher because the latter implies a bias caused by selection processes on the way to treatment.[42]

In Finnish community studies based on a twin register, incidence rates of 270 to 450 per 100,000 (depending on a narrow or broad definition) were found in 15- to 19-year-old females during the 1990s.[43] The incidence rates derived from primary care are shown in **Table 1**. Several studies were able to demonstrate that the highest incidence rates are found in this age group, with approximately 40% of all new cases appearing in this period.[5,42] In children between 5 and 12 years of age, the incidence rates for restrictive eating disorders (not all fulfilling DSM-IV criteria for AN) were estimated at 1 to 2.5,[44,45] although they seem to be on the increase.[46,47] While the incidence rates are stable in the adult group, they seem to be increasing in adolescents and children (for reviews see Smink and colleagues[42] and Favaro and colleagues[48]).

In adolescent samples, most studies found point and 12-month prevalence rates of AN, according to DSM-IV, of between 0.3 and 0.9[4,42,49] (including an epidemiologic

Table 1
Epidemiology of adolescent eating disorders

	AN		BN		BED (DSM-IV EDNOS)	
	Female	Male	Female	Male	Female	Male
Incidence[a]	40–100	1–4	40–50	2–3	70	10
12-month prevalence (%)	0.3–0.9	0.1–0.3	1–2.0	0.3–0.5	1.5–2.0	0.4–0.8

[a] Eating disorder per 100, 000 15–19-year-olds in primary care.
Data based on Refs.[4,5,51] and reviews by Refs.[42,89]

study investigating a nationally representative sample of 10,120 adolescents in the United States between 13 and 18 years and a median age at onset of 12.4 years). Point prevalence is defined by the prevalence at a given point in time and assessed according to the current standard of a 2-stage selection model. In this model, an epidemiologic sample is primarily investigated by means of a screening questionnaire to select for persons at risk. The at-risk individuals are then usually interviewed personally by a general or disorder-specific diagnostic instrument. The 12-month prevalence is the number of cases in a given year.

Bulimia Nervosa

Similarly to AN, community studies are scarce. In a Finnish epidemiologic study of BN, the incidence rate was measured at 200 per 100,000 females aged 16 to 20 years.[50] In studies based on primary care rates, incidence in adult individuals seemed to decrease, which can most likely be explained by an increasing number of treatment options in the community (eg, self-help group vs medical care). Alternatively, the initially high rates in the 1990s were due to the announcement and detection of the new diagnosis of "BN." Nevertheless, in young females and males the incidence rates of BN remain stable.[5,51] Some investigations even indicate that individuals with BN have been diagnosed at increasingly young ages.[48] Recent studies have reported controversial results as to whether the prevalence of BN is also decreasing (in accordance with incidence rates) (for a review see Smink and colleagues[42]).

Binge-Eating Disorder and Eating Disorder Not Otherwise Specified

To the author's knowledge there are no incidence studies in BED, as up to recently no DSM criteria existed. A recent study reports on the increasing incidence of EDNOS, including BED, in the United Kingdom between 2000 and 2009.[5] According to this study, EDNOS is the most prevalent eating disorder.

For BED, prevalence rates are also scarce; the prevalence data in adolescents according to the earlier proposed DSM-5 criteria are estimated to be approximately 1% to 5%.[4,52] In a longitudinal study, the prevalence of BED increased significantly in girls between 14 and 20 years of age.[52] The prevalence in males was lower than in females; however, the gap between the sexes was less pronounced than in AN and BN.

Changes in Epidemiology from Diagnostic and Statistical Manual of Mental Disorders, 4th edition to Diagnostic and Statistical Manual of Mental Disorders, 5th edition

Recent studies demonstrate that the revised version of eating disorders in DSM-5 alters the frequency of disorders previously reported according to DSM-IV. In all studies, AN and BN rates increased in children and adolescents when using DSM-5; in a clinical eating disorder sample, the proportions of AN and BN rose from 30% to 40% and from 7% to 12%, respectively.[53] An increase was also found in epidemiologic studies when comparing DSM-IV prevalence rates with the prevalence rates obtained according to DSM-5.[52,54] In the clinical sample by Ornstein and colleagues,[53] the percentage of EDNOS was reduced by nearly half when applying DSM-5 criteria. A significant reduction was also found in epidemiologic studies. All of the investigators agree that DSM-5 criteria effectively restricted the residual diagnosis of EDNOS and better assigned eating-disordered individuals to specific and homogeneous diagnostic categories.

COMORBIDITY
Medical Comorbidity

As already mentioned, eating disorders have a high rate of medical comorbidity. In a recent meta-analysis based on 36 studies, the standardized mortality rates (ratio of observed to expected deaths) were 5.86 for AN, 1.93 for BN, and 1.92 for EDNOS (according to DSM-IV criteria). The mortality rates for AN showed a significant association with age but not with BMI, underlining the danger of a long-lasting illness.[7] The severity and consequences of somatic sequelae depend on the extent and rapidity of weight loss, the current degree of underweight, the duration of the eating disorder, the intensity of purging, and the age of the patient. In general, because of a smaller amount of fat mass, children suffer from more medical comorbidities in comparison with adolescents. In contrast to adult patients, children and adolescents with AN experience severe effects on their pubertal development and growth. The most important somatic changes and dysfunctions are described in **Table 2**.

In AN, signs of malnutrition often make diagnosis easy, whereas BN patients are of normal weights and often deny their symptoms. AN patients present with emaciated limbs, a wasting of the subcutaneous fat tissue and muscles, bony prominences, and protruding ribs. Dental assessment might show erosion of dental

Table 2
Medical alterations in adolescent eating disorders

	AN	BN
Physical examination findings	Dry skin Lanugo hair formation (only with severe weight loss) Acrocyanosis Alopecia Low body temperature Dehydration Retardation of growth and pubertal development	Erosion of dental enamel Parotid/salivary gland enlargement Scars on the skin of the back of the hand resulting from inducing the gag reflex Dehydration
Cardiovascular system	Bradycardia ECG abnormalities (mostly prolonged QT interval) Pericardial effusion Edema (before or during refeeding)	ECG abnormalities (cardiac arrhythmia, prolonged QT interval)
Gastrointestinal system	Impaired gastric emptying Pancreatitis Constipation	Esophagitis Pancreatitis Delayed gastric emptying
Blood	Leukocytopenia, thrombocytopenia Anemia	
Biochemical abnormalities	Hypokalemia Hyponatremia Hypomagnesemia Hypocalcemia Hypophosphatemia (during refeeding) Low glucose levels AST ↑, ALT ↑ (with severe fasting or beginning of refeeding) Cholesterol	Hypokalemia Hyponatremia Hypomagnesemia (caused by diarrhea) Hypocalcemia Metabolic alkalosis (in case of severe purging) Metabolic acidosis (in case of severe laxative abuse)

Abbreviations: ALT, alanine aminotransferase; AST, aspartate aminotransferase; ECG, electrocardiographic.

Data from Herpertz-Dahlmann B. Adolescent eating disorders: definitions, symptomatology, epidemiology and comorbidity. Child Adolesc Psychiatr Clin N Am 2009;18(1):31–47.

enamel, which is a characteristic of vomiting in AN and BN patients. The effect of starvation on the heart and low thyroid hormones explain the bradycardia, low body temperature, hypotension, and orthostatic problems. Fluid and electrolyte abnormalities may be especially serious in binge/purge AN or BN patients. Hypokalemia is especially frequent in the latter disorder, and represents a harmful complication that might result in cardiac arrest. Gastrointestinal complications are also frequent in AN and BN, including dysfunctions of the pancreas and the liver and increased levels of amylase, lipase, and liver enzymes. The usually mild elevations described here may be the result of severe malnutrition or a consequence of refeeding. The hallmark of refeeding syndrome is hypophosphatemia associated with neurologic and cardiac adverse events. Renal dysfunction may be revealed by elevated levels of creatinine or blood urea nitrogen. Persistently elevated creatinine levels may point to a chronic renal abnormality. Many patients with AN, especially those who drink large amounts of water to appease their hunger, have problems concentrating their urine and exhibit disturbed osmoregulation. Recent studies have reported abnormalities in vitamin blood levels, such as vitamin D deficiencies and high levels of vitamin A.[55] Many patients complain of hair loss, brittle nails, constipation, headache, or fatigue (for a review see Katzman[56]). A full medical assessment is recommended (**Box 4**).

AN and, to a lesser degree, BN lead to endocrine changes. In general, these abnormalities are a consequence of semistarvation, abnormal eating behaviors, or both, and are regarded as adaptive mechanisms to conserve energy. The most important (but not all) of the changes are listed in **Table 3**.

Osteopenia and Osteoporosis

As shown later, AN (and, to a lesser degree, BN and OSFED) is characterized by widespread endocrinologic abnormalities, such as hypogonadotropic hypogonadism, hypercortisolemia, low level of insulin-like growth factor 1, deficits in adipocyte hormones, including leptin, and changes in gut hormones, including ghrelin. All of these contribute to the uncoupling of bone formation and bone resorption, resulting in an impaired bone structure and reduced bone strength (see **Box 4**). Low bone density is generally not completely reversible, even after weight rehabilitation. Several studies have demonstrated that adolescent AN is associated with a 2- to 7-fold higher fracture risk later in life (for a review see Fazeli and Klibanski[57]). Osteoporosis is not only a problem of females but also of male patients, owing to their deficits in gonadal hormones.[58]

Box 4
Medical assessment of eating disorders

- Physical assessment (heart rate, blood pressure, body temperature)
- Complete blood count
- Biochemical profile (sodium, potassium, calcium, chloride, magnesium, phosphate, creatinine, urea, serum proteins, glucose, liver enzymes, amylase, lipase)
- Electrocardiogram
- Electroencephalography, magnetic resonance imaging, computed tomography (in case of atypical eating disorder, eg, boys, children, or manifestation of seizures)

Data from Herpertz-Dahlmann B. Adolescent eating disorders: definitions, symptomatology, epidemiology and comorbidity. Child Adolesc Psychiatr Clin N Am 2009;18(1):31–47.

Table 3
Endocrinologic changes in AN and BN

	AN	BN
Thyroid axis	↓ fT3, n (↓) fT4	n (↓)
Gonadal axis	↓ FSH	n (↓)
	↓ LH pulsatility	n (↓)
	↓ Estrogens	n (↓)
	↓ Androgens	n (↓)
Adrenal axis	↑ Cortisol	n (↑)
	n DHEAS	n
Growth hormone	GH resistance (↑ GH/↓ IGF-1)	n (↑)
Appetite-regulating hormones	↓ Leptin	n (↓)
	↑ Ghrelin (fasting)	↑
	↑ (n) PYY (fasting)	n

Abbreviations: DHEAS, dehydroepiandrosterone; FSH, follicle-stimulating hormone; fT3, free triio-dothyronine; fT4, free thyroxine; GH, growth hormone; IGF-1, insulin-like growth factor type 1; LH, luteinizing hormone; n, normal; PYY, peptide YY; ↑, elevated; ↓, reduced.
   Data from Miller KK. Endocrine dysregulation in anorexia nervosa update. J Clin Endocrinol Metab 2011;96(10):2939–49; and Herpertz-Dahlmann B, Holtkamp K, Konrad K. Eating disorders: anorexia and bulimia nervosa. Handb Clin Neurol 2012;106:447–62.

Implications of Anorexia Nervosa for Brain Development

In the starved state, AN leads to reduced volumes of gray and white matter in the brain. Although these reductions do improve on weight restoration, the completeness of the brain-volume rehabilitation remains equivocal. Studies in adolescent AN have shown larger effects for brain-volume changes than in adult AN.[59,60] There is also recent evidence that long-lasting starvation-induced hormone deficits may be linked to the disturbed development of certain brain regions, especially the volumes of the amygdala and hippocampus.[61] These disruptions are most likely responsible for the neuropsychological deficits, such as impaired memory and learning and reduced cognitive flexibility that render psychotherapy difficult during acute stages of the illness (see later discussion on neuropsychological impairment).

Psychiatric Comorbidity

Eating disorders are often accompanied by other psychiatric disorders, either before or during the acute state of the illness or in the long-term course. Clinicians should conduct a thorough psychiatric assessment focusing on comorbid disorders, continuing through treatment. Onset patterns (eg, which disorder preceded the other) might also be important. The rates of concurrent affective and anxiety disorders are high in both females and males.[58] In an 18-year follow-up study of 51 former adolescents with AN, based on an epidemiologic sample, 1 in 4 did not have paid employment owing to psychiatric problems.[62]

Physical Comorbidity and Eating Disorders

Greater negative long-term outcomes of eating disorders seem to be associated with additional psychiatric disorders.

Anorexia Nervosa

In clinical and epidemiologic samples, the lifetime prevalence rates of at least 1 co-morbid condition according to DSM-IV range from 45% to 97%.[4,63] The most preva-lent disorders are mood and anxiety disorders, obsessive-compulsive disorder (OCD), substance abuse, and personality disorders. In general, adolescents with AN seem to display lower rates of comorbid disorders than do adults.[64]

The 2 subtypes of AN, the restricting type and the binge-purging type, display different patterns of comorbid conditions, with the binge/purge subtype more closely resembling the pattern of BN than that of the restricting type of AN.

In more recent studies, up to 60% of adolescent patients with AN display some type of mood disorder,[65–67] with usually higher rates in clinical than in epidemiologic sam-ples.[4] Patients complain of depressed mood, emotional emptiness, social withdrawal, anhedonia, loss of libido, and low self-esteem. In standard depression inventories, they usually score in the mild to moderate range, with the bingeing type scoring higher than the restrictive type. Several studies found an association between weight loss and depression; for example, patients with a high degree of starvation also felt more depressed. Mood is substantially affected by starvation; thus, clinicians should always question whether depressive states are primarily the result of acute AN and might thus be alleviated by nutritional rehabilitation, or whether depression preceded or outlasted the eating disorder.

Anxiety disorders other than OCDs are very common in AN. About one-fourth of patients with acute AN report 1 or more anxiety disorders, with no significant dif-ferences in clinical or epidemiologic samples.[4,65] The most frequent anxiety dis-orders are specific phobias, separation anxiety disorders, and social phobia. In many cases, the anxiety disorders begin in childhood and predate the eating disorder.[68]

In DSM-5, OCD is no longer subsumed among anxiety disorders but instead consti-tutes a separate entity. Its onset often occurs in childhood. OCD in AN mostly mani-fests as ordering or washing rituals, in addition to being obsessed with the thought that things are going wrong. These genuine OCD phenomena must be differentiated from eating disorder–related obsessions and compulsions, such as certain rituals or eating strictly at the same time of day. In addition, there are some traits in AN patients that are related to obsessive-compulsive personality disorder, such as perfectionism, rigidity, and scrupulosity. It remains undetermined whether OCD symptoms are more prevalent in restrictive or binge/purging AN.

A similar debate is ongoing regarding substance abuse. About one-fourth of AN pa-tients suffer from substance abuse, with a ratio between restricting AN and binge/ purging AN of 1:2.[69] Some investigators even go so far as to consider AN a protective factor against substance abuse.[70] The most prevalent substance abuse is amphet-amine and cocaine dependence, but many patients also abuse nicotine.[71,72]

As mentioned earlier, the most common personality disorders in adults with AN are Cluster-C personality disorders, which include OCD and avoidant personality disorder.[73]

Suicidality

Suicidality is one of the most important reasons for premature death in AN. Suicidal ideation is found in about half of adolescent AN patients, and suicidal attempts are observed in 3% to 7%. There are few studies on adolescent AN that investigate sui-cidal ideation. Although suicidality is much lower in adolescent AN than in adult AN, a strong association between depression, the binge/purge subtype of AN, and the duration of illness has been reported.[66,67]

Suicidal Ideation and Eating Disorders

Suicidal ideation should be carefully assessed in eating-disordered adolescent patients, especially in those with depressive mood, bingeing, and self-harm behavior.

Neuropsychological impairment

Several studies addressing flexibility have described an impaired set-shifting ability (ie, concrete and rigid behaviors in reaction to changing patterns) in adult patients with AN, which was found to be independent of nutritional and body-weight status (for review see Friederich and Herzog[74]). In adolescent patients, deficits in set shifting are less pronounced and are correlated with perfectionistic traits.[64] Poor achievement in set-shifting tasks has also been reported in patients with OCD and those with obsessive-compulsive personality traits, consistent with the personality model of anorexic patients who exhibit high perfectionism, harm avoidance, rigidity, and obsessive traits (see earlier discussion).

Hilde Bruch reported a "narrow range of emotional reactions" in her AN patients.[75] Some researchers have suggested an overlap between AN and autism spectrum disorder, indicating their corresponding cognitive styles, such as impaired weak central coherence, set shifting, and an impairment of theory-of-mind capacities. These impairments seem to be independent of the starved state and instead are stable characteristics of individuals with AN. In an 18-year follow-up study of adolescent AN subjects, difficulties in mentalizing tasks remained in several subjects after recovery and were independent of body-weight loss and the duration of the eating disorder.[76] In this study, autistic traits in childhood were found to be predictive of a poor global outcome in the eating disorder in adulthood.[62] Moreover, the author's own study of adolescent patients, hypoactivations in the brain networks supporting the theory of mind functions were associated with a poor clinical outcome 1 year later.[77]

Bulimia Nervosa

The prevalence rates of mood disorders are similar to those in AN (50%–70%).[61] In a large epidemiologic study, 50% of individuals with BN suffered from some type of mood disorder, and 66% from some type of anxiety disorder.[4] In this study, specific phobias were the most prevalent, followed by posttraumatic stress disorder and social phobia. Suicidality was high. More than half of the adolescents with BN recalled an instance of lifetime suicidality; more than a third had a history of suicide attempts. While some investigators argue that OCD is more strongly related to AN, others report similar prevalence rates.[78,79] Substance abuse also seems to affect a substantial proportion of patients with AN. In the aforementioned study, 20% of adolescents with BN reported some sort of substance abuse. In a meta-analysis, bulimic individuals with purging behaviors had the highest rates of abuse.[80]

Some more recent research supports an important association between BN and attention-deficit/hyperactivity disorder (ADHD). Blinder and colleagues[63] found that 9% of 882 patients with BN also had ADHD; however, this study did not use standardized tools to diagnose BN or ADHD. Yates and colleagues[81] examined 37 female inpatients with BN and 97 female inpatients with binge/purge AN, and found that 6.7% of all participants met a diagnosis of childhood-onset ADHD. In the author's own study, approximately 20% of adolescent and adult patients with BN met the criteria for previous childhood ADHD, compared with 2.5% of healthy controls. The risk for adult ADHD was also significantly higher than for healthy controls. Most importantly, patients with BN and previous childhood ADHD were more impulsive and inattentive than patients with BN alone. These patients also displayed more severely disordered eating patterns and more general psychopathological symptoms in comparison with those without ADHD.[82]

Comparable with ADHD, many bulimic patients display impulsive behavior. Thus, in addition to Cluster-C disorders, the most prevalent personality disorders in BN are Cluster-B disorders, including borderline personality disorder.[83]

Binge-Eating Disorder and Loss of Control of Eating

As mentioned earlier, LOC often precedes BED. In 10-year-old youths, LOC was associated with the development of BED 4 years later; in addition, these children developed more disordered eating attitudes and depressive symptoms than those without LOC, even after controlling for body mass growth.[25,84] LOC was also predictive of higher weight gain[39] and drug abuse.[25] Other studies have also reported of a higher risk of binge drinking.[85]

Because BED was only just established as a category of its own in DSM-5, studies on comorbidity are scarce.

Most studies have found an association between binge eating and purging on one side and feelings of depression and ineffectiveness, negative self-esteem, and somatic complaints on the other.[86,87] In a large epidemiologic study on more than 10,000 adolescents between 13 and 18 years of age, 45% of individuals with BED had a comorbid mood disorder; about one-third had an anxiety disorder; and one-fourth had a substance abuse disorder.[4] In approximately 10%, ADHD was diagnosed.

According to a recent meta-analysis, the most frequent personality disorders were Cluster-C and Cluster-B disorders.[88]

Evidence-based treatment strategies for adolescent eating disorders are limited. Family-based therapy is considered to be an effective treatment for adolescent AN. Given the expanding knowledge of the neurobiology and psychological mechanisms underlying the development of these disorders, clinicians should intensify efforts to generate more effective treatment interventions for this age group, keeping in mind that outcomes may be influenced by early diagnosis and support.

REFERENCES

1. Gonzalez A, Kohn MR, Clarke SD. Eating disorders in adolescents. Aust Fam Physician 2007;36(8):614–9.
2. American Psychiatric Association. Diagnostic and statistical manual of mental disorders, 5th edition (DSM-5). Washington, DC: American Psychiatric Press; 2013.
3. Fairburn CG, Harrison PJ. Eating disorders. Lancet 2003;361(9355):407–16.
4. Swanson SA, Crow SJ, Le Grange D, et al. Prevalence and correlates of eating disorders in adolescents. Results from the national comorbidity survey replication adolescent supplement. Arch Gen Psychiatry 2011;68(7):714–23.
5. Micali N, Hagberg KW, Petersen I, et al. The incidence of eating disorders in the UK in 2000-2009: findings from the general practice research database. BMJ Open 2013;3(5). pii:e002646.
6. Hudson JI, Hiripi E, Pope HG Jr, et al. The prevalence and correlates of eating disorders in the national comorbidity survey replication. Biol Psychiatry 2007; 61(3):348–58.
7. Arcelus J, Mitchell AJ, Wales J, et al. Mortality rates in patients with anorexia nervosa and other eating disorders. A meta-analysis of 36 studies. Arch Gen Psychiatry 2011;68(7):724–31.

8. Powers PS, Cloak NL. Failure to feed patients with anorexia nervosa and other perils and perplexities in the medical care of eating disorder patients. Eat Disord 2013;21(1):81–9.
9. Villarejo C, Fernandez-Aranda F, Jimenez-Murcia S, et al. Lifetime obesity in patients with eating disorders: increasing prevalence, clinical and personality correlates. Eur Eat Disord Rev 2012;20(3):250–4.
10. Bulik CM, Marcus MD, Zerwas S, et al. The changing "weightscape" of bulimia nervosa. Am J Psychiatry 2012;169(10):1031–6.
11. Lamerz A, Kuepper-Nybelen J, Bruning N, et al. Prevalence of obesity, binge eating, and night eating in a cross-sectional field survey of 6-year-old children and their parents in a German urban population. J Child Psychol Psychiatry 2005;46(4):385–93.
12. Pauli-Pott U, Becker K, Albayrak O, et al. Links between psychopathological symptoms and disordered eating behaviors in overweight/obese youths. Int J Eat Disord 2013;46(2):156–63.
13. Tanofsky-Kraff M, Yanovski SZ, Schvey NA, et al. A prospective study of loss of control eating for body weight gain in children at high risk for adult obesity. Int J Eat Disord 2009;42(1):26–30.
14. Tanofsky-Kraff M. Binge eating among children and adolescents. In: Jelalian E, Steele RG, editors. Handbook of Childhood and Adolescent Obesity. New York: Springer Science; 2008.
15. American Psychiatric Association. Diagnostic and statistical manual of mental disorders. Washington, DC: American Psychiatric Association; 1994.
16. American Psychiatric Association. Diagnostic and statistical manual of mental disorders. Text revision. 4th edition. Washington, DC: American Psychiatric Association; 2000.
17. Maier A, Ernst JP, Muller S, et al. Self-perceived stigmatization in female patients with anorexia nervosa—results from an explorative retrospective pilot study of adolescents. Psychopathology 2014;47(2):127–32.
18. Focker M, Knoll S, Hebebrand J. Anorexia nervosa. Eur Child Adolesc Psychiatry 2013;22(Suppl 1):S29–35.
19. Herpertz SH, Fichter M, Tuschen-Caffier B, et al. S3-Leitlinie Diagnostik und Behandlung von Essstörungen. Heidelberg (Germany): Springer-Verlag; 2011.
20. Hebebrand J, Himmelmann GW, Herzog W, et al. Prediction of low body weight at long-term follow-up in acute anorexia nervosa by low body weight at referral. Am J Psychiatry 1997;154(4):566–9.
21. Lock J, Le Grange D, Agras WS, et al. Randomized clinical trial comparing family-based treatment with adolescent-focused individual therapy for adolescents with anorexia nervosa. Arch Gen Psychiatry 2010;67(10):1025–32.
22. Beumont PJ, Touyz S. Relevance of a standard measurement of undernutrition to the diagnosis of anorexia nervosa: use of Quetelet's body mass index (BMI). Int J Eat Disord 1988;7:399–405.
23. Uher R, Rutter M. Classification of feeding and eating disorders: review of evidence and proposals for ICD-11. World Psychiatry 2012;11(2):80–92.
24. Wonderlich SA, Gordon KH, Mitchell JE, et al. The validity and clinical utility of binge eating disorder. Int J Eat Disord 2009;42(8):687–705.
25. Sonneville KR, Horton NJ, Micali N, et al. Longitudinal associations between binge eating and overeating and adverse outcomes among adolescents and young adults: does loss of control matter? JAMA Pediatr 2013;167(2):149–55.
26. Le Grange D, Crosby RD, Engel SG, et al. DSM-IV-defined anorexia nervosa versus subthreshold anorexia nervosa (EDNOS-AN). Eur Eat Disord Rev 2013;21(1):1–7.

27. Herpertz-Dahlmann B. Adolescent eating disorders: definitions, symptom-atology, epidemiology and comorbidity. Child Adolesc Psychiatr Clin N Am 2009;18(1):31–47.
28. Hebebrand J, Exner C, Hebebrand K, et al. Hyperactivity in patients with anorexia nervosa and in semistarved rats: evidence for a pivotal role of hypolep-tinemia. Physiol Behav 2003;79(1):25–37.
29. Holtkamp K, Herpertz-Dahlmann B, Hebebrand K, et al. Physical activity and restlessness correlate with leptin levels in patients with adolescent anorexia nervosa. Biol Psychiatry 2006;60(3):311–3.
30. Kostrzewa E, van Elburg AA, Sanders N, et al. Longitudinal changes in the physical activity of adolescents with anorexia nervosa and their influence on body composition and leptin serum levels after recovery. PLoS One 2013; 8(10):e78251.
31. Duclos M, Ouerdani A, Mormede P, et al. Food restriction-induced hyperactivity: addiction or adaptation to famine? Psychoneuroendocrinology 2013;38(6): 884–97.
32. Steinhausen HC, Grigoroiu-Serbanescu M, Boyadjieva S, et al. Course and pre-dictors of rehospitalization in adolescent anorexia nervosa in a multisite study. Int J Eat Disord 2008;41(1):29–36.
33. Bratland-Sanda S, Sundgot-Borgen J, Ro O, et al. "I'm not physically active - I only go for walks": physical activity in patients with longstanding eating disor-ders. Int J Eat Disord 2010;43(1):88–92.
34. Solenberger SE. Exercise and eating disorders: a 3-year inpatient hospital re-cord analysis. Eat Behav 2001;2(2):151–68.
35. Dalle Grave R, Calugi S, Marchesini G. Compulsive exercise to control shape or weight in eating disorders: prevalence, associated features, and treatment outcome. Compr Psychiatry 2008;49(4):346–52.
36. Strober M, Freeman R, Morrell W. The long-term course of severe anorexia nervosa in adolescents: survival analysis of recovery, relapse, and outcome predictors over 10-15 years in a prospective study. Int J Eat Disord 1997; 22(4):339–60.
37. Slade PD. Body image in anorexia nervosa. Br J Psychiatry Suppl 1988;2:20–2.
38. Legenbauer T, Thiemann P, Vocks S. Body image disturbance in children and adolescents with eating disorders. Z Kinder Jugendpsychiatr Psychother 2014;42(1):51–9.
39. Tanofsky-Kraff M, Marcus MD, Yanovski SZ, et al. Loss of control eating disorder in children age 12 years and younger: proposed research criteria. Eat Behav 2008;9(3):360–5.
40. Boutelle KN, Tanofsky-Kraff M. Treatments targeting aberrant eating patterns in overweight youth. New York: Guilford Press; 2011.
41. Czaja J, Rief W, Hilbert A. Emotion regulation and binge eating in children. Int J Eat Disord 2009;42(4):356–62.
42. Smink FR, van Hoeken D, Hoek HW. Epidemiology of eating disorders: inci-dence, prevalence and mortality rates. Curr Psychiatry Rep 2012;14(4):406–14.
43. Keski-Rahkonen A, Hoek HW, Susser ES, et al. Epidemiology and course of anorexia nervosa in the community. Am J Psychiatry 2007;164(8):1259–65.
44. Pinhas L, Morris A, Crosby RD, et al. Incidence and age-specific presentation of restrictive eating disorders in children: a Canadian paediatric surveillance pro-gram study. Arch Pediatr Adolesc Med 2011;165(10):895–9.
45. Nicholls DE, Lynn R, Viner RM. Childhood eating disorders: British national sur-veillance study. Br J Psychiatry 2011;198(4):295–301.

46. German Institute for Federal Statistics. Diagnosedaten der Krankenhäuser ab 2000. Available at: www.destatis.de, www.gbe-bund.de. Accessed May 29, 2013.
47. Health and Social Care Information Centre. Provisional monthly hospital episode statistics for admitted patient care. Outpatient and accident and emergency data—April to June 2012. Topic of interest: eating disorder. Available at: https://catalogue.ic.nhs.uk/publications/hospital/monthly-hes/prov-mont-hes-admi-outp-ae-apr-jun-12/prov-mont-hes-admi-outp-ae-apr-jun-12-toi-rep.pdf. Accessed May 29, 2013.
48. Favaro A, Caregaro L, Tenconi E, et al. Time trends in age at onset of anorexia nervosa and bulimia nervosa. J Clin Psychiatry 2009;70(12):1715–21.
49. Machado PP, Machado BC, Goncalves S, et al. The prevalence of eating disorders not otherwise specified. Int J Eat Disord 2007;40(3):212–7.
50. Keski-Rahkonen A, Hoek HW, Linna MS, et al. Incidence and outcomes of bulimia nervosa: a nationwide population-based study. Psychol Med 2009; 39(5):823–31.
51. Currin L, Schmidt U, Treasure J, et al. Time trends in eating disorder incidence. Br J Psychiatry 2005;186:132–5.
52. Allen KL, Byrne SM, Oddy WH, et al. Early onset binge eating and purging eating disorders: course and outcome in a population-based study of adolescents. J Abnorm Child Psychol 2013;41(7):1083–96.
53. Ornstein RM, Rosen DS, Mammel KA, et al. Distribution of eating disorders in children and adolescents using the proposed DSM-5 criteria for feeding and eating disorders. J Adolesc Health 2013;53(2):303–5.
54. Machado PP, Goncalves S, Hoek HW. DSM-5 reduces the proportion of EDNOS cases: evidence from community samples. Int J Eat Disord 2013;46(1):60–5.
55. Higgins J, Hagman J, Pan Z, et al. Increased physical activity not decreased energy intake is associated with inpatient medical treatment for anorexia nervosa in adolescent females. PLoS One 2013;8:e61559.
56. Katzman DF. Assessment of eating disorders in children and adolescents. New York: Guilford Press; 2011.
57. Fazeli PK, Klibanski A. Bone metabolism in anorexia nervosa. Curr Osteoporos Rep 2014;12(1):82–9.
58. Norris ML, Apsimon M, Harrison M, et al. An examination of medical and psychological morbidity in adolescent males with eating disorders. Eat Disord 2012;20(5):405–15.
59. Seitz J, Buhren K, von Polier GG, et al. Morphological changes in the brain of acutely ill and weight-recovered patients with anorexia nervosa. Z Kinder Jugendpsychiatr Psychother 2014;42(1):7–18.
60. Castro-Fornieles J, Bargallo N, Lazaro L, et al. A cross-sectional and follow-up voxel-based morphometric MRI study in adolescent anorexia nervosa. J Psychiatr Res 2009;43(3):331–40.
61. Mainz V, Schulte-Ruther M, Fink GR, et al. Structural brain abnormalities in adolescent anorexia nervosa before and after weight recovery and associated hormonal changes. Psychosom Med 2012;74(6):574–82.
62. Wentz E, Gillberg IC, Anckarsater H, et al. Adolescent-onset anorexia nervosa: 18-year outcome. Br J Psychiatry 2009;194(2):168–74.
63. Blinder BJ, Cumella EJ, Sanathara VA. Psychiatric comorbidities of female inpatients with eating disorders. Psychosom Med 2006;68(3):454–62.
64. Buhren K, Mainz V, Herpertz-Dahlmann B, et al. Cognitive flexibility in juvenile anorexia nervosa patients before and after weight recovery. J Neural Transm 2012;119(9):1047–57.

65. Salbach-Andrae H, Lenz K, Simmendinger N, et al. Psychiatric comorbidities among female adolescents with anorexia nervosa. Child Psychiatry Hum Dev 2008;39(3):261–72.
66. Fennig S, Hadas A. Suicidal behavior and depression in adolescents with eating disorders. Nord J Psychiatry 2010;64(1):32–9.
67. Buhren K, Schwarte R, Fluck F, et al. Comorbid psychiatric disorders in female adolescents with first-onset anorexia nervosa. Eur Eat Disord Rev 2014;22(1): 39–44.
68. Godart NT, Flament MF, Lecrubier Y, et al. Anxiety disorders in anorexia nervosa and bulimia nervosa: co-morbidity and chronology of appearance. Eur Psychiatry 2000;15(1):38–45.
69. Root TL, Pinheiro AP, Thornton L, et al. Substance use disorders in women with anorexia nervosa. Int J Eat Disord 2010;43(1):14–21.
70. Kaye WH, Wierenga CE, Bailer UF, et al. Nothing tastes as good as skinny feels: the neurobiology of anorexia nervosa. Trends Neurosci 2013;36(2):110–20.
71. Thompson-Brenner H, Eddy KT, Franko DL, et al. Personality pathology and substance abuse in eating disorders: a longitudinal study. Int J Eat Disord 2008;41(3):203–8.
72. Barbarich-Marsteller NC, Foltin RW, Walsh BT. Does anorexia nervosa resemble an addiction? Curr Drug Abuse Rev 2011;4(3):197–200.
73. Herpertz-Dahlmann B, Muller B, Herpertz S, et al. Prospective 10-year follow-up in adolescent anorexia nervosa–course, outcome, psychiatric comorbidity, and psychosocial adaptation. J Child Psychol Psychiatry 2001;42(5):603–12.
74. Friederich HC, Herzog W. Cognitive-behavioral flexibility in anorexia nervosa. Curr Top Behav Neurosci 2011;6:111–23.
75. Herpertz-Dahlmann B, Seitz J, Konrad K. Aetiology of anorexia nervosa: from a "psychosomatic family model" to a neuropsychiatric disorder? Eur Arch Psychiatry Clin Neurosci 2011;261(Suppl 2):S177–81.
76. Gillberg IC, Billstedt E, Wentz E, et al. Attention, executive functions, and mentalizing in anorexia nervosa eighteen years after onset of eating disorder. J Clin Exp Neuropsychol 2010;32(4):358–65.
77. Schulte-Ruther M, Mainz V, Fink GR, et al. Theory of mind and the brain in anorexia nervosa: relation to treatment outcome. J Am Acad Child Adolesc Psychiatry 2012;51(8):832–41.e1.
78. Swinbourne JM, Touyz SW. The co-morbidity of eating disorders and anxiety disorders: a review. Eur Eat Disord Rev 2007;15(4):253–74.
79. Kaye WH, Bulik CM, Thornton L, et al. Comorbidity of anxiety disorders with anorexia and bulimia nervosa. Am J Psychiatry 2004;161(12):2215–21.
80. Calero-Elvira A, Krug I, Davis K, et al. Meta-analysis on drugs in people with eating disorders. Eur Eat Disord Rev 2009;17(4):243–59.
81. Yates WR, Lund BC, Johnson C, et al. Attention-deficit hyperactivity symptoms and disorder in eating disorder inpatients. Int J Eat Disord 2009;42(4):375–8.
82. Seitz J, Kahraman-Lanzerath B, Legenbauer T, et al. The role of impulsivity, inattention and comorbid ADHD in patients with bulimia nervosa. PLoS One 2013; 8(5):e63891.
83. Lilenfeld LR, Stein D, Bulik CM, et al. Personality traits among currently eating disordered, recovered and never ill first-degree female relatives of bulimic and control women. Psychol Med 2000;30(6):1399–410.
84. Tanofsky-Kraff M, Shomaker LB, Olsen C, et al. A prospective study of pediatric loss of control eating and psychological outcomes. J Abnorm Psychol 2011; 120(1):108–18.

85. Field AE, Sonneville KR, Micali N, et al. Prospective association of common eating disorders and adverse outcomes. Pediatrics 2012;130(2):e289–95.
86. Pasold TL, McCracken A, Ward-Begnoche WL. Binge eating in obese adolescents: emotional and behavioral characteristics and impact on health-related quality of life. Clin Child Psychol Psychiatry 2013;19(2):299–312.
87. Glasofer DR, Tanofsky-Kraff M, Eddy KT, et al. Binge eating in overweight treatment-seeking adolescents. J Pediatr Psychol 2007;32(1):95–105.
88. Friborg O, Martinsen EW, Martinussen M, et al. Comorbidity of personality disorders in mood disorders: a meta-analytic review of 122 studies from 1988 to 2010. J Affect Disord 2014;152–154:1–11.
89. Smink FR, van Hoeken D, Hoek HW. Epidemiology, course, and outcome of eating disorders. Curr Opin Psychiatry 2013;26(6):543–8.

Correction

Simkin DR, Thatcher RW, Lubar J: Quantitative EEG and Neurofeedback in Children and Adolescents in Simkin DR and Popper CW: Alternative and Complementary Therapies for Children with Psychiatric Disorders, Part 2. Child and Adolescent Psychiatric Clinics of North America, July 2014, Volume 23, Issue 3.

Page 438 should state: Increases of information flow in the thalamic-cortical-thalamic pathway occurs when the rhythm increases from a theta (4–8 Hz) and low alpha (8–10 Hz) range to the faster rhythms in the high alpha (11–12 Hz) range and still faster beta (12.5–2.0 Hz) range.

Child Adolesc Psychiatric Clin N Am 24 (2015) 197
http://dx.doi.org/10.1016/j.chc.2014.09.007
1056-4993/15/$ – see front matter © 2015 Elsevier Inc. All rights reserved.

Index

Note: Page numbers of article titles are in **boldface** type.

Child Adolesc Psychiatric Clin N Am 24 (2015) 199–210
http://dx.doi.org/10.1016/S1056-4993(14)00106-0
1056-4993/15/$ – see front matter © 2015 Elsevier Inc. All rights reserved.